# Risks Associated with Smoking Cigarettes with Low Machine-Measured Yields of Tar and Nicotine

U.S. DEPARTMENT OF HEALTH
AND HUMAN SERVICES
Public Health Service
National Institutes of Health
National Cancer Institute

# Smoking and Tobacco Control Monographs Issued to Date

*Strategies to Control Tobacco Use in the United States: a blueprint for public health action in the 1990's.* Smoking and Tobacco Control Monograph No. 1. Bethesda, MD: U.S. Department of Health and Human Services, Public Health Service, National Institutes of Health, National Cancer Institute. NIH Publication No. 92-3316, December 1991.

*Smokeless Tobacco or Health: An international perspective.* Smoking and Tobacco Control Monograph No. 2. Bethesda, MD: U.S. Department of Health and Human Services, Public Health Service, National Institutes of Health. NIH Publication No. 92-3461, September 1992.

*Major Local Tobacco Control Ordinances in the Unites States.* Smoking and Tobacco Control Monograph No. 3. Bethesda, MD: U.S. Department of Health and Human Services, Public Health Service, National Institutes of Health. NIH Publication No. 93-3532, May 1993.

*Respiratory Health Effects of Passive Smoking: Lung cancer and other disorders. The Report of the U.S. Environmental Protection Agency.* Smoking and Tobacco Control Monograph No. 4. Bethesda, MD: U.S. Department of Health and Human Services, Public Health Service, National Institutes of Health, NIH Publication No. 93-3605, August 1993

*Tobacco and the Clinician. Interventions for Medical and Dental Practice.* Smoking and Tobacco Control Monograph No. 5. Bethesda, MD: U.S. Department of Health and Human Services, Public Health Service, National Institutes of Health. NIH Publication No. 94-3693, January 1994.

*Community-based Interventions for Smokers: The COMMIT Field Experience.* Smoking and Tobacco Control Monograph No. 6. Bethesda, MD: U.S. Department of Health and Human Services, Public Health Service, National Institutes of Health. NIH Publication No. 95-4028, August 1995.

*The FTC Cigarette Test Method for Determining Tar, Nicotine, and Carbon Monoxide Yields of U.S. Cigarettes. Report of the NCI Expert Committee.* Smoking and Tobacco Control Monograph No. 7. Bethesda, MD: U.S. Department of Health and Human Services, Public Health Service, National Institutes of Health. NIH Publication No. 96-4028, August 1996.

*Changes in Cigarette Related Disease Risks and Their Implication for Prevention and Control.* Smoking and Tobacco Control Monograph No. 8. Bethesda, MD: U.S. Department of Health and Human Services, Public Health Service, National Institutes of Health. NIH Publication No. 97-4213, February 1997.

*Cigars. Health Effects and Trends.* Smoking and Tobacco Control Monograph No. 9. Bethesda, MD: U.S. Department of Health and Human Services, Public Health Service, National Institutes of Health. NIH Publication No. 98-4302, February 1998.

*Health Effects of Exposure to Environmental Tobacco Smoke. The Report of the California Environmental Protection Agency.* Smoking and Tobacco Control Monograph No. 10. Bethesda, MD: U.S. Department of Health and Human Services, Public Health Service, National Institutes of Health, National Cancer Institute. NIH Publication No. 99-4645, August 1999.

*State and Local Legislative Action to Reduce Tobacco Use.* Smoking and Tobacco Control Monograph No. 11. Bethesda, MD: U.S. Department of Health and Human Services, National Institutes of Health, National Cancer Institute, NIH Publication No. 00-4804, August 2000.

*Population Based Smoking Cessation: Proceedings of a Conference on What Works to Influence Cessation in the General Population.* Smoking and Tobacco Control Monograph No. 12. Bethesda, MD: U.S. Department of Health and Human Services, National Institutes of Health, National Cancer Institute, NIH Publication No. 00-4892, November 2000.

# Preface

This monograph, *Risks Associated with Smoking Cigarettes with Low Machine-Measured Yields of Tar and Nicotine*, is the 13th report published in the National Cancer Institute's (NCI) Smoking and Tobacco Control Program Monograph Series. The concept for this series was formed by the late Dr. Joseph W. Cullen, former Deputy Director of the Division of Cancer Prevention and Control. On the inside front cover of this volume, appears a list of previously published monographs. In addition to the current monograph, there are two more under development. One will be entitled *Changing Adolescent Smoking Behavior: Where It Is and Why.* The other will be called *Is the Target Hardening?* The "target" refers to those long-term smokers who, in many cases, have tried to stop smoking and been unable to do so. Future monographs will address important and timely issues on tobacco control, and will reflect our continuing mission to reduce cancer risk, incidence, morbidity, and mortality caused by tobacco use, as well as enhance the quality of life of current and former users of tobacco.

The initial meeting of the authors for the Low Tar Monograph took place in November of 1999. At that meeting, each author presented a preliminary paper or outline. The group discussed each presentation and made suggestions as to which subtopics might be removed from or added to each chapter and determined the boundaries of the various chapters.

One feature of the this monograph is that it blends the old with the new. Monograph 7, *The FTC Cigarette Test Method for Determining Tar, Nicotine, and Carbon Monoxide Yields of U.S. Cigarettes,* covered the history of that protocol and recommended changes in its procedures. Chapter 2 of this publication cites this earlier monograph, brings us up to date on the FTC method, and provides additional suggestions as to what can be done to help alert the public to the dangers of smoking.

The examination of the scientific literature on low-tar and low-nicotine cigarettes is not unique to this monograph. Several of the earlier volumes devoted one or more chapters to discussions of the various health aspects of tar and nicotine levels. However, this monograph includes more than just the study of amounts of tar and nicotine. Chapter 5 includes a discussion on the continued health risks to smokers, even those who smoke a low-tar/low-nicotine cigarette, while Chapter 2 describes how changes in the cigarette design affect an individual's smoking habit. Chapter 7 points out how the tobacco companies' advertisements have changed to match the emerging public preference for low-tar/low-nicotine cigarettes.

This monograph is unique in another important aspect. For the first time, the authors who prepared the various chapters have had extensive access to the information gleaned from the internal documents of the tobacco companies. The tobacco industry files now open to the public and available on the Internet constitute some 33 million pages of formal and informal memos, meeting notes, research papers, and similar corporate documents. Included are marketing strategies that express the growing concern among the various tobacco companies of the potential loss of new recruits. This concern over the potential loss of market was due to the evolving public opinion that smoking is harmful to health and that it is related to many of the illnesses that smokers experience over the course of their lives.

The singular message that has been delivered to the public—smoking causes cancer—is gradually being accepted by more and more people of all ages. This message has been reported in many scientific papers over the last 50 years. In a historical context, however, the bellwether publication that galvanized the public opinion was the original 1964 Surgeon General Report, *Smoking and Health: Report of the Advisory Committee to the Surgeon General of the Public Health Service.* The fact that the public has slowly realized and, more importantly, accepted the danger of smoking undoubtedly concerned the tobacco companies.

Access to internal industry papers allowed monograph authors to cite a number of tobacco company documents that show a long-term trend altering the tar and nicotine content of cigarettes by various chemical and mechanical procedures. The documents further reveal the industry's efforts to produce cigarettes that could be marketed as acceptable to health-conscious consumers. Ultimately, these low-tar/low-nicotine cigarettes were part of the industry's plan to maintain and expand its consumer base.

The monograph authors show that the tobacco companies set out to develop cigarette designs that markedly lowered the tar and nicotine yield results as measured by the Federal Trade Commission (FTC) testing method. Yet, these cigarettes can be manipulated by the smoker to increase the intake of tar and nicotine. The use of these "decreased risk" cigarettes have not significantly decreased the disease risk. In fact, the use of these cigarettes may be partly responsible for the increase in lung cancer for long-term smokers who have switched to the low-tar/low-nicotine brands. Finally, switching to these cigarettes may provide smokers with a false sense of reduced risk, when the actual amount of tar and nicotine consumed may be the same as, or more than, the previously used higher yield brand.

This monograph compliments the recently released Institute of Medicine report entitled *Clearing the Smoke: Assessing the Science Base for Tobacco Harm Reduction.* Together, the documents reflect a growing body of research that has explored the impact of products intended to reduce harm in an environment where there is near universal recognition of tobacco's harmful effects. Both documents reflect the need for more research to better understand the feasibility and desirability of developing and marketing products intended to reduce risk, but both also conclude that there is currently no safe tobacco product.

We hope that this evidence-based review will inform any potential recommendations that the Department of Health and Human Services (DHHS) might make to the FTC regarding the cigarette testing method.

# Acknowledgements

This monograph, entitled *Risks Associated with Smoking Cigarettes with Low Machine-Measured Yields of Tar and Nicotine*, was prepared under the general editorship of **Donald R. Shopland**, former Coordinator for the Smoking and Tobacco Control Program (STCP), National Cancer Institute, Bethesda, Maryland.

The Senior Scientific Editor for this monograph was **David M. Burns**, M.D., Professor of Medicine, School of Medicine, University of California at San Diego, California. The Co-Scientific Editor was **Neal L. Benowitz**, M.D., Professor of Medicine, Chief Division of Clinical Pharmacology and Experimental Therapeutics, University of California at San Francisco, California. The Managing Editor for the monograph was **Richard H. Amacher**, Project Director, KBM Group Inc., Silver Spring, Maryland.

The editors and STCP staff members gratefully acknowledge the many researchers and authors who made this monograph possible through their many hours of writing and review. Contributors to each chapter are as follows:

| **Chapter 1** | **Overview and Summary** | David M. Burns, M.D.<br>Professor of Medicine<br>School of Medicine<br>University of California,<br>San Diego School of<br> Medicine<br>San Diego, CA |
|---|---|---|
| | | Neal L. Benowitz, M.D.<br>Professor of Medicine and<br> Chief<br>Division of Clinical<br> Pharmacology and<br> Experimental Therapeutics<br>University of California at<br> San Francisco<br>San Francisco, CA |

| | | |
|---|---|---|
| **Chapter 2** | **Cigarette Design** | Lynn T. Kozlowski, Ph.D.<br>Professor and Head<br>Department of Biobehavioral Health<br>The Pennsylvania State University<br>University Park, PA |
| | | Richard J. O'Connor, B.A.<br>Research Assistant<br>Department of Biobehavioral Health<br>The Pennsylvania State University<br>University Park, PA |
| | | Christine T. Sweeney, M.P.H., Ph.D.<br>Scientist<br>Pinney Associates, Inc.<br>Bethesda, MD |
| **Chapter 3** | **Compensatory Smoking of Low-Yield Cigarettes** | Neal L. Benowitz, M.D.<br>Professor of Medicine and Chief<br>Department of Clinical Pharmacology and Experimental Therapeutics<br>University of California at San Francisco<br>San Francisco, CA |
| **Chapter 4** | **Smoking Lower Yield Cigarettes and Disease Risks** | David M. Burns, M.D.<br>Professor of Medicine<br>University of California, San Diego School of Medicine<br>San Diego, CA |
| | | Jacqueline M. Major, M.S.<br>Statistician<br>Tobacco Control Policies Project<br>University of California at San Diego<br>San Diego, CA |

Thomas G. Shanks, M.P.H.,
M.S.
Principal Statistician
Tobacco Control Policies
 Project
University of California at
 San Diego
San Diego, CA

Michael J. Thun, M.D., M.S.
Vice President of
 Epidemiology and
 Surveillance Research
American Cancer Society
Atlanta, GA

**Chapter 5**  **The Changing Cigarette: Chemical Studies and Bioassays**

Dietrich Hoffmann, Ph.D.
Associate Director
American Health
 Foundation
Valhalla, NY

Ilse Hoffmann, B.Sc.
Editorial Coordinator
American Health
 Foundation
Valhalla, NY

**Chapter 6**  **Public Understanding of Risk and Reasons for Smoking Low-Yield Products**

Neil D. Weinstein, Ph.D.
Professor of Human Ecology
Rutgers, The State University
 of New Jersey
New Brunswick, NJ

**Chapter 7**  **Marketing Cigarettes with Low Machine-Measured Yields**

Richard W. Pollay, Ph.D.
Professor of Marketing,
 Faculty of Commerce
Curator of the History of
 Advertising Archives
University of British
 Columbia
Vancouver, Canada

Timothy Dewhirst, M.A.
 Ph.D. Candidate
University of British
 Columbia
Vancouver, Canada

The editors are indebted to a number of distinguished scientists, researchers, and others in the government, universities, and the private sector who contributed critical reviews during the formation of this final monograph. We are also grateful for the guidance and support provided by **Stephen Marcus**, Ph.D., who has been given the responsibility to continue the STCP monograph series in the future.

Jeffery Wigand, Ph.D.
President
Smoke-Free Kids
Charleston, SC

Diane Pettitti, M.D., M.P.H.
Director
Division of Research and Evaluation
Kaiser Permanente Medical Care
 Program
Southern California Region
Pasadena, CA

William Farone, Ph.D.
President
Applied Power Concepts, Inc.
Anaheim, CA

Brian Beech, M.S. (OEH), C.I.H.
 (CP), R.O.H.
Tobacco Strategy Branch
Ministry of Health
Government of British of Columbia
British Columbia, Vancouver

Joel B. Cohen, Ph.D.
Distinguished Service Professor and
 Director
Center for Consumer Research
Warrington College of Business
 Administration
University of Florida

Gary A. Giovino, Ph.D., M.S.
Department of Cancer Prevention,
 Epidemiology, and Biostatics
Roswell Park Cancer Institute
Buffalo, NY

David M. Mannino, M.D.
Medical Epidemiologist
National Center for Environmental
 Health
Centers for Disease Control and
 Prevention
Atlanta, GA

Patricia Richter, Ph.D.
Toxicologist
Centers for Disease Control and
 Prevention
Office on Smoking and Health
Atlanta, GA

Ralph Caraballo, Ph.D.
Epidemiologist
Centers for Disease Control and
 Prevention
Office on Smoking and Health
Atlanta, GA

Sir Richard Doll, C.H., F.R.S., F.R.C.P.
Emeritus Professor of Medicine
Nuffield Department of Clinical
 Medicine
Oxford University
Oxford, United Kingdom

Jesse L. Steinfeld, M.D.
Former Surgeon General

C. Everett Koop, M.D., Sc.D.
Former Surgeon General
Senior Scholar
The C. Everett Koop Institute at
 Dartmouth
Hanover, NH

Jonathan M. Samet, M.D., M.S.
Professor and Chairman
Department of Epidemiology
School of Hygiene and Public Health
Johns Hopkins University
Baltimore, MD

Dorothy K. Hatsukami, Ph.D.
Professor of Psychiatry
University of Minnesota Medical
 School
Minneapolis, MN

Jack E. Henningfield, Ph.D.
Associate Professor
Department of Psychiatry and
 Behavioral Sciences
Johns Hopkins University School of
 Medicine
Baltimore, MD

and

Vice President
Research and Health Policy
Pinney Associates, Inc.
Bethesda, MD

John M. Pinney, B.A.
President
Pinney Associates, Inc.
Bethesda, MD

John R. Hughes, M.D.
Professor
Department of Psychiatry,
 Psychology, and Family Practice
University of Vermont
Burlington, VT

Sir Richard Peto, F.R.S., Hon
 M.R.C.P.
Professor of Medical Statistics and
 Epidemiology
Nuffield Department of Clinical
 Medicine
Oxford University
Oxford, United Kingdom

David T. Sweanor, J.D.
Legal Counsel
Smoking and Health Action
 Foundation
Ottawa, Canada

Kenneth E. Warner, Ph.D.
Richard D. Remington Collegiate
 Professor of Public Health/Director
University of Michigan Tobacco
 Research Network
University of Michigan

The editors also acknowledge the following individuals at the **Tobacco Control Policies Project**, University of California at San Diego, San Diego, California, for their assistance in the preparation of the monograph:

**Robert W. Davignon, M.S.**
Production Editor

**Christy M. Anderson, B.S.**
Statistician

**Jerry W. Vaughn, B.S.**
Programmer/Analyst

**Sharon Buxton**
Administrative Assistant

**Don F. Harrell**
Administrative Assistant

Finally, the editors and STCP staff would like to acknowledge the contributions of the following staff members at **KBM Group, Inc.**, Silver Spring, Maryland, who provided technical and editorial assistance in the preparation of the monograph:

**Ann L. Kreske, M.S.**
Editor/Graphic Designer

**Catherine M. McDermott, B.S.**
Copy Editor

**Heidi S. Volf, B.A.**
Proof Reader/Graphic Designer

**Sarah W. Weinstein, B.A.**
Graphic Designer

**Yaa Nsia Opare-Phillips, B.S.**
Administrative Assistant

# Contents

# Public Health Implications of Changes in Cigarette Design and Marketing

David M. Burns, Neal L. Benowitz

**INTRODUCTION**    Cigarettes have changed dramatically over the last 50 years, but the data contained in this volume make it clear that the disease risks associated with smoking have not. Following the demonstration that cigarettes could cause cancer in the 1950s (Wynder and Graham, 1950; Doll and Hill, 1952, 1954; Hammond and Horn, 1958), cigarette manufacturers added filters to their products. They also embarked on an effort to lower the machine-measured tar and nicotine yields produced by their cigarettes when tested under a protocol specified by the Federal Trade Commission (FTC) (Pillsbury, 1996). These changes led to more than a 60-percent reduction in machine-measured tar yields of U.S. cigarettes over the last 50 years (see Figure 1-1).

However, it appears that many of the same changes in cigarette design that reduced machine-measured tar yields also led to a disassociation between the machine-measured yield of the cigarette and the amount of tar and nicotine actually received by the smoker (see Chapters 2 and 3). As a result, tar and nicotine measurements made by the FTC method for current cigarettes have little meaning for the smoker, either for how much he or she will receive from a given cigarette or for differences in the amount of tar and nicotine received when he or she smokes different brands of cigarettes.

The absence of meaningful differences in smoke exposure when different brands of cigarettes are smoked (see Chapter 3) and the resultant absence of meaningful differences in risk (see Chapter 4) make the marketing of these cigarettes as lower-delivery and lower-risk products deceptive for the smoker (see Chapters 6 and 7). The reality that many smokers chose these products as an alternative to cessation—a change that would produce real reductions in disease risks—makes this deception an urgent public health issue.

**HOW DID IT HAPPEN?**    Epidemiological studies established an increased risk of lung cancer among cigarette smokers in the 1950s (Wynder and Graham, 1950; Doll and Hill, 1952, 1954; Hammond and Horn, 1958). At the same time, it was discovered that painting tobacco tar on the backs of mice could produce cancers (Wynder et al., 1953). Widespread public dissemination of the results of these studies led many smokers to quit (Burns et al., 1997), but the majority of smokers were addicted and were unable to quit or unwilling to try. Faced with the continuing exposure of large numbers of smokers to the cancer-causing substances in tobacco smoke, public health authorities made the valid conclusion that cigarettes that delivered less tar

**Figure 1-1**
**Sales-Weighted Tar and Nicotine Values for U.S. Cigarettes as Measured Using the FTC Method 1954\*-1998**

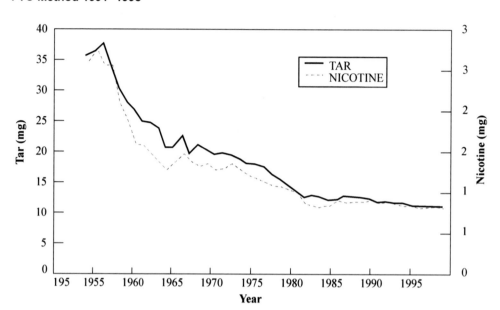

*\*Values before 1968 are estimated from available data, D. Hoffmann personal communication.*

to smokers would be likely to produce less cancer as well (U.S. Congress, 1967), and the effort to produce and market low-tar cigarettes began to gather momentum.

The recommendations by public health authorities to produce low-tar cigarettes failed to appreciate two important realities. First, smokers were powerfully addicted to the nicotine in cigarettes. They actively changed the way they smoked individual cigarettes (see Chapters 2 and 3)—and some smokers increased the number of cigarettes they smoked per day (see Chapter 4)—in order to preserve their moment-to-moment and daily intake of nicotine. Because cigarettes deliver smoke with a relatively fixed ratio of tar to nicotine, smokers also preserved their dose of tar when they preserved their dose of nicotine.

Second, public health authorities dramatically underestimated the ability of cigarette manufacturers to engineer cigarettes that would yield very low tar and nicotine values when machine smoked, but yielded much higher levels of tar and nicotine when smoked by the smoker. Cigarettes were designed with an elasticity of delivery that allowed smokers to get much higher yields of tar and nicotine by altering their pattern of puffing. Smokers may also obtain higher yields of tar and nicotine by blocking ventilation holes in the filters with their fingers or lips (see Chapter 2). Low-yield cigarettes were designed in such a way that the same alterations in puff profile (*e.g.*, larger, faster puffs) that resulted from a smoker's effort to compensate for a reduced nicotine delivery also generated much higher deliveries of tar and nicotine from the cigarette. In addition, the ventilation holes in cigarette filters were placed in locations where they could easily be blocked by smokers' lips or fingers. The combination of these two phenomena—compensation on the part of the smoker and elasticity of delivery in the cigarette—meant that most, perhaps nearly all, smokers who switched to these low-yield brands did not substantially alter their exposure to tar and nicotine and, correspondingly, did not lower their risk.

**COMPENSATION IN SMOKERS**   Nicotine intake is a principal reason why most smokers smoke (U.S. DHHS, 1988). In the absence of nicotine, smokers do not continue the compulsive use of cigarettes that characterizes addiction. Tobacco companies recognized early in the process of developing lower yield cigarettes that smokers would attempt to preserve the amount of nicotine derived from smoking (Wakeham, 1961). Compensation for reduced delivery of nicotine takes many forms and develops over time after shifting to lower yield cigarettes (see Chapter 3). Smokers may take larger puffs, inhale more deeply, take more rapid or more frequent puffs, block ventilation holes in the filters with their fingers or lips, or increase the number of cigarettes they smoke per day.

The most important question on compensatory smoking is the extent to which it occurs when smokers actually switch brands of cigarettes through their own choice. Unfortunately, this is also the most difficult circumstance under which to obtain detailed measurements of large numbers of smokers. Many studies have examined smokers when smoking in a laboratory setting or when asked to switch at specific points in time or to specific brands of cigarettes. These studies offer some insight into how smokers compensate, but may not reflect smokers' behavior when they are switching of their own volition to a brand of their choice.

Some compensatory smoking changes are evident immediately upon switching to lower yield cigarettes, but it is common for smokers to require some time to learn how to smoke lower yield cigarettes in ways that increase the delivery of nicotine to the smoker. Even under laboratory conditions, when smokers are rapidly switched to lower yield cigarettes, considerable compensation is evident. The extent of compensation increases in smokers who are allowed longer periods to adapt to smoking the new cigarettes or who are switched under conditions that more closely mimic the voluntary switching of smokers to lower yield cigarettes. When smokers of cigarettes with different machine-measured nicotine yields from the general population are examined, there is little or no relationship between the nominal nicotine yield of the cigarette smoked and measures of nicotine intake by the smoker, such as blood cotinine levels (Benowitz *et al.*, 1983: Benowitz, 1996; Jarvis *et al.*, 2001). These observations suggest that, at least when considering modern cigarettes, switching from higher to lower yield cigarettes per se is not likely to reduce tar intake and resultant disease risks.

**ELASTICITY OF DEMAND**    Early in the 1950s, cigarette manufacturers began to
**IN THE CIGARETTE**    place filters on the end of the cigarette rod. Many different filters were developed, but the most common type used in the United States was made of cellulose acetate. A variety of other approaches to tar reduction was also utilized, including "puffing" the tobacco to reduce the weight of tobacco in a cigarette, altering the blends of tobacco and porosity of the paper wrapper, changing the density of the tobacco rod, using tobacco stems and reconstituted tobacco sheet, and using a wide variety of filter materials (see Chapter 5).

In exploring these approaches, cigarette manufacturers recognized that approaches to reduction of tar yields that actually reduced the nicotine (and tar) delivery to smokers resulted in smokers discontinuing the use of those brands of cigarettes. This led to an effort to design into the cigarette an elasticity of delivery so that smokers could extract from the cigarette as much nicotine as they needed by changing the pattern of puffing on the cigarette (see Chapter 2). The goal of this effort was to develop cigarettes that would produce very low yields of tar when tested by machine smoking using the FTC protocol, but would deliver a much higher dose of nicotine when these cigarettes were smoked by actual smokers with the puffing profiles the companies knew they would use.

An important cigarette design feature allowing a low machine-measured yield with a higher actual yield is the use of ventilated filters. Holes are cut into the paper wrapping the filter in locations where they are not covered when the cigarettes are placed into the smoking machine. However, the lips or fingers of the smoker can easily cover the holes. When the holes are uncovered and the low draw rates specified by the FTC protocol are used, air is drawn into the smoking machine, diluting the smoke coming through the rod of tobacco and lowering the machine-measured tar values. When the holes are covered or when the smoker draws more rapidly on the cigarette, much more of the puff volume is composed of smoke drawn through the rod of tobacco and much less is composed of air drawn from the ventilation holes. The result is a dramatic rise in the tar and nicotine delivered to the smoker by the cigarette.

A given cigarette can be made to deliver any lower level of tar in machine measurements by increasing the size or number of the ventilation holes in the filter. The amount of nicotine in the unburned tobacco is similar for cigarettes with a wide range of machine-measured nicotine yields, as is the tar-to-nicotine ratios of the smoke from these cigarettes when they are smoked under conditions that mimic those of actual smokers (see Chapter 3). This combination of factors, plus the learned compensatory behaviors of the smoker, allows most cigarettes to deliver similar amounts of tar and nicotine to cigarette smokers without regard to the amount of tar and nicotine reported using the FTC method.

This effort by cigarette manufacturers to design cigarettes that could yield very low levels of tar when smoked by the machine while delivering full doses of tar and nicotine to smokers was not the only option available to the cigarette manufacturers. Internal tobacco company documents are replete with descriptions of filters that could selectively remove toxic smoke constituents, of treatments of tobacco with catalysts like palladium that reduced levels of carcinogens in the smoke, and of other promising modifications of cigarette toxicity. Many of the changes in cigarette design developed by cigarette manufacturers lowered levels of the toxic constituents in cigarette smoke, at least as the cigarettes were smoked using the FTC protocol. However, these paths were not pursued to the point of bringing products to market with scientifically established reductions in toxicity or carcinogenicity for smokers. The principal marketing advantage of a cigarette design scientifically established to cause less harm would be the reduced toxicity of the product. Because cigarette manufacturers persistently maintained that cigarette smoking did not cause any disease, they could not advertise a product as safer since it would be necessary to acknowledge the risks of their existing products.

One unfortunate outcome of the tobacco companies' position that cigarettes had not been established to cause any disease is the lost opportunity to develop cigarettes that have actual reductions in biological toxicity rather than simply the ability to reassure smokers concerned about the risk of smoking. The more unfortunate outcome of this position was the marketing of cigarettes with no real difference in disease risks as "safer" products.

**MARKETING OF LOW-YIELD CIGARETTES**  The link between tar and cancer risk also led to marketing of cigarettes with lower machine-measured tar yields as reduced-risk cigarettes. Terms such as 'Light' and 'Ultra-Light' were added to brand names, and substantial numbers of smokers switched to these brands in an effort to reduce their disease risks (see Chapter 6). Marketing this illusion of risk reduction would have been of concern even if the target for these brands had been confined to continuing smokers. Instead, these brands were targeted at those smokers who were thinking of quitting in an effort to intercept the smokers and keep them smoking cigarettes (see Chapter 7). The switch to low machine-measured-yield cigarettes with the illusion of risk reduction was, therefore, substituted for a real risk reduction that would have occurred had the smoker quit smoking altogether.

Beginning in the 1950s, filter cigarettes were advertised using claims of scientific discoveries, modern pure materials, and implied endorsements from medical and scientific organizations. These claims were not supported by testing that demonstrated lower deliveries of tar and nicotine to smokers or by studies of actual disease risks. However, the clear message delivered to smokers by the advertising was that these cigarettes were safer.

With the endorsement of lower tar cigarettes by public health authorities in the 1960s (U.S. Congress, 1967), cigarette marketing began to focus on machine-measured tar deliveries. Tobacco industry research and engineering efforts recognized that at least two directions were possible with the development of either a health-image (health reassurance) cigarette or a cigarette with minimal biological activity (one that would actually produce less disease) (Green, 1968). Unfortunately, the dominant direction taken was the production of health reassurance cigarettes engineered so that they

5

**Figure 1-2**
**Low Tar is Important to Me**

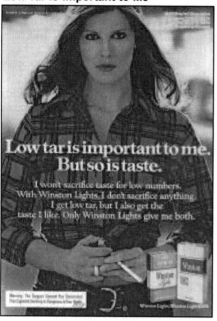

Low tar is important to me. But so is taste.

I won't sacrifice taste for low numbers. With Winston Lights, I don't sacrifice anything. I get low tar, but I also get the taste I like. Only Winston Lights give me both.

would deliver low yields of tar under FTC machine-smoking conditions. These low machine yields were touted in the advertisements and incorporated into cigarette brand names with terms such as 'Light' and 'Ultra-Light'. However, the promise of low tar delivery was only valid for the smoking machine. Smokers received a much higher dose of tar and enough nicotine to satisfy their addiction.

This dichotomy of delivery between smokers and machines was the intended result of the engineering effort to design elasticity of delivery into cigarettes. Testing of these design concepts on actual smokers revealed that Light and Regular cigarettes delivered the same levels of tar and nicotine when smoked by smokers (Goodman, 1975) and that advertising these cigarettes as low-tar-yield cigarettes was deceptive (Peeples, 1976). But these cigarettes satisfied the demand for cigarettes that could be marketed as low-tar cigarettes with full flavor or taste (See Figure 1-2). The low-tar claim presented in the ad only existed for machine smoking and the full flavor received by the smoker was accompanied by full yields of tar and full disease risks.

**DISEASE RISKS**    Having demonstrated that smokers derive similar amounts of nicotine from cigarettes with a wide variety of machine-measured nicotine yields because those cigarettes were designed to deliver a full dose of nicotine (and tar) to the smoker, one might expect that there would be little or no difference in disease risks among groups of smokers who smoke cigarettes with different machine-measured tar and nicotine yields. However, epidemiological studies have demonstrated that smokers of lower tar or filtered cigarettes had lower lung cancer risks (see Chapter 4). These findings, made in the late 1960s and 1970s, were particularly exciting since smokers had been smoking these reduced-yield cigarettes for only short periods of time. As more individuals used these products for longer periods of time, the reduction in disease risk would be expected to increase and national lung cancer death rates would fall.

Use of lower yield cigarettes grew until they were the dominant type of cigarette on the U.S. market, with 97 percent of the cigarettes currently sold in the United States being filtered cigarettes, but lung cancer rates continued to rise. Lung cancer death rates finally peaked in 1990 among White males; they continue to rise among women in spite of a higher prevalence of low-yield cigarette use among females. Examination of these trends show that they are explained by changes in smoking prevalence without postulating reductions in disease risks due to changes in cigarette design (Mannino et al., 2001; see Chapter 4).

In addition, prospective mortality studies examining smokers in the United States (Thun and Heath, 1997; Thun *et al.*, 1997) and the United Kingdom (Doll *et al.*, 1994) revealed an increase—rather than a decrease—in the risk of smoking over a period when tar and nicotine yields of cigarettes were declining. Data from two large prospective mortality studies conducted by the American Cancer Society (ACS) more than 20 years apart are particularly compelling (Thun and Heath, 1997). Machine-measured tar and nicotine yields of U.S. cigarettes declined dramatically in the interval between these two studies (see Figure 1-1), and the machine-measured yields of the cigarettes actually smoked by the participants in these two studies were dramatically different as a result (see Figure 1-3). Despite the substantive reduction in tar yield of the cigarettes smoked in CPS (Cancer Prevention Study)-II, lung cancer disease risks increased, rather than decreased, compared to CPS-I, even when controlled for differences between the two studies in number of cigarettes smoked per day and duration of smoking.

The risk reduction with use of lower yield cigarettes demonstrated in epidemiological studies and the absence of a risk reduction in U.S. lung cancer mortality trends or in the two ACS studies with changing cigarette design are observations that offer apparently conflicting interpretations of the likely disease consequences of smoking lower yield cigarettes. The epidemiological observation of lower risks with use of filtered and lower tar cigarettes has been reproduced in multiple populations and cannot be dismissed as an artifact of a single analysis or a single population. Similarly, national death rate trends are real observations not easily dismissed.

Epidemiological studies and national death rates both measure the impact of low-yield cigarettes in somewhat different ways. Epidemiological studies of disease risks compare disease rates among populations of smokers who use cigarettes with different characteristics. These studies can define whether the disease experiences of smokers of different types of cigarettes are different. However, attributing differences in disease experience to the type of cigarette smoked requires careful consideration of, and adjustment for, characteristics of the two groups that may influence disease risks other than the type of cigarette smoked.

National mortality rate trends are the cumulative result of all of the changes in smoking behavior over time, changes in cigarette design, demographic changes, and changes in smoking behavior. However, smokers of different types of cigarettes cannot be examined directly for their contribution to these trends.

The marketing of low-yield cigarettes as less risky (see Chapters 6 and 7) results in smokers switching from higher to lower yield cigarettes in an effort to reduce their disease risks (Cohen, 1996a & b; see Chapters 6 and 7), in an effort to quit, or in an effort to substantially reduce their smoking (Giovino *et al.*, 1996). Because of these health concerns and an ongoing interest in cessation, these same low-yield cigarette smokers may also have higher rates of successful long-term smoking cessation or may voluntarily reduce the amount that they smoke for health reasons. Risk reductions that

Figure 1-3
**Percentage Distribution of Tar Content, as Measured by Machine Smoking, of the Cigarette Brand Smoked at Enrollment**

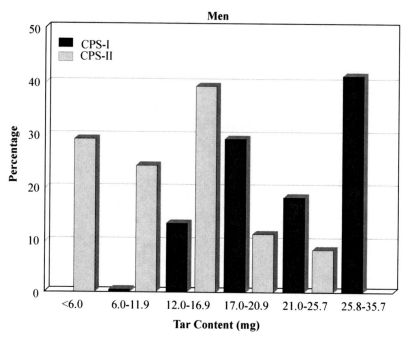

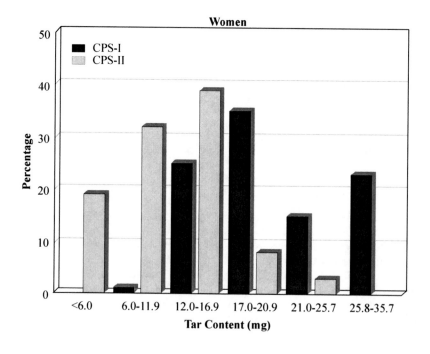

accompany cessation or lowered smoking intensity may appear to be related to the tar level of the cigarette smoked when a population is followed longitudinally for assessment of disease risk without repeated follow-up assessment of smoking status. This effect and other differences in health-related behaviors linked to low-yield cigarette use may confound the analysis of disease risk in prospective studies of low yield cigarettes.

Many published epidemiological studies of low-yield cigarettes have adjusted for the number of cigarettes smoked per day because it is the most readily available quantitative measure of smoking intensity. The potential for smokers to increase the number of cigarettes they smoke per day when they switch to lower yield cigarettes can confound analyses of disease risks among smokers of different types of cigarettes in both case-control and prospective epidemiological evaluations (see Chapter 4). Data presented in Chapter 4 show that smokers who switched to low-yield cigarettes in the ACS CPS-I increased the number of cigarettes that they smoked per day, and that smokers of ultralow-nicotine-yield cigarettes smoked more cigarettes per day in recent California tobacco surveys.

The differences between self-selected populations of smokers of different types of cigarettes and the potential for confounding between type of cigarette smoked and the number of cigarettes smoked per day may explain why epidemiological studies have demonstrated a risk difference when one has not appeared in national death rates.

However, it is clear that the expected lung cancer risk reduction offered by the reduction in lung cancer rates in epidemiological studies has not been realized in national lung cancer death rate trends. When all of the epidemiological evidence is considered in the context of what is currently known about cigarette design and compensation, it does not support the conclusion that a reduction in disease risks has occurred in the population of smokers due to the design changes that occurred in cigarettes over the last 50 years.

This report reviews evidence on the FTC method for measuring tar and nicotine yields and the disease risks of machine-measured low-tar cigarettes. The evidence is derived from research on human behavior and exposures, cigarette design and yields, smoke chemistry, epidemiological other and population-based data on human disease risk. In conducting this review, the objective was to determine whether the evidence taken as a whole shows that the cumulative effect of engineering changes in cigarette design over the last 50 years has reduced disease risks in smokers. Traditional scientific judgment requires compelling evidence of a difference before concluding that use of lower yield products reduces disease risk. These judgments are especially important for harm reduction claims, as they may deter smokers from cessation of tobacco use. Moreover, there have been previous public policy statements on the likely benefits of lower yield products. These prior statements may lead to confusion by creating an implication that the appropriate standard for judgment would require proof of the absence of an effect before the policy recommendations should be withdrawn. Given the consequences of being wrong on the advice given to smokers, the burden of proof should not be shifted from proving the presence of an effect. The perspective of this report is whether the existing evidence is sufficient to support claims that disease risks are reduced when smokers switch to lower yield cigarettes and policy recommendations that smokers who cannot quit should switch to these products. The answers to these questions are that current evidence does not support either claims of reduced harm or policy recommendations to switch to these products.

Many questions remain unanswered. For example, the disease risks of recently introduced cigarettes or cigarette-like products are not known. Similarly, the cancer risks for individuals who have only used low and ultra-low cigarettes, and who may have different intensities of smoking as a result, have yet to be fully described. Changes in age-specific lung cancer death rates at younger ages in the United Kingdom suggest that the future lung cancer experiences of these young smokers may differ from that of prior generations of smokers. In addition, the possibility exists that individual product design changes, or future changes in tobacco industry produced nicotine delivery devices, may reduce disease risks in the future. However, the burden of proof for these benefits must remain with those who would make the claims. The proof must integrate both measurements of dose and measures of actual biological effect. The very real probability that addicted smokers will seek out and rely upon the promised potential of reduced risk for products that allow continued smoking creates an obligation to require clear scientific proof of harm reduction claims before they are communicated to potential product users.

## CONCLUSIONS

1. Epidemiological and other scientific evidence, including patterns of mortality from smoking-caused diseases, does not indicate a benefit to public health from changes in cigarette design and manufacturing over the last fifty years.

2. For spontaneous brand switchers, there appears to be complete compensation for nicotine delivery, reflecting more intensive smoking of lower-yield cigarettes.

3. Widespread adoption of lower yield cigarettes in the United States has not prevented the sustained increase in lung cancer among older smokers.

4. Many smokers switch to lower yield cigarettes out of concern for their health, believing these cigarettes to be less risky or to be a step toward quitting. Advertising and marketing of lower yield cigarettes may promote initiation and impede cessation, more important determinants of smoking-related diseases.

5. Measurements of tar and nicotine yields using the FTC method do not offer smokers meaningful information on the amount of tar and nicotine they will receive from a cigarette. The measurements also do not offer meaningful information on the relative amounts of tar and nicotine exposure likely to be received from smoking different brands of cigarettes.

## REFERENCES

Benowitz, N.L. Biomarkers of cigarette smoking. *The FTC Cigarette Test Method for Determining Tar, Nicotine, and Carbon Monoxide Yields of U.S. Cigarettes. Report of the NCI Expert Committee.* Smoking and Tobacco Control Monograph No. 7. U.S. Department of Health and Human Services, National Institutes of Health, National Cancer Institute, NIH Publication No. 96-4028, 1996.

Benowitz, N.L., Hall, S.M., Herning, R.I., Jacob, P., Jones, R.T., Osman, A. Smokers of low-yield cigarettes do not consume less nicotine. *New England Journal of Medicine* 309(3):139-42, 1983.

Burns, D., Lee, L., Shen, Z., Gilpin, B., Tolley, D., Vaughn, J., Shanks, T. Cigarette smoking behavior in the United States. *Changes in Cigarette-Related Disease Risks and Their Implication for Prevention and Control.* Smoking and Tobacco Control Monograph No. 8. U.S. Department of Health and Human Services, National Institutes of Health, National Cancer Institute, NIH Publication No. 97-4213, 1997.

Cohen, J. B. Consumer/smoker perceptions of Federal Trade Commission tar ratings. *The FTC Cigarette Test Method for Determining Tar, Nicotine, and Carbon Monoxide Yields of U.S. Cigarettes. Report of the NCI Expert Committee.* Smoking and Tobacco Control Monograph No. 7. U.S. Department of Health and Human Services, National Institutes of Health, National Cancer Institute, NIH Publication No. 96-4028, 1996a.

Cohen, J. B. Smokers' knowledge and understanding of advertised tar numbers: Health policy implications. *American Journal of Public Health* 86(1):18-24, 1996b.

Doll, R., Hill, A.B. A study of the aetiology of carcinoma of the lung. *British Medical Journal* 2:1271-1286, 1952.

Doll, R., Hill, A.B. The mortality of doctors in relation to their smoking habits: A preliminary report. *British Medical Journal* 1(4877):1451-1455, 1954.

Doll, R., Peto, R., Wheatley, K., Gray, R., Sutherland, I. Mortality in relation to smoking: 40 years' observations on male British doctors. *British Medical Journal* 309(6959):901-911, 1994.

Giovino, G.A., Tomar, S.L., Reddy, M.N., Peddicord, J.P., Zhu, B.P., Escobedo, L.G., Eriksen, M.P. Attitudes, knowledge, and beliefs about low-yield cigarettes among adolescents and adults. *The FTC Cigarette Test Method for Determining Tar, Nicotine, and Carbon Monoxide Yields of U.S. Cigarettes. Report of the NCI Expert Committee.* Smoking and Tobacco Control Monograph No. 7. U.S. Department of Health and Human Services, National Institutes of Health, National Cancer Institute, NIH Publication No. 96-4028, 1996.

Goodman, B. to Meyer, L.F. September 17, 1975. Memo by Barboro Goodman. Marlboro—Marlboro Lights study delivery data. Bates No. 2021544486.

Green, S.J. Research conference held at Hilton Head Island, S.C. September 24th-30th, 1968. University of California San Francisco Tobacco Archive Document I.D. No. 1112.01, 1968.

Hammond, E.C., Horn, D. Smoking and death rates—Report on forty-four months of follow-up of 187,783 men. II. Death rates by cause. *Journal of the American Medical Association* 166:1294-1308, 1958.

Jarvis, M.J., Boreham, R., Primatesta, P., Feyerabend, C., Bryant, A. Nicotine yield from machine-smoked cigarettes and nicotine intakes in smokers: Evidence from a representative population survey. *Journal of the National Cancer Institute* 93(2):134-138, 2001.

Mannino, D.M., Ford, E., Giovino, G.A, Thun, M. Lung cancer mortality rates in birth cohorts in the United States from 1960 to 1994. *Lung Cancer* 31(2-3):91-99, 2001.

Pepples, E. Industry response to cigarette/health controversy. Memo dated February 4, 1976. University of California San Francisco Tobacco Archive Document I.D. No. 2205.01, 1976.

Pillsbury H.C. Review of the Federal Trade Commission Method for determining cigarette tar and nicotine yield. *The FTC Cigarette Test Method for Determining Tar, Nicotine, and Carbon Monoxide Yields of U.S. Cigarettes. Report of the NCI Expert Committee.* Smoking and Tobacco Control Monograph No. 7. U.S. Department of Health and Human Services, National Institutes of Health, National Cancer Institute, NIH Publication No. 96-4028, 1996.

Thun, M.J., Heath, C.W. Changes in mortality from smoking in two American Cancer Society prospective studies since 1959. *Preventive Medicine* 26(4):422-426. 1997.

Thun, M., Myersm D., Day-Lallym C., Myers, D.G., Calle, E., Flanders, W.D., Zhu, B.P., Namboodiri, M., Heath, Jr, C. Trends in tobacco smoking and mortality from cigarette use in Cancer Prevention Studies I (1959 through 1965) and II (1982 through 1988). *Changes in Cigarette-Related Disease Risks and Their Implications for Prevention and Control.* Smoking and Tobacco Control Monograph No. 8. U.S. Department of Health and Human Services, National Institutes of Health, National Cancer Institute, NIH Publication No. 97-4213, 1997.

U.S. Congress. Hearings before the Consumer Subcommittee of the Committee on Commerce. Senate, 90th Congress, August 23-24, 1967.

U.S. Department of Health and Human Services. *The Health Consequences of Smoking: Nicotine Addiction. A Report of the Surgeon General.* Washington, D.C.: U.S. Department of Health and Human Services, Public Health Service, Centers for Disease Control and Prevention, Center for Health Promotion and Education, Office on Smoking and Health, DHHS Publication No. (CDC) 88-8406, 1988.

Wakeham, H. to Cullman, H. March 24, 1961. Memo by Hugh Wakeham. Trends in tar and nicotine deliveries over the last 5 years. Bates No. 1000861953.

Wynder, E.L., Graham, E.A. Tobacco smoking as a possible etiologic factor in bronchogenic carcinoma. A study of six hundred and eighty-four proved cases. *Journal of the American Medical Association* 143:329-336, 1950.

Wynder, E.L., Graham, E.A., Croninger, A.B. Experimental production of carcinoma with cigarette tar. *Cancer Research* 13:855-864, 1953.

# Cigarette Design

Lynn T. Kozlowski, Richard J. O'Connor, Christine T. Sweeney

**CIGARETTE-YIELD TESTING BY SMOKING MACHINE USING THE FTC PROTOCOL** The modern low-yield cigarette is defined by a standardized smoking-machine test commonly referred to as the FTC method (Peeler, 1996), based on the Federal Trade Commission protocol. This smoking-machine procedure simulates a precise manner of smoking by fixing puff size (35 ml), puffing rate (once per minute), puff duration (2 seconds), and butt length to which the cigarette is smoked (23 mm on an unfiltered cigarette or overwrap, plus 3 mm on a filtered cigarette). The number of puffs to be taken is not specified. The standard yields of tar and nicotine measured are reported in cigarette advertising (according to a cooperative agreement) and on some very low-tar cigarette packs (as measured by the FTC method) at the manufacturer's discretion (Peeler, 1996; Kozlowski *et al.*, 1998c). Carbon monoxide (CO) is also measured, but is not reported in advertising. The same basic methodology is used for cigarette testing in Canada, Australia, and the United Kingdom. In the United States, cigarette brands yielding approximately 1-5 or 6 mg tar by this standard method are generally called 'Ultra-Light'; brands yielding between approximately 6 or 7-15 mg tar are called 'Light'; and brands yielding more than 15 mg tar are called 'Regular' or 'Full Flavor'. By convention, cigarettes yielding 15 mg tar by the FTC method are called 'low tar'.

The origins of the FTC method can be found in the early efforts of tobacco industry researchers to compare cigarettes of the day. They arbitrarily selected the smoking parameters of a 35-ml puff volume, a 2-second puff duration, and a one-puff-per-minute frequency (Bradford *et al.*, 1936). At the time, nearly all cigarettes were unfiltered, lacked overwraps, and were of similar length, weight, and circumference; presumably, most had similar burn times, a characteristic closely related to the number of puffs taken. The past 30 years has seen dramatic growth of variation in the physical characteristics of cigarettes, with differences in circumference ('slims' to 'wides'), length (70-120 mm), and weights.

**CHANGES IN FTC MACHINE-SMOKED YIELDS OVER TIME** Each year since 1968, the FTC has reported sales-weighted yields of tar and nicotine based on the FTC protocol (Table 2-1). Average sales-weighted standard tar yield decreased from 21.6 mg in 1968 to 12.0 mg in 1997 (44.4 percent), while average sales-weighted nicotine yield decreased from 1.35 mg to 0.89 mg (34.1 percent). Though standard tar and nicotine yields have the status of official FTC data, it would be wrong to assume that these numbers have any bearing on smoker exposure to tar and nicotine.

13

Table 2-1
**Sales-Weighted Tar and Nicotine Yields: 1968-1997**

| Year | Tar(mg) | Nicotine (mg) | Tar/Nicotine |
|------|---------|---------------|--------------|
| 1968 | 21.6 | 1.35 | 16.00 |
| 1969 | 20.7 | 1.38 | 15.00 |
| 1970 | 20.0 | 1.31 | 15.27 |
| 1971 | 20.2 | 1.32 | 15.30 |
| 1972 | 19.9 | 1.39 | 14.32 |
| 1973 | 19.3 | 1.32 | 14.62 |
| 1974 | 18.4 | 1.24 | 14.84 |
| 1975 | 18.6 | 1.21 | 15.37 |
| 1976 | 18.1 | 1.16 | 15.60 |
| 1977 | 16.8 | 1.12 | 15.00 |
| 1978 | 16.1 | 1.11 | 14.50 |
| 1979 | 15.1 | 1.07 | 14.11 |
| 1980 | 14.1 | 1.04 | 13.56 |
| 1981 | 13.2 | 0.92 | 14.35 |
| 1982 | 13.5 | 0.89 | 15.17 |
| 1983 | 13.4 | 0.88 | 15.23 |
| 1984 | 13.0 | 0.89 | 14.61 |
| 1985 | 13.0 | 0.95 | 13.68 |
| 1986 | 13.4 | 0.93 | 14.41 |
| 1987 | 13.3 | 0.94 | 14.15 |
| 1988 | 13.3 | 0.94 | 14.15 |
| 1989 | 13.1 | 0.96 | 13.65 |
| 1990 | 12.5 | 0.93 | 13.44 |
| 1991 | 12.6 | 0.94 | 13.40 |
| 1992 | 12.4 | 0.92 | 13.48 |
| 1993 | 12.4 | 0.90 | 13.78 |
| 1994 | 12.1 | 0.90 | 13.44 |
| 1995 | 12.0 | 0.87 | 13.79 |
| 1996 | 12.0 | 0.88 | 13.64 |
| 1997 | 12.0 | 0.89 | 13.48 |

**DESIGN CHANGES THAT REDUCE STANDARD YIELDS** Changes in cigarette design have produced the reductions in standard yields of tar and nicotine measured over the past several decades. Although it is unlikely that decreases in FTC tar yields of only a few milligrams are toxicologically consequential, cigarette manufacturers can manipulate variables that combine to make small changes in yields or in the sensory effects of cigarettes. Such reformulations can have important policy implications. For example, changing a cigarette slightly to reduce the standard tar yield from 16 mg to 15 mg would increase the percentage of low-tar cigarettes on the market, and thereby reduce sales-weighted tar levels. However, even without compensatory smoking, such a small change would likely have negligible effects on health.

Cigarette design manipulations intended to decrease standard yields can be divided into those having two broad functional effects: 1) reducing the number of puffs per cigarette, and 2) reducing the tar and nicotine concentration in smoke per puff (Kozlowski, 1983). Table 2-2 provides a summary

Table 2-2
**Main Ways to Reduce Standard Tar and Nicotine Yields**

**A. Reduce the number of puffs taken by:**
  1) decreasing the length of the available tobacco column with
        a. longer filter overwraps,
        b. longer filters;
  2) increasing the burn rate of the column with
        a. chemical additives in paper or tobacco,
        b. higher porosity paper,
        c. less tobacco (by weight),
        d. lower diameter tobacco column.

**B. Reduce concentration of tar and nicotine per puff by:**
  1) increasing filter efficiency with
        a. ventilated filters (by reducing tobacco amount/puff),
        b. longer filters,
        c. denser filters,
        d. 'active' filters;
  2) increasing air dilution of mainstream smoke with
        a. ventilated filters,
        b. higher porosity paper;
  3) decreasing the density of tobacco with
        a. reconstituted sheet tobacco,
        b. puffed or expanded tobaccos,
        c. flavorings (casings) and additives,
        d. smaller circumference cigarettes;
  4) tobacco blending with
        a. use of lower nicotine yield tobacco strains,
        b. flue-cured, burley, oriental tobaccos,
        c. different parts/leaf positions of plants.

of these factors. Manufacturing cigarettes that produce lower FTC tar and nicotine yields is a complex, multi-factorial process—a complicated recipe. Manipulating one variable also affects other variables. Cigarette design involves alteration of elements within a complex system. For example, if one simply increased filter ventilation greatly, this would cause less tobacco to be consumed with each standard puff, and thereby cause an increased number of puffs. Altering design to increase the inter-puff burn rate (*e.g.*, chemical treatments of the cigarette paper or using less tobacco) deals with this issue (Philip Morris, 1980).

The design features listed in Table 2-2 should not be considered 'secrets' of cigarette manufacture. Many of these design characteristics were discussed in a classic book on tobacco and tobacco smoke by Wynder and Hoffman (1967) and more recently by Browne (1990). Journals such as *Beitrage Zur Tabakforschung* and *Tobacco Science* have been available in research libraries for decades. Research articles on such design features have been published by various industry scientists (*e.g.*, Parker and Montgomery,

1979; Shoffner and Ireland, 1982). What is secret, however, is the exact for-mulation of a particular brand at any given time. Even if details are sup-plied in some of the formerly secret tobacco company documents, there is no guarantee, for example, that the Marlboro Light® brand of 1985 is the same in all attributes as the same named brand in 2000.

Three design features that can influence standard yield will be dis-cussed. They are: available length of tobacco (which relates to burn rate), tobacco column nicotine content, and filter ventilation.

**Available Length of Tobacco**  Because the last few puffs on a cigarette have higher deliveries than the first few puffs, eliminating the last puff by increasing the burn rate has a relatively large effect on reducing tar and nicotine yields. The FTC test method has never required the recording or reporting of the number of puffs taken by the smoking machine, yet industry testing of cigarettes has routinely done so. The official Canadian cigarette testing laboratory (Labstat Incorporated, Kitchener, Ontario) has customarily col-lected the number of puffs taken by the machine for each cigarette smoked. In one study, 12 best-selling Canadian cigarette brands were shown to have decreased from 9.8 to 8.8 puffs per cigarette (a 10 percent reduction) between 1969 and 1974; during the same period, tar yield decreased 13.6 percent, from 22 mg to 19 mg (Kozlowski *et al.*, 1980b).

There is some evidence that increases in the length of the overwrap (the distinctive paper wrap covering the outside of the filter) have been used to decrease the number of puffs taken (Grunberg *et al.*, 1985). Other things being equal, a longer "filter plus overwrap" will result in a longer butt being left in the smoking machine. However, tobacco exists under the overwrap that is still available to be smoked by the human smoker. This additional tobacco would not be burned in the FTC test, resulting in a lower standard yield, but a potentially higher yield for the actual smoker.

**Nicotine Content of Tobacco**  Different types of tobacco can contain different amounts of nicotine, with burley being the highest and flue-cured tobacco being somewhat lower. Oriental tobaccos and reconstituted tobacco sheet have substantially lower nicotine contents. Different parts of the same tobacco plant can contain different nicotine levels based on stalk position, soil nitrogen, and the curing process. Blends of tobacco strains and tobacco from particular segments can contribute to the blend of a particular ciga-rette brand. These blends, combined with the use of fillers, additives, and reconstituted sheet tobacco in the tobacco column of cigarettes, can lead to differences in nicotine contents among brands. Kozlowski and colleagues (1998b) measured the nicotine content of the "tobacco column" (a complex of tobacco, reconstituted sheet, flavorings, and casings) in American, British, and Canadian cigarette brands. On the whole, American cigarette brands contained less nicotine per cigarette (10.2 mg ± 0.25 SEM) than either British (12.5 mg ± 0.33 SEM) or Canadian (13.5 mg ± 0.49 SEM) brands (p < 0.008). Among American brands, nicotine contents ranged from a high of 13.4 mg (Newport Full-Flavor®) to a low of 7.3 mg (GPC Lights®). The nicotine content of Canadian brands ranged from a high of 18.3 mg (Players Extra Light®) to a low of 8.0 mg (Players Full Flavour®), while

British brands ranged from a high of 15.9 mg (Knightsbridge® Super King) to a low of 9.0 mg (Dorchester®). Brands with the lowest standard nicotine yield (0.1 mg), such as Carlton®, Carlton® 100, Merit Ultima®, and Craven Ultra-Mild®, contained between 8.7-11.2 mg nicotine per cigarette (Kozlowski *et al.*, 1998b).

These same authors found a significant positive correlation ($r = 0.51$ [95% CI = 0.20–0.73]) between brand FTC nicotine yield and the nicotine content of tobacco. In 1997, the state of Massachusetts required testing of the best-selling cigarettes ($N = 15$ brand groups) for nicotine content of whole tobacco (American Cancer Society, 2000). This testing showed no significant differences between brand categories (Full Flavor, Light, or Ultra-Light). This discrepancy in the relationship between standard yields and nicotine content may be due to the exclusion of poor-selling, very low FTC tar brands from the Massachusetts sample. But substantial differences in nicotine content of tobacco were nonetheless found between some brands. Values ranged from a low of 8.3 mg for GPC Lights® King Size to a high of 15.48 mg for Marlboro® 100 Soft Pack (an 87 percent difference—low to high), which cannot be viewed as a small difference. Note that Kozlowski and associates (1998b) found an 84 percent difference between the lowest and highest nicotine content observed (see above).

**Filter Ventilation**     Although each of the manufacturing changes listed in Table 2-2 (including those intended to reduce the number of puffs per cigarette) has contributed to the development of lower tar and nicotine cigarettes, filter ventilation has been the major innovation behind the modern low-yield cigarette (Kozlowski, 1983; Kozlowski *et al.*, 1998b). Filter vents, which usually are one or more rings of small holes or perforations, serve to dilute smoke with air, thereby reducing standard yields of tar, nicotine, and CO.

A 1956 Philip Morris memo to the company's most senior executives maintained that ventilation could serve as a "counter-attack" to negative health claims about smoking because it reduced "smoke solids," CO, and irritation (DuPuis, 1956).

Vents are placed in the filter by one of three main processes: electrostatic perforation, mechanical perforation, or laser perforation (Helms, 1983; Helms and Lorenzen, 1984). The method of perforation can influence actual tar and nicotine delivery to the smoker (this issue will be addressed further in the next section). Whatever the method of perforation, the location of filter vents generally ranges from 11 to 15 mm from the mouth end of the filter. In a recent study, the filter ventilation levels of 32 U.S. cigarette brands were tested and found to range from 0 to 83 percent (Kozlowski *et al.*, 1998b). A cigarette with 0 percent filter ventilation would produce a puff of smoke undiluted by air from filter vents. A cigarette with 83 percent filter ventilation would produce a puff that is 83 percent air from vents and 17 percent smoke undiluted by air from vents.

Increases in ventilation appear to have been important in meeting the tar-yield maximum in the European Economic Community. Internal Philip Morris documents indicated that the company's strategy for reducing the

17

smoke deliveries of its Marlboro® brands in Europe rested primarily on increasing filter ventilation (Stolt, 1977). Tests have shown that Full-Flavor Marlboro® cigarettes are now twice as ventilated in the United Kingdom as in the United States (19.5 versus 10.2 percent); similar differences are seen for Marlboro Light® (44.9 versus 22.5 percent) (Kozlowski *et al.*, 1998b).

## COMPENSATION AND CIGARETTE DESIGN: DIFFERENCE IN YIELD WITH DIFFERENT SMOKING PATTERNS

The observed decreases in standardized yields of tar and nicotine that have occurred since 1968 do not seem to translate into reduced exposures for smokers. Smokers can consciously or unconsciously compensate for lower standard yields in a number of easy and effective ways.

**Increasing Puff Number**    Of course, smokers are not limited in the number of puffs they may take from a cigarette. Smokers can counteract yield reduction methods that reduce puff number simply by taking more puffs per cigarette. If smokers receive less tar and nicotine per puff from lower yield products, they can easily compensate by taking more puffs or, of course, smoking more cigarettes per day. Across 32 studies cited by the Surgeon General (U.S. DHHS, 1988), the average of the mean inter-puff intervals was 34 seconds, with a range of 18-64 seconds. This contrasts with the 58-second inter-puff interval used with the FTC method. Naturally, the actual range of inter-puff intervals would be much larger than this range of means. Results from a recent laboratory study revealed that smokers of low-yield ($\leq$ 0.8 mg nicotine by FTC method) and high-yield (0.9-1.2 mg nicotine by FTC method) cigarette brands had significantly shorter inter-puff intervals (about 20 seconds) than those of the FTC protocol (Djordjevic *et al.*, 2000). Clearly, smokers often take more than one puff per minute and can thereby increase their actual yield.

**Increasing Puff Volume**    A major and easy way for the smoker to increase smoke intake is to increase the volume of each puff. Total puff volume per cigarette is a function of puff number and volume per puff. In terms of overall exposure, total volume per cigarette is a better index and gives insight into how much 'work' the smoker performed in smoking the cigarette. Smokers are free to take large or small puffs on their cigarettes. The 32 studies summarized in the Surgeon General report (U.S. DHHS, 1988) confirmed that puff volumes often deviate from the FTC standard. The average of mean puff volumes across the studies was 43 ml, with a range of 22-66 ml. Again, because these represent ranges of means, the actual ranges of individual scores would be broader.

Published studies confirm that smokers will change their puff sizes in response to the type of cigarette that they smoke. Herning and associates (1981) studied smokers who were smoking the first cigarette of the day. These smokers showed larger puff volumes on the low-nicotine cigarettes (47.8 ml) than on either the medium- or high-nicotine cigarettes (35.9 ml and 36.9 ml, respectively). Among 10 participants studied by Tobin and Sackner (1982), larger puff volumes were taken from the low-tar cigarettes (52 ml) than from the high-tar cigarettes (39 ml) ($P < 0.001$). A study by Moody (1980) reported a mean puff volume of 43.5 ml. Djordjevic and colleagues (2000) recently reported that the average volumes of smoke per puff for smokers of low-yield and medium-yield cigarette brands were 48.6 ml and 44.1 ml, respectively. Other investigators have noted similar findings (*e.g.*, Zacny *et al.*, 1986, 1987; Zacny and Stitzer, 1988). These studies showed that the FTC test underestimates the volume of smoke taken from lower tar cigarettes. Industry studies show that smokers often take far more in total volume of smoke than is predicted by the FTC test. In two separate Philip Morris studies, smokers (one in each study) independently took nearly 1,400 ml of smoke from Carlton® cigarettes, in both cases nearly five times the expected FTC value for a whole cigarette (Wakeham, 1974; Kelley, 1977).

Additionally, unpublished industry research revealed that puff volumes increase as standard yields decrease (see Norman and Ihrig, 1980a & b, at Lorillard, discussed later in the chapter). Clearly, puff volume changes represent a significant and easy mode of compensation for low-yield products.

**Dilution and Puff Volume**    As discussed earlier, filter ventilation dilutes smoke with air. One way for the smoker to compensate for the reduced nicotine delivery that results from air dilution is to increase puff volume. If a smoker increases puff volume, he or she will receive more smoke from the cigarette along with more air. This larger puff might feel 'lighter' to the smoker than if they had taken a smaller, more concentrated puff of equivalent yield from an unventilated or less-ventilated cigarette. This effect of 'softening' the taste or reducing the harshness of taste may be an important reason for the perception of 'lightness' in lower standard-yield cigarettes (Kozlowski *et al.*, 1998a, 1999, 2000).

Consider a simplified model of ventilation and puff volume. A curvilinear relationship exists between the level of dilution and the puff volume needed to compensate for reduced yield (Sutton *et al.*, 1978). The formula for puff volume percentage increase needed to compensate is as follows: percentage increase in puff volume = (% dilution/[100 − % dilution]) x 100. As dilution increases, puff volume to compensate increases exponentially. According to Kozlowski and colleagues (1998b), for a cigarette with 13 percent dilution (*e.g.*, Marlboro® Full Flavor), a small puff volume increase (15 percent, from 35 ml to 40 ml) would provide full compensation for the dilution. To compensate fully for a 40 percent diluted cigarette (*e.g.*, Virginia Slims Light® 100), a puff volume of 58 ml (a 67 percent increase) would be needed. In contrast, with a highly ventilated cigarette such as Carlton® 100 (83 percent diluted), a large and generally impractical puff volume of 206 ml would be required. These estimates assume a 35 ml base puff (the base puff is what is assumed to occur with no ventilation). For those with a 45 ml base puff, a heroic puff of 265 ml would be required to compensate for the 83 percent dilution on the 1 mg tar cigarette. The best-selling Marlboro Light® cigarette is just 23 percent diluted, and an easy puff of about 60 ml (from a 45 ml base) or only 45 ml (from a 35 ml base) would fully compensate. Increased puff volume is a very likely mode of compensation when it can be performed without significant additional effort (*i.e.*, for a Light cigarette with low-to-moderate air dilution). For a heavily ventilated cigarette (*e.g.*, 83 percent diluted, 1 mg tar), increasing per-puff volume within acceptable bounds of comfort and effort alone will not generally provide full or even substantial compensation. (Of course, smokers are not constrained to simply take bigger puffs; they may also take more puffs; for more, see Kozlowski *et al.*, 1998b.)

The phenomenon of compensating with bigger puffs is well known to industry scientists. For example, Norman and Ihrig (1980a) of Lorillard conducted a series of studies concerning puff volumes and puff velocities on lower tar cigarettes being greater than those for higher tar cigarettes. These authors assumed that ultralow-tar brands were more palatable to the smoker if compensatory smoking required a modest amount of additional effort. To describe this effort, they derived the "puffing power function" (Norman and Ihrig, 1980b), defined as the product of the flow rate through the cigarette and pressure drop required to produce that flow.

These authors examined the relationship between puffing power functions (expressed in 'puffing power units' or PPU) and puffing regimens (at standard FTC 35 ml as well as 50 ml puffs). The increase in PPU represented the "extra effort needed to obtain a given amount of additional [tar] from the cigarette" (Norman and Ihrig, 1980b). They thought that an understanding of puffing effort is critical for very low-yield brands, since these are most likely to be smoked with extra effort to obtain more smoke.

Increasing puff volume can have additional effects, especially if puff velocity also increases. Other things being equal, a higher velocity puff (*i.e.*, > 17.5 ml/sec) will reduce filter efficiency (*i.e.*, the percentage of what enters the filter that remains in the filter). Further, filter tip ventilation decreases as flow rate increases. If the cigarette is ventilated with high-porosity paper, however, the opposite is true—dilution increases with increasing flow rate:

> ". . . [A] cigarette constructed with low paper porosity but with filter tip ventilation would more readily allow a smoker to take a higher delivery of smoke by increasing the velocity of puffing. Such a cigarette construction would provide a marketing opportunity to offer a LOW to LOW TO MIDDLE delivery product when smoked by machine, which could be a LOW TO MIDDLE to MIDDLE delivery product when smoked by the smoker."

> . . . "Alternatively, if a cigarette is manufactured to have no filter tip ventilation, but high paper porosity, the smoker would not be able to compensate for reduced delivery by puffing harder; in fact, the higher the velocity of the puff, the lower the delivery. Theoretically the smoker would be able to increase delivery by reducing his puffing velocity and increasing the duration of the puff. This is unlikely to occur to any marked extent as it would require a marked change of habit that would probably feel uncomfortable to the smoker." (See Creighton, 1978a.)

Air drawn through the vents dilutes the smoke, but also generally reduces the draw resistance through the filter and tobacco rod (Creighton, 1978a). For example, Zacny and associates (1986) found that the average "resistance to draw" (RTD—the amount of pressure that must be exerted on the filter for inhalation) of an unblocked (*i.e.*, fully ventilated) Now® cigarette was 92.5 mm H2O (for Kozlowski *et al.*, 1998b, Now® was 66.3 percent diluted). In contrast, the same cigarette fully blocked (*i.e.*, unventilated) had an RTD of 184.4 mm H2O, a 100 percent increase. This lower RTD for the ventilated cigarette means the smoker can easily take a larger puff on the cigarette with little added effort and receive more smoke from the cigarette. Lower RTD, in effect, promotes the use of increased puff volume as a compensation method. Industry studies bear this observation out (Long, 1955; Goodman, 1977; Creighton and Watts, 1972; Mendell, 1983). The air-diluted smoke would also be less irritating than the same smoke undiluted, and thereby would also facilitate increased puff volumes because inhibitory oral and respiratory cues would be milder.

Additional industry research has looked at interactions between the type of ventilation used and puff volume. A. B. Norman and others at R. J. Reynolds Tobacco Co. compared laser, mechanical, and electrostatic perforation types (Norman *et al.*, 1984). Laser perforations were found to promote compensation with increased puff volumes. That is, as puff volumes increased, filter air dilution decreased most significantly with laser perforations. W. I. Casey (1994) at R. J. Reynolds explored yields from different tobacco blends with perforations as "holes" versus "slots" (hole versus slot is not defined). Cigarettes were tested according to FTC procedures as well as "50/30" procedures (50 ml puff, every 30 seconds); brands had approximately equal air-dilution levels (80-85 percent). Two rows of slots gave the same nicotine (0.11 mg) as did two rows of holes under FTC conditions, but gave more nicotine under the 50/30 condition: 0.67 versus 0.53 mg. Ventilation holes increased yield by 382 percent and ventilation slots increased yield by 509 percent over FTC estimates, simply by increasing puff volume and puff number. This effect of slots versus holes was not found for another tobacco blend. Here, one can see that design features (*e.g.*, filter ventilation and tobacco blend) can interact dramatically with smoker behavior (puff volume/puff interval) to produce more elastic products (*i.e.*, giving low values to the smoking machine, but higher values to smokers).

**Blocking Filter Vents**    Another technique smokers can use to increase smoke concentration is the blocking of filter vents. Research has found that the majority of smokers are unaware of the presence of vents in general or even on their own brands (Kozlowski *et al.*, 1996, 1998d). At best, filter vents are placed just millimeters from lips or fingers, and they are often not noticed by smokers (Kozlowski *et al.*, 1998d). Smokers can and do obstruct the vents with either their lips or fingers, thereby diminishing or defeating the air-dilution effect. The ease with which smokers can unknowingly compensate for low standard yields by interfering with this important design feature has long been known within the cigarette industry. Internal company documents from the British American Tobacco Co. indicate that the industry acknowledges the importance of filter ventilation for designing products to be compensatable or elastic. For example, in one document, this question was asked—"Which product/design properties influence elasticity?" The answer—"1. Tip ventilation: bigger effects at higher degree of ventilation. . . 2. Delivery of the blend . . ." (Brown & Williamson, 1984).

**Effects of Vent Blocking on Smoke Exposure** The earliest of the published studies to examine the effects of vent blocking used smoking machine estimates to simulate the effect of vent blocking. Blocking half the vents of a 4 mg tar cigarette, for example, increased the smoking-machine yields of tar by 60 percent (from 4.40 to 7.03 mg), nicotine by 62 percent (from 0.45 to 0.73 mg), and CO by 73 percent (from 4.50 to 7.80 mg) (Kozlowski *et al.*, 1980a & b). Blocking all of the filter vents of these same cigarettes with tape increased yields of tar by 186 percent (from 4.40 to 12.60 mg), nicotine by 118 percent (from 0.45 to 0.98 mg), and CO by 293 percent (from 4.50 to 17.70 mg). In another study, Kozlowski and colleagues (1982) completely tape-blocked the vents on different brands of 1 mg tar cigarettes from Canada, the United States, and the United Kingdom. Cigarettes were smoked more intensely in the blocked condition (2.4 second puff duration; 44 second puff interval; 47 ml puff volume). Tar yield increased from 1,360 percent (Cambridge® [0.8-11.7 mg]) to 3,800 percent (Viscount No. 1® [0.3-11.7 mg]). Nicotine yield increased from 720 percent (Cambridge® [0.1-0.82 mg]) to 1,767 percent (John Player Ultra Mild® King Size [0.12-2.24 mg]). Similarly, CO yield increased from 870 percent (Cambridge® [1.8-17.5 mg]) to 4,180 percent (John Player Ultra Mild® King Size [0.50-21.4 mg]) under the more intense smoking conditions. Compare this to an unventilated reference cigarette, which saw yield increases of 46 percent for tar, 35.8 percent for nicotine, and 35.7 percent for CO under these intense conditions.

In a 1983 study, Rickert and associates tested 36 brands of Canadian cigarettes (including 28 brands that had ventilated filters) on a smoking machine under three experimental conditions to simulate how smokers' exposure to toxic substances would be affected by smoking patterns of different intensities. In the 'moderate' condition (which was used to represent more typical smoking behavior), puff volume was increased to 48 ml, puff duration was increased to 2.4 seconds, and puff interval was reduced to 44 seconds. The parameters of the 'intense' condition were exactly the same as the 'moderate' condition, except that 50 percent of the vent holes were covered with tape. Comparing yields obtained under the moderate and intense conditions, then, shows the effect of blocking 50 percent of filter vents (Rickert *et al.*, 1983).

A secondary analysis of these data was performed on the 28 ventilated-filter brands. These were divided into three standard yield bands: 1-2 mg tar (*n* = 4), 3-5 mg tar (*n* = 11), and 6-14 mg tar (*n* = 13), roughly corresponding to Lowest Tar, Ultra-Light, and Light designations. Lowest Tar cigarettes showed a nicotine yield increase of 0.22 mg (130 percent), Ultra-Light cigarettes showed an increase of 0.31 mg (57 percent), and Light cigarettes showed an increase of 0.43 mg (36 percent). Lowest Tar cigarettes showed an increase of 2.5 mg tar (160 percent), compared to a 4.0 mg tar (63 percent) increase in Ultra-Light and a 5.5 mg tar (38 percent) increase in Lights. CO yields in Lights were increased by 4.7 mg (36 percent), while Ultra-Light brands increased 4.9 mg (75 percent) and Lowest Tar brands increased 2.6 g (150 percent).

Baker and colleagues (1998) presented an industry experiment on the effects of differing degrees of vent blocking on smoke yields. Both Light (9.3 mg tar, 0.89 mg nicotine, 8.7 mg CO at FTC conditions) and Ultra-Light (4.1 mg tar, 0.35 mg nicotine, 4.0 mg CO at FTC conditions) cigarettes were tested for the effect of vent blocking on yield under the FTC protocol. The Light cigarette showed an increase of 0.8 mg tar (8.6 percent), 0.08 mg nicotine (9.0 percent), and 1.4 mg CO (16 percent) when smoked with 50 percent of the vents blocked. The Ultra-Light cigarette showed an increase of 1.1 mg tar (27 percent), 0.09 mg nicotine (26 percent), and 2.3 mg CO (57.5 percent) with 50 percent vent blockage (Baker *et al.*, 1998).

Baker and Lewis (1997) provided the results of previously unreleased industry reports in which smoking machines were used to simulate the effect of vent blocking with lips and fingers on tar yields. These estimates were calculated assuming that the maximum coverage of filter vents is approximately 50 percent for lips and 25 percent for fingers. These researchers reported that blocking filter vents with fingers would increase the total particulate matter (TPM—tar plus nicotine, minus water) of a 1.3 mg tar cigarette by 23 percent to 1.6; blocking vents on the same brand with lips would increase the TPM by 92 percent to 2.5. Blocking filter vents with fingers would increase the TPM of a 2.2 mg tar cigarette by 32 percent to 2.9; blocking vents on the same brand with lips would increase the TPM by 59 percent to 3.5. Blocking filter vents with fingers would increase the TPM of a 6.7 mg tar cigarette by 10 percent to 7.4; blocking vents on the same brand with lips would increase the TPM by 21 percent to 8.1. Note that a negative relationship exists between tar yield and percentage of increase in TPM (Baker and Lewis, 1997).

Interestingly, the yield increases seen as a result of 50 percent blocking were significantly different between the Rickert and associates' (1983) and the industry's (Baker and Lewis, 1997; Baker *et al.*, 1998) studies. For example, nicotine yield in Ultra-Light cigarettes increased 57 percent in the Rickert and associates (1983) study, but only 26 percent in the Baker and colleagues (1998) study. Similarly, Rickert and associates found a 63 percent increase in tar, while Baker and colleagues found only a 27 percent increase. Baker and Lewis (who downplayed the effects of vent blocking) found that blocking 50 percent of vents caused a TPM increase of 59 percent, comparable to the Rickert results. However, they found a smaller effect for Lights (38 percent versus 22 percent increase in tar).

Why are there such discrepancies in the effects of vent blocking in these studies? Perhaps smoking conditions contribute to the effect of vent blocking. In the Rickert and associates (1983) study, cigarettes were smoked at a larger puff volume with shorter intervals than the FTC conditions used by Baker and colleagues (1998) and Baker and Lewis (1997). For example, to approach the 57 percent increase in nicotine yield at 50 percent blockage of

23

Ultra-Lights seen by Rickert and associates, Baker and colleagues tested their Ultra-Lights with 100 percent of vents blocked, and even here the yield increase was only 51 percent. An alternative explanation is that the cigarette designs selected for use in the Baker and colleagues study may be more resistant to the effect of vent blocking.

Zacny and associates (1986) evaluated the effect of vent blocking on smoke exposure in smokers. They found that blocking 0 percent, 50 percent, and 100 percent of the filter vents on a 1 mg tar cigarette with tape, while holding all other smoking parameters as constant as possible, increased CO exposure in an orderly fashion. Mean CO boosts (post-cigarette expired air CO level minus pre-cigarette expired air CO level) were 0.83 ppm, 2.87 ppm, and 7.07 ppm when 0 percent, 50 percent, and 100 percent of the filter vents were blocked.

This research was extended by Kozlowski and colleagues (1996b) to assess the effect of a behavioral vent blocking maneuver (*i.e.*, blocking vents with lips) on smoke exposure from the 1 mg tar Ultra-Light brand, Now®. Blocking filter vents with lips (estimated to be about 50 percent blockage) more than doubled the CO exposure from these cigarettes: CO boosts for the unblocked, lip-blocked, and 100 percent tape-blocked conditions averaged 2.7 ppm (SE = 0.52), 6.7 ppm (SE = 1.0), and 12.9 ppm (SE = 2.2), respectively.

Sweeney and Kozlowski (1998) examined the effect of blocking the filter vents of the best-selling cigarette brand, Marlboro Light®. CO boosts for the unblocked, lip-blocked, tape-blocked (50 percent coverage), and finger-blocked conditions were remarkably similar: 5.0 ppm (SE = 0.47), 4.9 ppm (SE = 0.86), 4.8 ppm (SE = 0.47), and 4.9 ppm (SE = 0.50), respectively. This "no-effect" finding for Marlboro Light® was subsequently replicated in a second study comparing the effects of finger-blocking and not blocking: the mean CO boosts for the unblocked and finger-blocked conditions were nearly identical: 6.3 ppm (SE = 0.50) and 6.5 ppm (SE = 0.52). In this same study, finger-blocking the vents on the 1 mg tar brand Now® led to a significantly higher (P = 0.0004) CO boost (5.4 ppm, SE = 0.64) than when filter vents were not blocked (2.8 ppm, SE = 0.34).

Puff number, puff duration, and puff interval were all controlled in these studies to examine the independent effects of vent blocking on smoke exposure. What type of an effect does vent blocking have on smoke exposure under more naturalistic conditions when parameters such as puff number and puff duration are free to vary? Zacny and associates (1986) explored this question with five smokers who smoked 1 mg tar cigarettes ad lib (*i.e.*, puff and inhalation parameters were free to vary) under each of three vent blocking conditions: 0 percent of the filter vents blocked; 50 percent of filter vents blocked with tape; and 100 percent of filter vents blocked with tape. Participants took significantly more puffs with significantly shorter interpuff intervals from cigarettes with unblocked filter vents than from cigarettes with blocked filter vents. Puff durations were similar across conditions, but puff volumes were larger when subjects smoked cigarettes with unblocked filter vents than when smoking cigarettes with blocked filter vents. Smokers were trying to compensate for smoke dilution by smoking the unblocked cigarettes more intensely. Nevertheless, participants still had greater CO exposure when smoking vent-blocked as compared with unblocked cigarettes, indicating that compensation was not complete. Mean CO boosts were 4.32 ppm, 6.44 ppm, and 8.96 ppm, when 0 percent, 50 percent, and 100 percent of filter vents were blocked, respectively (standard errors of the mean were not reported).

The two most recent studies in this area (Sweeney and Kozlowski, 1998; Sweeney *et al.*, 1999) further extended this research by examining the effects of behavioral vent-blocking maneuvers under ad lib smoking conditions. In the first study, participants smoked cigarettes from the brands Now® (1 mg tar by FTC method) and Marlboro Light® (10 mg tar by FTC method) under each of two vent-blocking conditions: unblocked and finger blocked. Blocking filter vents with fingers led to an 85 percent increase in CO exposure from Now®, but had no added effect on CO exposure from Marlboro Light®. The generalizability of these findings to all brands of Ultra-Light and Light cigarettes is limited, however, given that only one brand from each category was examined. A second study examined the effects of vent blocking using several cigarette brands of varying ventilation levels and standard tar yields. In a repeated-measures study with female daily cigarette smokers, the effect of lip-blocking on CO exposure was examined using four cigarette brands: Carlton® (1 mg FTC tar; 83 percent ventilated), Now® (2 mg FTC tar; 66 percent ventilated), Virginia Slims Ultra-Light® (5 mg FTC tar; 56 percent ventilated), and Virginia Slims Light® (8 mg FTC tar; 40 percent ventilated). Results showed that behavioral blocking caused all four brands to produce similar CO exposures. Blocking vents increased smokers' exposure to CO by 239 percent when smoking Carlton® and by 44 percent when smoking Now®. No significant increases in CO exposure with blocking were found for either of the Virginia Slims® brands.

The previous studies have used CO measures as an index of vent blocking because they are more practical and easy to obtain. However, one study has obtained salivary cotinine levels from self-selected 1 mg tar cigarette smokers (Kozlowski *et al.*, 1989). Here, large cotinine values were found in smokers who blocked the vents of 1 mg tar cigarettes; these values are larger than would be expected given the standard yield of their product and appear to compensate fully for that reduced yield. No other studies have been identified that investigated the effects of vent blocking on nicotine or cotinine levels. Obviously, further studies must be conducted on nicotine intake before concluding that vent blocking in Light cigarettes is inconsequential to exposure.

**Prevalence of Vent Blocking**  Published, peer-reviewed research has shown that a substantial proportion of smokers block vents. Using an unobtrusive indicator of vent blocking (stain pattern; discussed below), one study found that 58 percent of 135 cigarette filters from various Ultra-Light brands (4 mg tar or less) gave evidence of at least some vent blocking (Kozlowski *et al.*, 1988). Using similar procedures, another study found evidence of vent blocking in

53 percent of 158 filters of Light brands that were collected (Kozlowski *et al.*, 1994). In a study of 'high-risk' smoking practices used by the homeless, Aloot and colleagues (1993) found that 24 percent reported blocking filter vents (Aloot *et al.*, 1993).

The stain pattern technique for determining vent-blocking is straight-forward. Trained raters observe the mouth ends of cigarette butts and judge whether or not vent blocking has occurred based on the extent of the tar stain on the filter. A "bull's eye" pattern on the filter indicates that little or no vent blocking occurred, while a more uniform pattern across the filter would indicate that filter vents had been blocked. This technique has been validated and has been shown reliable on a number of brands (*e.g.*, Carlton®, Now®, Merit Ultima®, Camel Light®) through numerous refinements (Kozlowski *et al.*, 1980a & b; Pillitteri *et al.*, 1994; Sweeney, 1998). It must be stressed that this technique detects the presence or absence of any vent blocking with either fingers or lips. It should not be used to indicate the extent of vent blocking.

Industry scientists have objected to the use of the stain pattern technique (Baker and Lewis, 1997). They criticize raters' accuracy in judging the presence or absence of blocking and allege that the properties of laser-perforated filter vents produce variant patterns. Instead, the industry touts saliva-based measurements of lip placement around the ventilation zone as a better gauge of vent blocking. These techniques use ninhydrin and other biochemical stains to detect remnants of saliva in filters. These saliva-based techniques can detect vent blocking, but are impaired by factors such as lip dryness and so may underestimate its extent. Advocates of saliva-based measures admit that the technique often can fail to give a lip imprint stain for up to 20 percent of butts (Baker *et al.*, 1998). Another limitation of the saliva-based measures is that they will only detect lip blocking, totally ignoring finger blocking (unless the fingers have saliva on them).

During more than 15 years of published research on vent blocking, no formal response from the industry was put forth. In 1997, Baker and Lewis, two industry scientists, published their critique of peer-reviewed work on the subject. Their assertions were that: 1) vent blocking is not a significant mode of compensation because it does not occur often; 2) when vent blocking does occur, it hardly increases yields; and 3) mouth insertion depths of cigarettes do not differ greatly for ventilated and unventilated cigarettes.

Between 1974 and 1997, 10 studies were conducted by the tobacco industry in an attempt to measure the depth to which smokers insert cigarettes into their mouths by examining spent cigarette filters from public areas, such as shopping malls (Baker and Lewis, 1997). In these studies, a visible imprint of the lip marks on the filter was obtained by spraying the filter with either iodine or ninhydrin solutions to detect certain enzymes and amino acids in dried saliva on the filter. Across 10 studies, insertion depth measures ranged from 3 to 25 mm, with mean values ranging between 10.1 and 11.5 mm. Using both mouth insertion data based on 2,232 cigarette butts from a pair of 1997 Canadian studies, as well as information on ventilation zone location for leading U.S. brands, Baker and

Lewis (1997) estimated the proportion of smokers that would cover filter vents while smoking. They concluded that 36 percent of smokers will cover vents for at least one puff when they are placed at 11 mm, versus 6 percent of smokers who will cover the vent holes in at least one puff with ventilation zones positioned 17 mm from the mouth end of the filter.

Brands vary greatly in the placement of vents on the filter, and vent placement can bear little relationship to the standard yield of the cigarette. For example, a Marlboro® Full Flavor (16 mg tar) has vents at 12.5 mm from the mouth end, whereas a Carlton® (1 mg tar) has vents at 15 mm. Merit Ultima® (1 mg tar) has vents at 11.0 mm, whereas Camel® Full Flavor (17 mg tar) has vents at 14.5 mm (Kozlowksi *et al.*, 1997).

In an unpublished study by Röper (cited in Baker and Lewis, 1997), an attempt was made to assess more directly the prevalence of lip blocking by having 52 smokers take 1 puff on 5 cigarettes from each of 3 ventilated-filter brands. Of the 735 visible lip imprints that were obtained, 48 percent had at least some coverage of the ventilation zone.

Baker and colleagues (1998) examined 900 British smokers' filters for evidence of vent blocking using saliva-based techniques. They report that 15 percent of butts had at least partial vent coverage, while 85 percent showed no vent zone coverage. More interesting, however, are differences in coverage and insertion depth among standard (unventilated), Light, and Ultra-Light cigarettes. Light cigarettes showed partial coverage in 11.5 percent of cases and complete coverage in 1.5 percent of cases. In contrast, Ultra-Light cigarettes showed partial coverage in 9.6 percent of cases and complete coverage in 6.5 percent of cases. Further, standard cigarettes were inserted a mean of 7.8 mm (SD = 3.6) into a smoker's mouth, whereas Ultra-Light cigarettes were inserted a mean of 9.5 mm (SD = 5.0) into the mouth; in these cigarettes, the vents were placed 13.5-14.5 mm from the mouth end (Baker *et al.*, 1998).

Porter and Dunn (1998) of Imperial Tobacco examined butts collected in Montreal, Toronto, and Vancouver, Canada, for signs of vent blocking by examining mouth insertion depths. They found that the difference in insertion depths between ventilated and unventilated cigarettes was negligible (10.6 ± 3.6 mm versus 11.0 ± 3.6 mm). Further, they found that between 14 percent and 20 percent showed some evidence of partial vent coverage, whereas between 4 and 10 percent showed evidence of complete blockage (Porter and Dunn, 1998). In a similar study, McBride (1985), also of Imperial Tobacco, found that there were no significant differences in insertion depths between ventilated and unventilated cigarettes. However, McBride noted that "insertion depths were greatest for cigarettes in the very low delivery category." (McBride, 1985)

A study by British American Tobacco/Suisse (1984) examined the depths to which smokers inserted cigarettes into their mouths. Baker and Lewis (1997) cited this study along with several others as evidence that insertion depths are not large enough to interfere with ventilation in most cases. However, further examination of the results revealed that an interesting effect was obscured—insertion depths were greatest for the lowest yield cigarettes. The researchers concluded that "highly ventilated cigarettes are inserted deeply into the smokers mouth and consequently the ventilation level is reduced during normal smoking" (British American Tobacco/Suisse, 1984). For example, an Ultra-Low delivery cigarette (1 mg tar, 0.1 mg nicotine, 78 percent diluted) showed 43 percent of insertions beyond the vents, whereas a Full-Flavor brand (16 mg tar, 1.2 mg nicotine, 17 percent diluted) had only 22 percent of insertions beyond the vents; both brands had vents at 11-13 mm. By this technique, lip imprints beyond the vents were taken as evidence of vent blockage.

Large insertion depths seem to be about twice as common among less-popular 1 mg tar cigarettes. Given the relative disparity in sales (much greater for higher yield cigarettes), the 'few' blocked 1 mg tar cigarettes can be 'hidden' among the shallow insertion depths of more popular higher yielding brands. This causes average insertion depths to appear low enough not to interfere very much with vents. Furthermore, this permits the industry to argue (based on average insertion depths) that vent hole covering is not a major problem, when, in fact, their data suggest it is a significant problem for the lowest yield cigarettes. Porter and Dunn (1998) cited McBride's prior work, but made no mention of that researcher's finding of greater insertion depths for lower yield cigarettes (McBride, 1985), nor did they address the similar findings of the British American Tobacco/Suisse study (1984).

Ferris of the British American Tobacco Co. (cited by Baker and Lewis, 1997) conducted a study in 3 British cities in which 133 smokers of ventilated-filter cigarettes were videotaped. A total of 798 puffs were individually assessed from the video recordings: during 12 percent of the puffs, smokers' fingers were in contact with the cigarette for all or part of a puff. During 81 percent of the puffs, there was no finger contact with the cigarette. Ten percent of the puffs could not be assessed. During 29 percent of the final puffs, however, smokers' fingers were at least partially in contact with the cigarette. Eleven percent of participants had their fingers in contact with the cigarette for one or more puffs. However, since finger and lip blocking are mutually exclusive, it is noteworthy that lip blocking was not included in this study.

Baker and Lewis (1997) noted that when smoking an Ultra-Light cigarette (2.2 mg FTC tar), 45 percent of smokers blocked vents to some degree with their lips. Further, 21 percent of smokers (or nearly half of those who blocked vents) increased tar yields to at least 3.3 mg tar (50 percent). It was estimated that approximately 1 in 10 smokers doubled their tar yield from lip blocking alone; this is not insignificant, yet Baker and Lewis seemed to downplay these results.

Table 2-3 outlines the conditions under which different modes of compensation will be likely to occur. Reviewing the literature, vent blocking appears to be a significant mode of compensation for reduced yield among smokers of Lowest Tar cigarettes (*e.g.*, 1 mg FTC tar), but not likely among most smokers of Light and Ultra-Light cigarette brands.

Brand selection is usually not forced upon smokers. The self-selected choice of brands is due to many factors. It should be noted that some

Table 2-3

**Major Compensatory Behaviors in Relation to Cigarette Designs That Increase Total Smoke Volume per Cigarette**

**A. For more-popular lightly and moderately diluted cigarettes (*i.e.*, <60% ventilated, >4 mg FTC tar yield—"Light" and "Ultra-Light")**

    1) Increase volume per puff.

        Probably the easiest, most common method; for example, the smoke intake from a 45 ml puff on a 23% ventilated cigarette can be equivalent to the smoke intake from a 35 ml puff on an unventilated cigarette.

    2) Increase number of puffs taken.

    3) Reduce air dilution (as in Section B below).

        This likely will be a lesser-to-negligible compensation mode because (a) the effect is relatively small for these brands, and (b) increased puff volume and number can achieve all needed/desired compensation.

**B. For less-popular heavily diluted cigarettes (*i.e.*, 60-85% ventilated, 1-2 mg FTC tar yield— "Ultra-Low Tar")**

    1) Reduce air dilution by blocking filter vents with lips or fingers.

        Filter designs that promote ventilation 'compromise' (*e.g.*, Actron®) avoid the need to behaviorally block vents.

    2) Increase volume per puff.

        This technique would be more effective when coupled with some dilution reduction. Laser filter vents become relatively less effective with increased puff volumes.

    3) Increase number of puffs taken.

smokers of the lowest yield cigarettes appear to have very low nicotine needs and are disinclined to over-smoke these cigarettes, while other smokers of the lowest yield cigarettes have high nicotine needs and can fully compensate using these brands (Kozlowski *et al.*, 1989).

In summary, published, peer-reviewed research has shown that a substantial proportion of smokers block vents and that it is a common mechanism used by smokers to compensate for the reduced nicotine yield of ventilated cigarettes.

**Tar/Nicotine Ratios Depend on Smoking Conditions** During the period 1968-1997, the average sales-weighted ratio of tar to nicotine (T/N ratio) decreased 15.8 percent. Generally, the higher the yield, the higher the T/N ratio (see Figure 2-1). However, compensatory smoking behaviors (taking more frequent puffs, taking larger puffs, or vent blocking) can have dramatic effects on T/N ratios (Creighton and Lewis, 1978; Kozlowski *et al.*, 1980b; Rickert *et al.*, 1983). Given that some researchers have indicated an interest in using these ratios in the governmental regulation of cigarettes (*e.g.*, Russell, 1976; Gori, 1990; Bates *et al.*, 1999), this issue takes on greater importance.

In their study, Rickert and associates (1983) demonstrated that as intensity of smoking increased, T/N ratios increased. Intensely smoked Ultra-Light cigarettes provided a nearly identical T/N ratio (12.2) as Light ciga-

**Figure 2-1**
**FTC Tar/Nicotine Ratios for 2,052 Brands Tested as a Function of FTC Tar Yield Categories (FTC, 1999)**

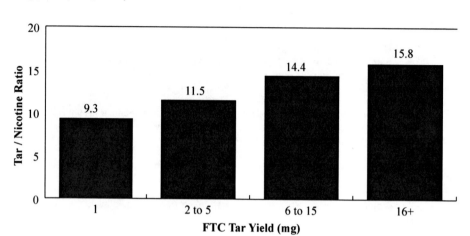

*Note: Figure 2-1 shows the T/N ratios for all 2,052 brands tested by the FTC method in 1997 (FTC, 1999) as a function of FTC tar yield categories. One-way analysis of variance shows that T/N ratios increase as tar yield increases (P<0.0001, all pairwise comparisons significant P<0.001, Bonferroni t-tests) (Ns, SEMs: 15, 0.50; 159, 0.22; 922, 0.07; 156, 0.17).*

rettes smoked under standard conditions (11.9). The difference between standard and intense condition T/N ratios across all brands is significant (P< 0.0001). The blocking of vents has a greater effect on the change in T/N ratios in Lowest Tar brands (1.90 or 20.5 percent) than in Lights (0.78 or 6.5 percent) (P = 0.0146).

Internal tobacco company studies revealed that there is great variability in the T/N ratios of otherwise equivalent cigarettes. An R. J. Reynolds study tested the yields of Now® brand cigarettes and comparable experimental cigarettes (both 1 mg tar/FTC) smoked under two conditions, the standard FTC method and the previously mentioned "50/30" condition (a 50 ml puff taken every 30 seconds) (Casey, 1994). The T/N ratio of the Now® blend under standard conditions was 8.33; however, under 50/30 conditions, the ratio rose to 10.98 (an increase of 31.8 percent). At the same time, an experimental blend saw its T/N ratio increase from 6.36 at standard conditions to 6.72 at 50/30 conditions (an increase of only 5.7 percent) (Casey, 1994). It would appear that the trends for reduced "standardized smoking-machine" T/N ratios may have little relation to the ratios delivered to actual smokers. Empirical evidence for this proposition is presented in Chapter 3.

**Elastic Cigarette Designs** The rules or constraints of the FTC measurement regimen can be viewed as obstacles to be overcome by manufacturers that wish to design cigarettes that deliver lower yields during the course of the standardized smoking-machine test, while enabling smokers to achieve yields higher than would be predicted by smoking machines. A design that gives a low value to smoking machines but can potentially give higher values to smokers is termed 'elastic'. Internal tobacco industry documents revealed a concern for cigarette elasticity:

"Smokers have disappointed us in that they have not chosen to smoke twice as many 10mg cigarettes if they changed from 20mg products. Thus in order to reinforce the primary pleasures of smoking, I have proposed to make it easier for smokers to take what they want from a cigarette which might well have a low delivery when smoked by machine which overcomes current legal constraints and to enhance the sensations from the first few puffs." (See Creighton, 1980s.)

"Irrespective of the ethics involved, we should develop alternative designs (that do not invite obvious criticism) which will allow the smoker to obtain significant enhanced deliveries should he so wish" (See British American Tobacco Company, 1984.)

"Compensation - It exists; most smokers practice it, but we need to understand it better before advantage can be taken in the marketplace. Here, I believe designing to the subconscious is preferred to requiring the smoker to commit a conscious act." (See Sandford, 1985.)

In a presentation given to marketers at the British American Tobacco Co., scientist D. E. Creighton described advances in the design of "compensatable" filter products:

"The design of a cigarette with a compensatable filter will have a high taste to tar ratio. . . . This [the HH filter] was designed in BAT Hamburg and has been tested on consumers, who found the cigarettes too strong. As the sample cigarettes had a machine smoked delivery of about 1mg tar, the product must be very compensatable. Our own tests both subjective and objective suggested that it is a compensatable filter, when smoked against conventionally constructed controls. The objective test we have used is to smoke at 35 and 50ml puff volumes and to see if the increase in delivery at the higher puff volume is pro-rata or more. With HH, the delivery was more than pro-rata." [This paper goes on to compare the HH filter to the Actron filter used in Barclay®, discussed below.] (See Creighton, 1980s.)

The ventilated Actron filter makes use of plastic channels to feed air from vent holes back to the end of the filter. It appears that this channel system dramatically increased the likelihood of vent blocking because, in addition to blocking air intake holes, one could also subvert the ventilation system by either causing the fragile plastic channels to collapse or by blocking air exit holes with lips. This filter design caused competing manufacturers to complain to the FTC that this cigarette design was classified as 1 mg but gave much higher actual deliveries. The courts ruled that the FTC test could not properly provide tar and nicotine numbers for this type of filter (FTC v. Brown & Williamson Tobacco Corporation, 1985). The Actron filter can still be found on Brown & Williamson's Barclay® and Kool Ultra® brands.

With some brands, elasticity arose from the ease with which a smoker could alter their smoking patterns on the product. Internal tobacco company documents show an industry aware that some lower yield products were smoked more intensely than higher yield products:

> "The smoker profile data reported earlier indicated that Marlboro Lights cigarettes were not smoked like regular Marlboros. In effect, the Marlboro 85 smokers in this study did not achieve any reduction in smoke intake by smoking a cigarette (Marlboro Lights) normally considered lower in delivery." (See Goodman, 1975.)

> "Numerous experiments have been carried out in Hamburg, Montreal and Southampton within the company, as well as many other experiments by research workers in independent organisations, that show that generally smokers do change their smoking patterns in response to changes in the machine smoked deliveries of cigarettes." (See Creighton, 1978b.)

**Cigarette Length**    In the late 1960s, Philip Morris undertook the Smoke Exposure Study, termed SEX-1 in their internal documents. While the actual report is currently unavailable in the company's Internet document archive, references to the results are available in other documents. In a memo discussing reasons to publish the SEX-1 report, the effect of cigarette length on exposure is discussed. It appears that smokers of 100 mm cigarettes showed an increased intake of tar and nicotine compared to 85 mm cigarette smokers. However, it is noted that this increase was "not as great as would have been predicted from the increase in available tar" (Dunn, 1971). This issue of cigarette length and exposure was evidently significant, because the design of a subsequent study (SEX-2) was modified to include smokers who switched from 85 mm to 100 mm cigarettes to determine changes in daily smoke intake (Dunn, 1969). While the results of the SEX-1 study are far from clear, no other findings related to cigarette length are known to exist. Interestingly, the percentage of cigarettes sold ranging in length from 94 to 101 mm increased from 9 to 39 percent during the period 1967-1997 (FTC, 1999).

In summary, the tobacco industry has a stake in smokers' continued use of their products. Cigarette designs that promote compensation and/or elasticity of yield have been used, both in the research and development laboratories and in the marketplace. These designs allow the smoker to obtain more smoke (tar, nicotine, and CO) from each cigarette than would be indicated by the FTC testing method.

**MORE EVIDENCE FROM INDUSTRY DOCUMENTS RELATED TO COMPENSATION, CIGARETTE DESIGN, AND THE FTC TESTING METHOD** As shown in previous sections, considerable evidence exists in tobacco industry documents of knowledge regarding compensation and elasticity. Also revealed in industry documents are discussions about whether smokers might be misled by FTC tar and nicotine ratings used in advertisements and league tables. Particularly of concern were those customers who switched to a lower yield brand due to health concerns:

"Should we market cigarettes intended to re-assure the smoker that they are safer without assuring ourselves that indeed they are so or are not less safe? For example should we 'cheat' smokers by 'cheating' League Tables? If we are prepared to accept that government has created league tables to encourage lower delivery cigarette smoking and further if we make league table claims as implied health claims—or allow health claims to be so implied—should we use our superior knowledge of our products to design them so that they give low league table positions but higher deliveries on human smoking?"

. . . "Are smokers entitled to expect that cigarettes shown as lower delivery in league tables will in fact deliver less to their lungs than cigarettes shown higher?" (See British American Tobacco Company, 1977.)

"It is difficult to ignore the advice of Health Authorities who advise smokers to give up smoking or change to a lower delivery brand but there is now sufficient evidence to challenge the advice to change to a lower delivery brand, at least in the short term. In general a majority of habitual smokers compensate for changed delivery, if they change to a lower delivery brand." (See Creighton, 1978b.)

"1) Some concern has been expressed concerning the moral obligation of Philip Morris (and perhaps the tobacco industry) to reveal to the FTC the fact that some cigarette smokers may be getting more tar than the FTC rating of that cigarette. . . . 2) I believe that there need be no such concern, at least from a position of morality. It is obvious that HEW [Department of Health, Education, and Welfare; now the Department of Health and Human Services] knows that smokers vary their intake. Otherwise they would not urge smokers to take fewer puffs. There are published papers which show that different puffing patterns on the same cigarette will yield different amounts of tar." (See Fagan, 1974)

**SUMMARY** Many smokers switch to cigarette brands advertised as delivering lower yields out of concerns for their health, believing them to be less risky or a step toward quitting (Kozlowski *et al.*, 1998a, 1999; Giovino *et al.*, 1996). These decisions are often based on the FTC tar ratings, which can be inaccurate in assessing human smoking conditions. Through compensation behaviors (*i.e.*, vent blocking on Ultra-Low FTC tar cigarettes, larger puff volumes, or more frequent puffs), many smokers can obtain adequate nicotine from their new lower yield brand to sustain their addiction.

Published research results, supplemented by previously unavailable industry data, show that the 44 percent reduction in standard tar yield and 34 percent reduction in standard nicotine yield seen since 1968 do not necessarily mean that smokers have been receiving less tar and nicotine from their cigarettes with each passing year. Smokers can and do compensate for reduced tar and nicotine yield by altering their smoking patterns. Compensation behaviors can range from simple maneuvers such as taking more puffs per cigarette, to increasing volume per puff, to blocking filter vents with fingers or lips. Changes in cigarette design have engineered cigarettes that have an elasticity of delivery, which allows smokers to derive markedly different amounts of nicotine from the same cigarette by changing the way that they smoke it. This designed elasticity is intrinsic to the process of compensation when smokers switch to lower yield cigarettes. Elastic products such as the Actron filter, laser-perforated filters, and invisible filter vents on cigarettes facilitate compensation behaviors in smokers. Larger puff volumes, increasing puff frequency, and other changes in smoking behavior allow smokers to derive doses of nicotine from cigarettes with low machine-measured yields sufficient to fully satisfy their addiction. Smokers are increasingly likely to engage in compensation as the machine-measured yields of cigarettes fall and the percentages of ventilation increase.

## CONCLUSIONS

1. Several design changes in the way that cigarettes are manufactured have led to a substantial reduction in the machine-measured tar and nicotine yields of U.S. cigarettes over the last several decades.

2. Many of the same design changes that have reduced machine-measured tar yields, particularly placing ventilation holes in the cigarette filters, also create an elasticity of delivery for the cigarette, allowing a wide range of tar and nicotine deliveries from the same cigarette when a smoker alters his or her smoking behavior.

3. Increasing puff volume and frequency, covering the ventilation holes with fingers or lips, and other changes in smoking behavior known to occur with use of low machine-measured-tar cigarettes can dramatically increase the tar and nicotine delivery of low- and ultralow-yield brands.

4. Variations in the tar and nicotine delivery that result from the known compensatory alterations in smoking behaviors make the current U.S. cigarette tar and nicotine yields as measured by the FTC method not useful to the smoker either for understanding how much tar and nicotine he or she is likely to inhale from smoking a given cigarette or for comparing the tar and nicotine intake that is likely to result from smoking different brands of cigarettes.

# REFERENCES

Aloot, C.B., Vredevor, D.L., Brecht, M. Evaluation of high-risk smoking practices used by the homeless. *Cancer Nursing* 16(2):123-130, 1993.

American Cancer Society. Nicotine content of whole tobacco. *1997 Cigarette Nicotine Closure Report.* Available at http://www.cancer.org/tobacco/nicotine report/content.html.

Baker, R.R., Dixon, M., Hill, C.A. The incidence and consequences of filter vent blocking amongst British smokers. *Beitrage zur Tabakforschung International* 18(2):71-91. 1998.

Baker, R.R., Lewis, L.S. Filter ventilation—Has there been a "cover-up"? *Recent Advances in Tobacco Science* 23:152-196, 1997.

Bates, C., McNeill, A., Jarvis, M., Gray, N. The future of tobacco product regulation and labelling in Europe: Implications for the forthcoming European Union directive. *Tobacco Control* 8(2):225-235, 1999.

Bradford, J.A., Harlan, W.R., Hanmer, H.R. Nature of cigarette smoke. Technique of experimental smoking. *Industrial and Engineering Chemistry* 28(7):836-839, 1936.

British American Tobacco Company. Research and Development views on potential marketing opportunities. September 12, 1984. Minnesota Trial Exhibit 11,275.

British American Tobaco Company. Suggested Questions for JH CAC.III, August 26, 1977. Minnesota Trial Exhibit 11,390.

British American Tobacco Suisse. Insertion depth study on Swiss cigarettes. BAT Suisse, 1989. Bates No. 2501268539. Available at www.pmdocs.com.

Brown & Williamson. Proceedings of the Smoking Behaviour Marketing Conference, July 9th-12th 1984, Session III. (Minnesota Trial Exhibit 13,431.)

Browne, C.L. *The Design of Cigarettes, 3rd Edition.* Hoechst Celanese Corporate, 1990.

Casey, W.J. Data related to very high air dilution cigarettes. R.J. Reynolds Tobacco Company, 1994. Bates No. 512480043. Available at www.rjrtdocs.com.

Creighton, D.E. Measurement of the degree of ventilation of cigarettes at various flow rates. British American Tobacco Company, 1978a. Available at www.cdc.gov/tobacco/industrydocs.

Creighton, D.E. Compensation for changed delivery. British American Tobacco Company. June 27, 1978b. Minnesota Trial Exhibit 11,089.

Creighton, D.E. Structured creativity group presentation. British American Tobacco Company, 1980s. BAT No. 102690336-3501. Available at www.tobaccopapers.org.

Creighton, D.E., Lewis, P.H. The effect of different cigarettes on human smoking patterns. In: *Smoking Behavior: Physiological and Psychological Influences.* R.E. Thornton (Editors.). Edinburgh, Scotland: Churchill Livingstone, 1978.

Creighton, D.E., Watts, R.M. The effect of introducing pinholes in front of the filter on human smoking pattern. British American Tobacco, 1972. Bates No. 650316736. Available at www.cdc.gov/tobacco.

Djordjevic, M.V., Stellman, S.D., Zang, E. Doses of nicotine and lung carcinogens delivered to cigarette smokers. *Journal of the National Cancer Institute* 92(2):106-111, 2000.

Dunn, W.L. to Charles, J.L., Cohen, M., Daylor, F., Eichorm, P., Filias, G., Forest, B., Ikeda, R., Johnston, M., Osmalov, J., Ryan, F., Tamol, R., Thomson, R., Tindall, J., Wakeham, H. April 8, 1969. Memo by W.L. Dunn. Modified design of SEX-2. Philip Morris, Inc. Bates No. 1003287567. Available at www.pmdocs.com.

Dunn, W.L. to Wakeham, H. February 11, 1971. Memo by W.L. Dunn. SEX-1. Philip Morris, Inc. Bates No. 2055083000A. Available at www.pmdocs.com.

DuPuis, R.H. Untitled memo—CONFIDENTIAL. Philip Morris, Inc., 1956. Bates No. 1001809856. Available at www.pmdocs.com.

Fagan, R. to Wakeham, H. March 7, 1974. Memo by R. Fagan. Moral issue on FTC tar. Bates No. 1000211075.

Federal Trade Commission. *"Tar", nicotine, and carbon monoxide of the smoke of 1262 varieties of domestic cigarettes for the year 1996.* Federal Trade Commission, Washington, D.C., 1999.

Federal Trade Commission v. Brown & Williamson Tobacco Corporation, 250 U.S. App DC 162; 778 F2d 35 (10 and 18 December, 1985). SCB: 580 F Suppl 981.

Giovino, G.A., Tomar, S.L., Reddy, M.N., Peddicord, J.P., Zhu, B.P., Escobedo, L.G., Eriksen, M.P. Attitudes, knowledge, and beliefs about low-yield cigarettes among adolescents and adults. *The FTC Cigarette Test Method for Determining Tar, Nicotine, and Carbon Monoxide Yields of U.S. Cigarettes. Report of the NCI Expert Committee.* Smoking and Tobacco Control Monograph No. 7. U.S. Department of Health and Human Services, National Institutes of Health, National Cancer Institute, NIH Publication No. 96-4028, 1996.

Goodman, B. to Meyer, L.F. September 17, 1975. Memo by B. Goodman. Marlboro—Marlboro Lights study delivery data. Trial Exhibit 11,564.

Goodman, B.L. to Meyer, L.F. New product development summary of human smoker simulator program. Philip Morris, 1977. Bates No. 1003728025. Available at www.pmdocs.com.

Gori, G.B. Cigarette classification as a consumer message (Review). *Regulatory Toxicology and Pharmacology* 12:253-262, 1990.

Grunberg, N.E., Morse, D.E., Maycock, V.A., Kozlowski, L.T. Changes in overwrap and butt length of American filter cigarettes. An influence on reported tar yields. *New York State Journal of Medicine* 85:310-312, 1985.

Helms, A. The concentration of tar, nicotine and carbon monoxide in the smoke of ventilated filter cigarettes—Comparison of different types of filter ventilations. Hamburg, Germany: Hauni-Werke Kurbar & Co. KG, 1983. Bates No. 2028562439. Available at www.pmdocs.com.

Helms, A., Lorenzen, H.C. Latest developments in the field of cigarette perforation (post-perforation) by laser. Hamburg, Germany: Hauni-Werke Kurbar & Co. KG, 1984. Available at www.rjrtdocs.com.

Herning, R.I., Jones, R.T., Bachman, J., Mines, A.H. Puff volume increases when low-nicotine cigarettes are smoked. *British Medical Journal (Clin Res Ed)* 283:187-189, 1981.

Kelley, M.F. Project Change-2001: Evaluation of a PM 2 mg experimental cigarette versus Now and Carlton 70. Philip Morris, 1977. Bates No. 1000364294. Available at www.pmdocs.com.

Kozlowski, L.T. Perceiving the risks of low-yield ventilated-filter cigarettes: The problem of hole-blocking. *Proceedings of the International Workshop on the Analysis of Actual vs. Perceived Risks.* Covello, V., Flamm, W.G., Rodericks, J., Tardiff, R. (Editors.). New York: Plenum, 1983.

Kozlowski, L.T., Frecker, F.C., Khouw,V., Pope, M.S. The misuse of 'less-hazardous' cigarettes and its detection: Hole-blocking of ventilated filters. *American Journal of Public Health* 70:1202-1203, 1980a.

Kozlowski, L.T., Goldberg, M.E., Sweeney, C.T., Palmer, R.F., Pillitteri, J.L., Yost, B.A., White, E.L., Stine, M.M. Smoker reactions to a "radio message" that light cigarettes are as dangerous as regular cigarettes. *Nicotine and Tobacco Research* 1:67-76, 1999.

Kozlowski, L.T., Goldberg, M.E., Yost, B.A., Ahern, F.M., Aronson, K.R., Sweeney, C.T. Smokers are unaware of the filter vents now on most cigarettes: Results of a national survey. *Tobacco Control* 5(4):265-270, 1996a.

Kozlowski, L.T., Goldberg, M.E., Yost, B.A., White, E.L., Sweeney, C.T., Pillitteri, J.L. Smokers' misperception of light and ultra-light cigarettes may keep them smoking. *American Journal of Preventive Medicine* 15(1):9-16, 1998a.

Kozlowski, L.T., Heatherton, T.F., Frecker, R.C., Nolte, H.E. Self-selected blocking of vents on low-yield cigarettes. *Pharmacology, Biochemistry, & Behavior* 33(4):815-819, 1989.

Kozlowski, L.T., Mehta, N.Y., Sweeney, C.T. Filter ventilation levels in selected U.S. cigarettes—1997. *Morbidity and Mortality Weekly Report* 46(44):1043-1047, 1997.

Kozlowski, L.T., Mehta, N.Y., Sweeney, C.T., Schwartz, S.S., Vogler, G.P., Jarvis, M.J., West, R.J. Filter ventilation and nicotine content of tobacco in cigarettes from Canada, the United Kingdom, and the United States. *Tobacco Control* 7(4):369-375, 1998b.

Kozlowski, L.T., O'Connor, R.J. Official cigarette tar tests are misleading: Use a two-stage, compensating test. *The Lancet* 355(9221):2159-61, 2000.

Kozlowski, L.T., Pillitteri, J.L., Sweeney, C.T. Misuse of "light" cigarettes by means of vent blocking. *Journal of Substance Abuse* 6(3):333-336, 1994.

Kozlowski, L.T., Pillitteri, J.L., Yost, B.A., Goldberg, M.E., Ahern, F.M. Advertising fails to inform smokers of official tar yields of cigarettes. *Journal of Applied Biobehavioral Research* 3:55-64, 1998c.

Kozlowski, L.T., Pope, M.A., Lux, J.E. Prevalence of the misuse of ultra-low-tar cigarettes by blocking filter vents. *American Journal of Public Health* 78(6):694-695, 1988.

Kozlowski, L.T., Rickert, W.S., Pope, M.A., Robinson, J.C., Frecker, R.C. Estimating the yield to smokers of tar, nicotine, and carbon monoxide from the 'lowest yield' ventilated filter cigarettes. *British Journal of Addiction* 77(2):159-165, 1982.

Kozlowski, L.T., Rickert, W.S., Robinson, J.C., Grunberg, N.E. Have tar and nicotine yields of cigarettes changed? *Science* 209(4464):1550-1551, 1980b.

Kozlowski, L.T., Sweeney, C.T., Pillitteri, J.L. Blocking cigarette filter vents with lips more than doubles carbon monoxide intake from ultra-low tar cigarettes. *Experimental and Clinical Psychopharmacology* 4:404-408, 1996b.

Kozlowski, L.T., White, E.L., Sweeney, C.T., Yost, B.A., Ahern, F.A., Goldberg, M.E. Few smokers know their own cigarettes have filter vents. *American Journal of Public Health* 88(4):681-682, 1998d.

Kozlowski, L.T., Yost, B., Stine, M.M., Celebucki, C. Massachusetts advertising against light cigarettes appears to change beliefs and behavior. *American Journal of Preventive Medicine* 18(4):339-342, 2000.

Long, L.L. Summary of results on ventilated cigarettes. Philip Morris, 1955. Bates No. 1001900842. Available at www.pmdocs.com.

McBride, C. A study to determine the maximum cigarette insertion depth used by Canadian smokers [Abstract]. Imperial Tobacco, Ltd, 1985. Bates No. 109874617. Available at www.tobaccopapers.org/documents/psc71e.pdf.

Mendell, S. 2001 New Product Development. The relationship between dilution/RTD ratios and consumer perception. Philip Morris, 1983. Bates No. 1003638145. Available at www.pmdocs.com.

Moody, P.M. The relationships of quantified human smoking behavior and demographic variables. *Social Science Medicine* 14A(1):49-54, 1980.

Norman, A.B., Newsome, J.B., Reynolds, J.H. Effects of tipping perforation method and vent location on filter ventilation during smoking. R.J. Reynolds Tobacco Company, 1984. Bates No. 504017981. Available at www.rjrtdocs.com.

Norman, V., Ihrig, A.M. A study of human smoking patterns of ultra-low yield cigarettes. Lorillard Tobacco Company, 1980a. Bates No. 00782382. Available at www.lorillarddocs.com.

Norman, V., Ihrig, A.M. The concept of a power function to describe smoking effort. Lorillard Tobacco Company, 1980b. Bates No. 00303446. Available at www.lorillarddocs.com.

Parker, J.A., Montgomery, R.T. Design criteria for ventilated filters. *Beitrage zur Tabakforschung International* 10:1-6, 1979.

Peeler, C.L. Cigarette testing and the Federal Trade Commission: A historical overview. *The FTC Cigarette Test Method for Determining Tar, Nicotine, and Carbon Monoxide Yields of US Cigarettes. Report of the NCI Expert Committee.* U.S. Department of Health and Human Services, National Institutes of Health, National Cancer Institute, NIH Publication No. 96-4028, 1996.

Philip Morris. Cigarettes a la carte or how to play with filter efficiency, filter dilution and expanded tobacco in designing low- and very-low-tar cigarettes. 1980. Bates No. 2501224987. Available at www.pmdocs.com.

Pillitteri, J.L., Morse, A.C., Kozlowski, L.T. Detection of vent blocking on light and ultralight cigarettes. *Pharmacology, Biochemistry, & Behavior* 48:539-542, 1994.

Porter, A., Dunn, P. Mouth insertion depths in Canadian smokers. *Beitrage zur Tabakforschung International* 18:85-91, 1998.

Rickert, W.S., Robinson, J.C., Young, J.C., Collishaw, N.E., Bray, D.F. A comparison of the yields of tar, nicotine, and carbon monoxide of 36 brands of Canadian cigarettes tested under three conditions. *Preventive Medicine* 12(5):682-694, 1983.

Russell, M.A. Low-tar medium-nicotine cigarettes: A new approach to safer smoking. *British Medical Journal* 1(6023):1430-1433, 1976.

Russell, M.A.H., Sutton, S.R., Iyer, R., Feyerabend, C., Vesey, C.J. Long-term switching to low-tar low-nicotine cigarettes. *British Journal of Addiction* 77(2):145-158, 1982.

Sandford, R.A. to Kohnhorst, E.E. June 28, 1985. Internal memo by R.A. Sandford. Brown & Williamson, Research Development and Engineering. Minnesota Trial Exhibit 13,250.

Shoffner, R.A., Ireland, M.S. Rapid analysis of menthol and nicotine in smoke and the effects of air dilution on delivery. *Tobacco Science* 26:109-112, 1982.

Stolt, P. Update on program for the reduction of Marlboro smoke deliveries in Europe by means of filter dilution. Philip Morris Incorporated, 1977. Bates No. 2024270885. Available at www.pmdocs.com.

Sutton, S.R., Feyerabend, C., Cole, P.V., Russell, M.A. Adjustment of smokers to dilution of tobacco smoke by ventilated cigarette holders. *Clinical Pharmacology and Therapeutics* 24(4):395-405, 1978.

Sweeney, C.T. Experimental Research on the Behavioral Blocking of Filter Vents on Low-Yield Cigarettes. Doctoral dissertation, Pennsylvania State University, 1998.

Sweeney, C.T., Kozlowski, L.T. Blocking filter vents increases carbon monoxide levels from ultralight but not light cigarettes. *Pharmacology, Biochemistry, & Behavior* 59(3):767-773, 1998.

Sweeney, C.T., Kozlowski, L.T., Parsa, P. Effect of filter vent blocking on carbon monoxide exposure from selected lower tar cigarette brands. *Pharmacology, Biochemistry, & Behavior* 63(1):167-173, 1999.

Tobin, M.J., Sackner, M.A. Monitoring smoking patterns of low and high tar cigarettes with inductive plethysmography. *American Review of Respiratory Disease* 126(2):258-264, 1982.

U.S. Department of Health and Human Services. *The Health Consequences of Smoking: Nicotine Addiction. A Report of the Surgeon General.* U.S. Department of Health and Human Services, Public Health Service, Centers for Disease Control and Prevention, Center for Health Promotion and Education, Office on Smoking and Health. DHHS Publication No. (CDC) 88-8406, 1988.

Wakeham, H. Some unexpected observations on tar and nicotine and smoker behavior. Philip Morris, 1974. Bates No. 1000260471. Available at www.pmdocs.com.

Wynder, E.L., Hoffman, D. *Tobacco and Tobacco Smoke.* New York: Academic Press, 1967.

Zacny, J.P., Stitzer, M.L. Cigarette brand-switching: Effects on smoke exposure and smoking behavior. *The Journal of Pharmacology and Experimental Therapeutics* 246:619-627, 1988.

Zacny, J.P., Stitzer, M.L., Brown, F.J., Yingling, J.E., Griffiths, R.R. Human cigarette smoking: Effects of puff and inhalation parameters on smoke exposure. *The Journal of Pharmacology and Experimental Therapeutics* 240(2):554-564, 1987.

Zacny, J.P., Stitzer, M.L., Yingling, J.E. Cigarette filter vent blocking: Effects on smoking topography and carbon monoxide exposure. *Pharmacology, Biochemistry, & Behavior* 25:1245-1252, 1986.

# Compensatory Smoking of Low-Yield Cigarettes

Neal L. Benowitz

**INTRODUCTION** Most smokers are addicted to nicotine (U.S. DHHS, 1988). Nicotine addiction results in smokers seeking to take in a constant level of nicotine from smoking each day (Benowitz, 1988; U.S. DHHS, 1988). Consequently, when faced with low-yield cigarettes, smokers tend to take in more nicotine and other tobacco smoke constituents from these cigarettes than would be predicted by machine testing in order to sustain optimal levels of nicotine intake. This phenomenon of taking in similar levels of nicotine from day to day has been termed 'regulation' or 'titration' of nicotine intake. The behavior of smoking cigarettes of different machine yields more or less intensively, and/or smoking more or fewer cigarettes to achieve a particular intake of nicotine, has been called 'compensation'. If regulation of nicotine intake is precise, that is, compensation is complete, then switching to low-yield cigarettes would not be expected to reduce exposure to tobacco toxins, nor to reduce the risk of disease from smoking.

Earlier chapters have described the nature of low-yield cigarettes and the ways in which smokers can modify their smoking behaviors to take in more tobacco smoke from their cigarettes than predicted by the standard smoking-machine test. In brief review—when faced with lower yield cigarettes, smokers can smoke more cigarettes per day, can take more and deeper puffs, can puff with a faster draw rate, and/or can block ventilation holes. Using these last four techniques, a smoker can increase his or her smoke intake from a particular cigarette several fold above the machine-predicted yields.

This chapter will review nicotine addiction and the evidence that smokers regulate their intake of nicotine from cigarettes. The focus will be on primarily studies in which human exposure has been biochemically assessed. Evidence from both experimental and cross-sectional studies will be examined. The question of whether or not tar exposure might be reduced despite compensation for nicotine itself when switching to low-yield cigarettes will also be examined.

**ROLE OF NICOTINE IN MAINTAINING TOBACCO ADDICTION** Nicotine is the main determinant of tobacco use and addiction. Detailed reviews of the pharmacology of nicotine and the evidence that nicotine is addictive have been published in Surgeon General's reports (for example, the 1988 Surgeon General's report, *The Health Consequences of Smoking: Nicotine Addiction*), as well as in a number of other reviews (Benowitz, 1988, 1999b; U.S. DHHS, 1988).

Nicotine is delivered to the smoker in particulate matter and, to some extent, in the gaseous phase of tobacco smoke. It is rapidly absorbed from the lungs into the arterial circulation, from which it goes to various organs, including the brain. Rapid delivery of nicotine to the brain is particularly important to the issue of compensation because it provides rapid feedback to the smoker on the dose of nicotine absorbed, and allows minute-to-minute titration of nicotine effects.

In the brain, nicotine binds to and activates nicotinic cholinergic receptors. There are a variety of nicotinic cholinergic receptor subtypes, which are believed to mediate different actions of nicotine in different parts of the brain (Picciotto *et al.*, 2000). Nicotinic receptor activation works, at least in part, by facilitating the release of neurotransmitters, including acetylcholine, norepinephrine, dopamine, beta endorphin, glutamate, gamma aminobutyric acid (GABA), and others. Nicotine also releases growth hormone, prolactin, and adrenocorticotropic hormone (ACTH). Most of the behavioral effects of nicotine in people are believed to be mediated by its actions on central nervous system receptors.

Nicotine self-administration appears to be motivated both by positive and negative reinforcement. Positive reinforcement includes pleasure, arousal, relaxation, reduced stress, enhanced vigilance, improved cognitive function, mood modulation, and lower body weight. With prolonged exposure to nicotine, there is an increase in the number of nicotinic cholinergic receptors in the brain that occurs in association with the development of tolerance to the effects of nicotine (Collins *et al.*, 1994; Breese *et al.*, 1997). In the tolerant state, nicotine is necessary to maintain normal brain functioning. In the absence of nicotine, brain functioning becomes abnormal and the individual experiences nicotine withdrawal symptoms, reflecting physical dependence. Withdrawal symptoms include nervousness, restlessness, irritability, anxiety, impaired concentration, impaired cognitive function, increased appetite, and weight gain. Negative reinforcement refers to the relief of withdrawal symptoms by nicotine intake. It is difficult to separate positive reinforcement from relief of withdrawal symptoms in smokers. However, it is clear that nicotine is used by smokers to modulate their levels of arousal, mood, and performance.

The cigarette is a drug delivery system for nicotine. Smokers tend to take in similar doses of nicotine on a day-to-day basis (Benowitz, 1988; U.S. DHHS, 1988), presumably to optimize the levels of arousal and mood. A variety of experimental studies support the theory that smokers regulate daily intake of nicotine. In addition to studies of changed smoking behavior in response to different brands of cigarettes (which was discussed in detail in Chapter 2), smokers have been shown to change smoking behavior in response to other interventions that alter nicotine availability. For example, when the excretion of nicotine from the body is accelerated by acidification of the urine, smokers will increase their smoking to take in more nicotine (Benowitz and Jacob, 1985). Conversely, when nicotine is administered intravenously or by administration of nicotine patches, smokers reduce their nicotine intake from smoking (Benowitz and Jacob, 1990; Benowitz *et al.*, 1998).

In summary, cigarettes smoking can be viewed as a process of delivering nicotine to the body. Daily smoking can be viewed as a situation in which nicotine is taken initially for pleasure, for arousal, and/or for mood modulation. As the day progresses for the smoker, tolerance develops to many of the effects of nicotine, and further nicotine may be taken to primarily relieve withdrawal symptoms that emerge between cigarettes. Smokers appear to have particular desirable levels of nicotine intake throughout the day that result in optimal functioning. The need for a particular level of nicotine is central to the concept of compensation for low-yield cigarettes.

**BIOMARKERS OF TOBACCO SMOKE EXPOSURE** As discussed previously, there is considerable individual variability in the way smokers smoke their cigarettes. Therefore, neither the number of cigarettes smoked per day, nor the machine-determined yield, nor even a combination of the two can provide complete information on the intake by an individual smoker of tobacco smoke toxins. To determine intake most accurately, one must measure human exposure to chemicals in tobacco smoke.

The tobacco smoke constituents that have been most widely used in quantitating human exposure to smoke are nicotine and carbon monoxide (CO) (Benowitz, 1996, 1999a). Nicotine can be measured directly in blood, but more commonly nicotine intake is estimated by measuring levels of its proximate metabolite, cotinine. Cotinine has a much longer half-life than nicotine; therefore, cotinine levels in the body vary much less throughout the day than do nicotine levels. Thus, sampling time for cotinine with respect to when the last cigarette was smoked is less critical. In addition, cotinine can be readily measured in blood, saliva, and urine. Measurement of the sum of nicotine and its metabolites in urine can also be used to assess nicotine exposure from smoking.

CO is present in high concentrations in tobacco smoke and is a useful marker of exposure to the gaseous fraction of tobacco smoke, but the short half-life of CO excretion makes it a measure that is predominantly influenced by smoking within the most recent several hours. There is no reason to believe that smokers adjust their smoking to regulate CO levels in the body. Therefore, discrepancies between CO levels measured in smokers and those predicted on machine yields are most likely a result of attempts to regulate nicotine intake. Changes in CO levels in response to different smoking behaviors may differ from changes in nicotine levels, because CO absorption is more heavily influenced by depth of inhalation than is nicotine. CO is absorbed across alveolar surfaces, whereas nicotine can be absorbed across the mucosa in the upper and lower airways, as well as across the alveolar surface. Levels of CO can be measured in expired air or in the blood, the latter as carboxyhemoglobin (COHb). CO is a widely used measure of cigarette smoke exposure, although its level can be influenced by environmental exposures and the rate of its elimination is markedly influenced by the level of physical activity.

Hydrogen cyanide is another component of tobacco smoke. In the body, cyanide is metabolized to thiocyanate, which can be measured in blood or saliva. Thiocyanate has been used as a marker of tobacco smoke exposure in many studies. Its main limitation is that there are many dietary sources of thiocyanate, and thiocyanate levels in nonsmokers are substantial. Thus, measurement of thiocyanate yields relatively poor sensitivity and specificity for tobacco smoke exposure, particularly at low levels of cigarette smoking.

In considering smoking-related cancer risks, it would be most appropriate to measure exposure to tobacco smoke carcinogens. Such carcinogens in tobacco smoke include polycyclic aromatic hydrocarbons (PAHs), various nitrosamines, naphthylamines, polonium-210, and others. The carcinogen biomarker that has shown the most promise has been a measurement of nicotine-derived nitrosamines (Hecht, 1998). The nicotine-derived nitrosamine, 4-(methylnitrosamino)-1-(3-pyridyl)-1-butanone (NNK), is specific for tobacco smoke exposure and is metabolized to a butanol metabolite, 4-(methylnitrosamino)-1-(3-pyridyl)-1-butanol (NNAL) and its glucuronide (NNAL-GLUC). Urine levels of NNAL + NNAL-GLUC are elevated in smokers (Hecht *et al.*, 1993). The assay for NNAL is technically demanding. As yet, studies of NNAL levels in smokers of different yields of cigarettes have not been published.

Other potential markers of carcinogen exposure include adducts of 4-aminobiphenyl to hemoglobin in red blood cells (Bartsch *et al.*, 1990); adducts of benzo(a)pyrene and other potential carcinogens to DNA in white blood cells (Jahnke *et al.*, 1990; van Maanen *et al.*, 1994); adducts of PAHs to plasma albumin (Mooney *et al.*, 1995); and urinary hydroxyproline or N-nitrosoproline excretion (Adlkofer *et al.*, 1984). None of these markers has been used to date in studying smokers of different yields of cigarettes.

One indirect measure of carcinogen exposure that has been used is the measurement of mutagenic activity of the urine (Yamasaki and Ames, 1977). This is commonly done using the Salmonella histadine auxotroph reversion assay. In vitro studies indicate that the mutagenic components of cigarette smoke are found primarily in the tar rather than in the gaseous fraction (Florin *et al.*, 1980). It is known that the urine of cigarette smokers is mutagenic. For an individual smoker, mutagenic activity of the urine tends to be constant from day to day and there is a relationship between mutagenic activity and the number of cigarettes smoked per day (Sorsa *et al.*, 1984; Benowitz, 1989). The test is limited in that it is not specific for exposure to particular carcinogens, there is considerable variability in results from assay to assay and from person to person, and dietary and environmental chemical exposures can influence mutagenic activity. However, for within-subject comparisons when assays are compared for the same individual, the test provides a quantitative estimate of exposure to tar and, thus, potential carcinogen exposure.

**NICOTINE ABSORPTION FROM** The intake of nicotine from a single cigarette
**CIGARETTE SMOKING** or while smoking cigarettes throughout the
day can be estimated by measuring blood levels of nicotine at frequent time intervals. If the clearance (a measure of the rate of metabolism and excretion) of nicotine is known, then blood level data can be converted to actual intake of nicotine from smoking. Nicotine clearance can be measured by

measuring blood levels during and after an intravenous infusion of a known dose. This technique has been used in the laboratory or on smokers in a research ward to determine the intake of nicotine from smoking (Benowitz and Jacob, 1984a; Feyerabend *et al.*, 1985; Benowitz *et al.*, 1991). On average, smokers take in about 1 mg of nicotine per cigarette. The intake of nicotine is quite variable from person to person, appears to be largely independent of machine-determined yield, and can increase three-fold or more in response to restricted cigarette availability (Benowitz and Jacob, 1984a; Benowitz *et al.*, 1986a).

As noted previously, cotinine can be used as a measure of nicotine intake from cigarette smoking (Benowitz, 1996). On average, 70-80 percent of nicotine is metabolized to cotinine. Cotinine has a half-life averaging 16 hours, such that levels are relatively stable throughout the day in smokers. There is some individual variation in the quantitative relationship between cotinine levels in blood, saliva, or urine, and the intake of nicotine. This is because different people convert different percentages of nicotine to cotinine (usual range is 55-92 percent) and because different people metabolize cotinine itself at different rates (Benowitz and Jacob, 1994).

The relationship between nicotine intake and cotinine levels can be expressed mathematically as:

$$\text{Intake of nicotine} = \frac{C_{ss}(CL_{COT})}{\%Conv_{NIC \to COT}}$$

where $C_{ss}$ is the steady-state blood cotinine concentration, $CL_{COT}$ is the clearance of cotinine, and $\%Conv_{NIC \to COT}$ is the percent conversion of nicotine to cotinine.

Rearranging the equation,

$$\text{intake of nicotine} = \left[ \frac{CL_{COT}}{\%Conv_{NIC \to COT}} \right] C_{ss} = K\,(C_{ss})$$

In adult smokers, the conversion factor K averages 0.08 mg/24 hours/ng/ml (Benowitz and Jacob, 1994). Thus, a cotinine level of 300 ng/ml in a typical smoker corresponds to a daily nicotine intake of 24 mg. Although cotinine screening levels do not precisely predict nicotine intake for an individual because of individual variability in the conversion factor, cotinine levels in groups of smokers are expected to predict average group exposure to nicotine. Thus, the K factor can be used in population studies to relate cotinine levels to overall intake of nicotine from particular brands of cigarettes.

Another way to estimate nicotine intake from cigarette smoking is to measure urinary excretion of nicotine and its metabolites (Byrd *et al.*, 1995, 1998). Measurement of all currently known metabolites of nicotine can account for approximately 90 percent of a dose of nicotine (Benowitz *et al.*, 1994). Assuming a steady level of smoking from day to day, the sum of nicotine and its metabolites (as measured in 24-hour urine samples) reflects the dose of nicotine taken in each day. A related but less precise way to assess nicotine intake is to measure nicotine and its metabolites in urine using a nonspecific colorimetric assay (Peach *et al.*, 1985). This assay does not distinguish particular nicotine metabolites and is less quantitative, but allows a semi-quantitative comparison of nicotine exposure in populations of smokers.

**ESTIMATING THE EXTENT OF COMPENSATION**  The analysis of biochemical markers after cigarette brand switching is often expressed as degree of percentage of compensation. Complete compensation means that the same amount of nicotine or other tobacco smoke constituents is taken in before and after a switch to a cigarette with a different nominal yield. No compensation means the intake changes in direct proportion to the change in machine-determined yields relative to the new brand.

Compensation, defined as the degree to which proportional changes in a smoker's intake of a smoke constituent make up for the same proportional change in the machine-determined yield of that constituent, can be expressed mathematically in the following equation (Alison *et al.*, 1989):

$$C = 1 - \left[ \frac{\log(\text{marker}_2) - \log(\text{marker}_1)}{\log(\text{yield}_2) - \log(\text{yield}_1)} \right]$$

where C = extent of compensation, $\text{marker}_1$ and $\text{yield}_1$ represent the levels of biomarker and yield before the brand change, and $\text{marker}_2$ and $\text{yield}_2$ represent the levels in the changed brand condition.

The Zacny and Stitzer (1988) data, which will be described in more detail later, were used to illustrate the use of this equation. Smokers were switched from their usual cigarettes with an average nicotine yield of 1.0 mg to cigarettes with an average nicotine yield of 0.4 mg. The average plasma cotinine concentrations were 252 ng/ml while smoking the higher yield and 188 ng/ml while smoking the lower yield cigarettes. Using the equation above,

$$C = 1 - \left[ \frac{\log(189) - \log(252)}{\log(0.4) - \log(1.0)} \right]$$

where data are available, the degree of compensation will be reported for the various studies discussed in subsequent sections.

**STUDIES OF SMOKING CIGARETTES WITH DIFFERENT MACHINE-DETERMINED YIELDS: METHODOLOGICAL CONSIDERATIONS**  The remainder of this chapter will review studies of human exposure to tobacco smoke chemicals that have used three main types of research designs. The first design is the experimental forced-switching study, in which smokers are asked to switch to brands of higher or lower machine-determined yield compared to their usual brand. These experimental studies have been separated into short term (up to 4 weeks) and long term (more than 4 weeks). Forced-switching studies are particularly useful in that smoking behavior and exposure can be assessed under close observation. The limitations of such studies include the fact that smokers are switching only for the purpose of the research. Motivation and cigarette acceptability are dissimilar from the natural situation of brand switching. These studies are performed over periods of time that may not provide adequate duration to adjust to the taste or puffing characteristics of the new cigarettes. Many of the short-term studies have been performed in laboratories or on research wards, environments in which individuals may not smoke cigarettes as they normally do. Longer term forced-switching studies do allow more time to become accustomed to the new cigarette and are conducted in the smoker's natural environment, but they still do not measure the effect of self-determined brand switching. Nonetheless, experimental switching studies have provided useful information on the mechanism and extent of compensation that can occur.

A second study design is one that follows smokers who smoke self-selected cigarette brands. These are cross-sectional studies of chemical exposures in smokers who have selected the brand of cigarette that they find satisfying. Data from this type of study provide the best estimate of chemical exposure in smokers smoking different brands of cigarettes, but do not address the question of what happens if a person switches brands—for example, if someone switches from high- to low-yield cigarettes.

The third type of study design is one that examines spontaneous brand switching. These are studies of smokers who have chosen to switch from higher to lower machine-determined yield cigarettes, or vice versa. In these studies, the brand of cigarettes has been selected by the smoker, not by the researchers. Such studies are more informative of smokers' exposure in the real world when switching from higher to lower yield cigarettes.

**SHORT-TERM EXPERIMENTAL SWITCHING STUDIES** A number of studies have examined the effects of switching from high- to low-yield cigarettes over a short period of time, defined for the purposes of this report as up to one month. The effects of short-term switching to low-yield cigarettes on how a cigarette is puffed and on vent hole blocking are discussed elsewhere in this volume. This section will focus on switching studies in which biomarkers of tobacco smoke exposure were measured.

Russell and coworkers (1975) studied 10 smokers on different days when they were smoking their usual brand (average yield, 1.34 mg nicotine), or when they were switched to higher yield (2.3 mg nicotine) or to lower yield (0.14 mg nicotine) cigarettes. The subjects were studied in the morning while smoking their usual brands, and then again after 5 hours of smoking either their usual, high-, or low-yield brands. Plasma nicotine concentrations were measured 3 minutes after smoking a cigarette as the indicator of nicotine exposure. Plasma nicotine concentrations were similar while smoking the usual and high-yield cigarettes (30.1 and 29.2 ng/ml, respectively) and significantly lower (8.5 ng/ml) while smoking the low-yield cigarette. The extent of compensation is estimated to be 96 percent for the high-yield and 20 percent for the low-yield cigarettes, respectively. The number of cigarettes smoked in the 5 hours of ad libitum smoking showed a 38 percent reduction while smoking the high-yield cigarettes and an increase from an average of 10.7 to 12.5 cigarettes per day for low-yield cigarettes (the latter comparison was not statistically significant).

Benowitz and Jacob (1984b) studied 11 smokers in a hospital research ward. They were smoking their own brand of cigarettes (average yield, 16.3 mg tar, 1.1 mg nicotine), or were switched to either Camel® (15.4 mg tar, 1.0 mg nicotine) or True® (4.6 mg tar, 0.4 mg nicotine) for 4 days each. Cigarette brands were assigned in a balanced order. Nicotine intake was determined by measuring blood nicotine concentrations throughout the day. When switched from their usual brand to either Camel® or True®, the smokers showed an approximately one-third decline in nicotine exposure. However, the intakes of nicotine and CO were similar when smoking Camel® or True®. Thus, using Camel®s as a comparator, the degree of compensation when smoking True® was 100 percent. Similar findings were obtained for CO exposure (based on measurements of COHb) or mutagenic activity in a 24-hour urine collection (a measure of exposure to potentially carcinogenic chemicals).

A similarly designed study was performed where 11 subjects were switched from their usual brand (average yield, 14.7 mg tar, 1.1 mg nicotine) to Camel® (15.4 mg tar, 1.0 mg nicotine) or to ultra-low Carlton® (tar 0.8 mg, nicotine 0.1 mg) cigarettes (Benowitz *et al.*, 1986b). Compared to the high-yield Camel® cigarette, when the participants smoked the Carlton® brand, their nicotine, CO, and mutagenic activity levels were reduced by 56, 36, and 49 percent, respectively. The percent compensation based on nicotine exposure was estimated to be 74 percent.

West and associates (1984) randomized 26 smokers of high-yield cigarettes (average yield, 14.2 mg tar, 1.3 mg nicotine) who either continued their own brand or switched to an ultra-low-yield cigarette (1 mg tar, 0.1 mg nicotine) for 10 days. Subjects smoked a similar number of cigarettes in the two conditions. The trough plasma nicotine level averaged 22.8 mg/ml for the usual brand condition versus 9.4 ng/ml for the ultra-low-yield brand condition. The latter is consistent with 36 percent compensation. A similar degree of compensation was estimated based on expired CO levels.

Zacny and Stitzer (1988) studied 10 smokers of high-yield cigarettes (average, 1.0 mg nicotine) who smoked five different brands of cigarettes— their own and cigarettes with yields of 0.1, 0.4, 0.7, and 1.1 mg nicotine— each for 5 days, in random order. Subjects smoked significantly more cigarettes per day of the two brands with the lowest yields compared to the three higher yield cigarettes. When smoking low-yield cigarettes, larger and more frequent puffs were taken as well. The plasma cotinine levels at the end of each smoking period averaged 152, 188, 221, 252, and 259 ng/ml for the 0.1, 0.4, 0.7, 1.0, and 1.1 mg nicotine brands, respectively. The cotinine levels measured when smoking the two lowest yield cigarettes were significantly lower than for the three others. Based on group average data, compensation was estimated to be 56, 58, and 60 percent for the 0.1, 0.4, and 0.7 mg nicotine brands, respectively.

A Benowitz study mentioned previously allowed a comparison of tar-to-nicotine ratios as predicted by the smoking machine and as experienced by the smoker (Benowitz *et al.*, 1986a). The machine-determined tar-to-nicotine ratios for low-yield cigarettes are generally lower than those for high-yield cigarettes. For example, the tar-to-nicotine ratios for cigarettes in this study were 15.4 for Camel®, 11.5 for True®, and 7.3 for Carlton®. Assuming that urinary mutagenicity is a quantitative measure of tar exposure (which is reasonable, since most mutagenic activity comes from tar), changes in the ratio of urinary mutagenicity to the area under the plasma nicotine concentration time curve over 24 hours can be used as an indicator of changes in the ratio of actual tar-to-nicotine exposure in the smoker. While urinary mutagenicity did decline when smokers were switched to ultra-low-yield cigarettes, the ratio of mutagenic activity to nicotine exposure did not differ for any of the cigarette types. This observation is consistent with smoking-machine studies in which vent-hole blocking and/or more intensive smoking of low-yield cigarettes resulted in increased tar-to-nicotine ratios (Rickert *et al.*, 1983). It has been suggested that low-yield cigarettes may be less hazardous, even if full compensation for nicotine occurs, because the lower tar-to-nicotine ratio would lead to less intake of tar for any given level of intake of nicotine. However, based on the urinary mutagenicity data, one must question whether predictions about lower exposure to tar based on machine-determined tar-to-nicotine ratios are valid.

In summary, these short-term switching studies demonstrated that smokers compensate for reduced nicotine deliveries, but the extent of compensation varied in different studies—from 20 percent to 100 percent. The degree of compensation is likely to be less in short-term switching studies compared to longer term switching studies, or studies in which smokers have selected their own brand of cigarettes. This is because 1) smokers have not chosen to smoke the particular brand of cigarette they are switched to, 2) they often find the low-yield cigarettes to be unsatisfying, and 3) they may not be smoking the cigarettes long enough to develop effective compensatory smoking behaviors. These short-term switching studies demonstrated that compensation occurs by a combination of smoking more cigarettes per day and by taking in more tobacco smoke per cigarette compared to smoking-machine predictions. The one study that estimated tar-to-nicotine ratios delivered to the smoker suggested that this ratio is much higher than is predicted by smoking-machine tests in smokers of low-yield cigarettes, consistent with smoking-machine studies that showed that intensive puffing increases tar-to-nicotine ratios.

**LONG-TERM EXPERIMENTAL SWITCHING STUDIES** Several studies have biochemically assessed the extent of compensation after switching from higher to lower yield cigarettes for periods of more than a few weeks. Russell and associates (1982) studied 12 smokers who typically smoked an average of 38 'middle-tar' cigarettes per day with an average yield of 17.4 mg tar and 1.3 mg nicotine. These subjects were switched to a low-tar ciga-rette (yield of 10.9 mg tar and 0.7 mg nicotine) for 10 weeks. Compared to baseline, the average cigarette consumption increased by about three ciga-rettes per day while smoking the low-yield cigarette, although this was not statistically significant. Plasma nicotine concentration (measured 2 minutes after smoking a test cigarette) and plasma cotinine concentrations declined by an average of 30 percent. There was no change in plasma thiocyanate or blood COHb. The percentage compensation based on plasma nicotine or plasma cotinine levels was 36 percent.

Robinson and colleagues (1983) switched a group of smokers of high-nicotine cigarettes (average yield, 1.8 to 1.1 mg nicotine) to lower yield brands over two stages. Six of the subjects, who served as controls, were switched to cigarettes similar to their usual brand. Sixteen subjects were switched initially to brands with 33 percent, then to brands with 61 percent reduction of nicotine yields over 8 weeks. The average serum cotinine level did not significantly decrease in those who decreased their brand yield (284 versus 244 ng/ml). Likewise, there was no significant reduction in plasma thiocyanate or blood COHb levels. Thus, the Robinson study demonstrated nearly complete compensation when switching to lower yield cigarettes. Some smokers in this study achieved compensation by smoking more ciga-rettes per day, but for most smokers the main mechanism was smoking cig-arettes more intensively and/or blocking ventilation holes.

Peach and associates (1986) studied 183 smokers of middle-tar cigarettes who were randomized to switch from their own brand to cigarettes of a similar yield (average, 15.5 mg tar, 1.5 mg nicotine) or a lower yield (9.0 mg tar, 0.9 mg nicotine). Test cigarettes could be purchased at a discount. The subjects were followed for 5 weeks and smoked an average of 20 cigarettes per day, a rate that did not differ between middle- and low-tar cigarettes. However, urine nicotine metabolite excretion was no different for individu-als smoking the two types of cigarettes, indicating 100 percent compensa-tion.

Guyatt and colleagues (1989) studied 29 smokers who smoked their usual brand for 4 months and then were switched to a lower tar brand for 9 months. The usual cigarette brand had an average yield of 15.6 mg tar and 1.3 mg nicotine. Subjects were switched to cigarettes of at least 3 mg lower tar than the usual brand—the average switch was to 9.3 mg tar and 0.9 mg nicotine. Smokers on average smoked a greater number of low-yield ciga-rettes compared to the usual brand (28.5 versus 24.9 cigarettes per day), but the difference was not statistically significant. Smokers did take more puffs and larger puff volumes when smoking the lower yield cigarettes. Plasma cotinine and COHb levels declined by 18 percent. Compensation was esti-mated by the authors to be 61 percent based on cotinine and 56 percent based on COHb levels. The main mechanism for compensation was judged to be more intensive puffing rather than greater cigarette consumption.

Frost and associates (1995) studied 434 smokers of high-yield cigarettes who were switched to cigarettes of approximately 50 percent lower yield compared to their usual brands. One group was switched to the cigarettes immediately, and another was switched gradually over several months. A third group, the control group, was switched to cigarettes of 10 percent lower yield than their usual cigarettes. Subjects were allowed to select the brand that they would smoke within the specified yield range. The follow-up was over 6 months. Compared to the preswitching value, levels of serum cotinine in the fast yield-reduction group declined by an average of 11 percent and COHb declined by 14 percent. In the slow yield-reduction group, there was a decrease of 6 percent in cotinine and 16 percent in COHb. For the two groups combined, the extent of compensation was estimated by the authors to be 79 percent based on cotinine and 65 percent based on COHb. There was no significant difference in the extent of compensation based on how fast the yields were reduced. On average, smokers reduced the number of cigarettes they smoked after switching, which was interpreted by the authors to reflect the desire of this group of smokers to reduce their smoking in general. The high degree of compensation despite smoking fewer cigarettes per day further demonstrates the point that cigarette yields are substantially increased by smoking lower yield cigarettes more intensively.

In summary, the data from these experimental long-term switching studies indicated that there was some reduction in smoke exposure, but that the magnitude of that reduction was small. The larger studies indicated that the extent of compensation based on nicotine intake was about 80 percent. Compensation occurred primarily by increasing the intensity with which cigarettes were smoked, in addition to the variable contribution of increased numbers of cigarettes smoked per day in the different studies. It is possible that voluntary efforts to cut down on smoking by subjects in some of these studies may have limited the increase in cigarette consumption that has been observed in response to switching to lower yield cigarettes in other studies.

## STUDIES OF SMOKERS SMOKING SELF-SELECTED BRANDS

### Studies of Nicotine Exposure

Cross-sectional population studies can provide data on exposure to tobacco smoke constituents in people who have selected the brand of cigarettes they find satisfying. While these studies may supply valuable data on tobacco smoke chemical exposure in smokers of different brands, there are limitations in extrapolating such data to brand switching. For example, the acceptability of nicotine delivery from a particular cigarette may influence brand selection, and a highly dependent smoker would choose only those cigarettes that would provide adequate doses of nicotine. Cross-sectional studies will also include some people who are in transition—that is, transition to regular smoking, to cessation, or in the process of relapsing from a previous cessation attempt. Health concerns may also affect brand selection. All these factors would be expected to affect the relationship between self-selected brand and measures of intensity of smoking. Therefore, self-selected brand studies are not a perfect model for studying compensation in response to brand switching.

The biomarkers used in cross-sectional studies include markers of nicotine exposure (blood nicotine, blood or saliva cotinine, or urinary nicotine metabolites) and markers of gas-phase exposure, such as CO and thiocyanate. This section focuses on studies that measured nicotine intake. Table 3-1 summarizes a number of studies in which nicotine intake was estimated in people who smoked cigarettes with different nominal yields. Most studies found either weak or no significant correlations between nominal yields and nicotine intakes.

Three large studies, which involved general populations of smokers, warrant particular discussion. Gori and Lynch (1985) recruited 865 smokers from shopping malls in different areas of the United States. Plasma nicotine and cotinine concentrations were weakly correlated with the Federal Trade Commission (FTC) method for machine-measuring nicotine yield (see Figure 3-1). Woodward and Tunstall-Pedoe (1992) studied 2,754 smokers as part of the baseline assessment in the Scottish Heart Health Study, which was conducted between 1984 and 1986. Their main analysis presented plasma cotinine data based on categories of yield: low tar (less than 13 mg/cigarette), middle tar (14-15 mg), and high tar (greater than 14 mg). The mean cotinine values were no different across categories for males (276, 294, and 278 ng/ml for low-, middle-, and high-tar groups, respectively). For females, the cotinine level was 26 percent lower in the low-tar group (199 ng/ml) but similar for the middle- and high-tar groups (270 and 270 ng/ml, respectively). Woodward and Tunstall-Pedoe (1993) performed another analysis of the same data with comparison of the cotinine concentrations to specific yields of tar, nicotine, and CO (see Figure 3-2). Multiple regression analysis—which included tar, nicotine, and CO yields as well as cigarette consumption and gender—found that tar was the best predictor of cotinine level, with an interaction for gender as previously discussed. However, the best regression model accounted for only 19 percent of the variance in cotinine levels.

Jarvis and colleagues (2001) conducted a study of 2,031 adult smokers in the United Kingdom as part of the 1998 Health Survey for England. Smokers were defined as anyone who reported current smoking and included those who smoked only occasionally. Saliva cotinine concentrations correlated weakly with machine-determined nicotine yield (r = 0.19, P < 0.001). After controlling for confounders, machine-determined yield accounted for 0.79 percent of the variance in saliva cotinine. Using the conversion factor for estimating nicotine intake from cotinine level as described earlier, Jarvis and associates estimated a nicotine intake per cigarette of 1.17 mg in smokers of brands with machine yields of less than 0.4 mg (average, 0.14 mg), 1.22 mg nicotine for cigarettes with yields of 0.4-0.75 mg (average, 0.57 mg), and 1.31 mg for brands with yields greater than 0.75 mg (average, 0.91 mg). The authors did not find that smokers of low-yield cigarettes smoked more cigarettes than smokers of higher yield cigarettes. However, in their analysis, most of the occasional smokers fell into the low-yield cigarette group. Thus, the low-yield group contained a mixture of addicted and nonaddicted smokers, whereas the higher yield groups included a greater proportion of addicted smokers (Jarvis *et al.*, 2001).

Table 3-1
**Studies of Nicotine Intake Compared with Machine Nicotine Yield**

| Study | Population | Nicotine Yields (mg) | Results |
|---|---|---|---|
| Russell *et al.*, 1980 | 330 from smokers' clinics or research volunteers | 0.5-3.5 | PNIC vs. Mach-N<br>$r = 0.21^*$ |
| Rickert and Robinson, 1981 | 84 during routine medical exams | 0.25-1.3 | PCOT vs. Mach-N<br>$r = 0.08$ |
| Benowitz *et al.*, 1983 | 272 seeking smoking cessation therapy | <0.1-1.9 | BCOT vs. FTC-N<br>$r = 0.15$ (n = 137)<br>$r = 0.06$ (n = 123) |
| Ebert *et al.*, 1983 | 76; mix of smoking cessation, hospital employees, and ambulatory patients | 0.1-1.5 | PNIC vs. FTC-N<br>$r = 0.25^*$ |
| Gori and Lynch, 1985 | 865 recruited from shopping malls; 10 or more cigarettes per day | 0.1-1.6 | PNIC vs. FTC-N<br>$r = 0.37^*$<br>PCOT vs. FTC-N<br>$r = 0.23^*$ |
| Benowitz *et al.*, 1986b | 248 seeking smoking cessation (137 from previous study) | 0.1-1.9 | BCOT values similar for FTC-N 0.21 to >1.0<br>BCOT 2/3 of others for FTC-N < 0.20 |
| Russell *et al.*, 1986 | 392 from smokers' clinics | — | BCOT vs. Mach-N<br>$r = 0.13^*$<br>BNIC vs. Mach-N<br>$r = 0.26^*$ |
| Rosa *et al.*, 1992 | 125 attending military medical center | 0.38-1.38 | BCOT vs. Mach-N<br>$r = 0.30$ |
| Coultas *et al.*, 1993 | 298 from Hispanic household survey | — | SCOT vs. FTC-N<br>$r = 0.12$ |
| Woodward and Tunstall-Pedoe, 1993 | 2,754 from Scottish Heart Health Study (1984-1986) | 0.1-1.7 | BCOT vs. Mach Tar, N, and CO and gender (multiple regression); accounted for 19% variance |
| Byrd *et al.*, 1995 | 33 volunteers | 0.13-1.3 | UNIC + metabolites vs. FTC-N<br>N/24 hr: $r = 0.68^*$<br>N/cig: $r = 0.79^*$ |

Table 3-1 (continued)

| Study | Population | Nicotine Yields (mg) | Results |
|-------|-----------|----------------------|---------|
| Hee *et al.*, 1995 | 108 volunteers; 5 or more cigarettes per day | 0.09-1.19 | UNIC, UCOT vs. Mach-N; NS |
| Byrd *et al.*, 1998 | 72 volunteers | 0.1-1.4 | UNIC + metabolites vs. FTC-N N/24 hr: $r = 0.19$ N/cig: $r = 0.31$* SCOT vs. FTC-N $r = 0.15$ |
| Jarvis *et al.*, 2001 | 2,031 from 1998 Health Survey for England | 0.04-1.06 | SCOT vs. Mach-N $r = 0.19$* |

*$P < 0.05$.

Key: PCOT = plasma cotinine concentration; Mach-N = smoking-machine-determined nicotine yield; PNIC = plasma nicotine concentration; BCOT = blood cotinine concentration; FTC-N = machine yield by Federal Trade Commission method; BNIC = blood nicotine concentration; SCOT = saliva cotinine concentration; UNIC = urine nicotine concentration; UCOT = urine cotinine concentration; N = nicotine; CO = carbon monoxide.

Figure 3-1

**Plasma Cotinine and Nicotine Concentrations in Cigarette Smokers According to the FTC Nicotine Yield**

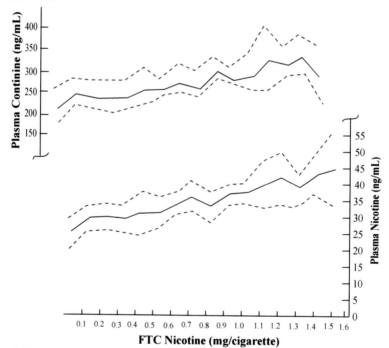

Note: Solid line indicates mean; dashed line indicates 95% confidence intervals (from Gori and Lynch, 1985).

Figure 3-2
**Mean Values for Expired Carbon Monoxide v. CO Yield, Serum Thiocyanate v. Tar Yield, and Serum Cotinine Against Machine-Determined Yields for Men and Women**

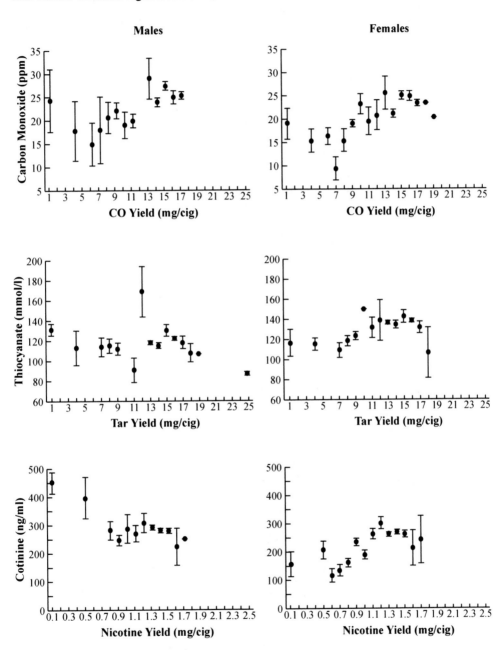

Note: Bars indicate one standard error (from Woodward and Tunstall-Pedoe, 1993).

53

Another study by Gori and Lynch (1983) warrants particular discussion with respect to ultra-low-yield brands of cigarettes. They studied 288 smokers of two ultra-low-yield cigarette brands (1 mg tar). The subjects were recruited in shopping malls, and plasma cotinine levels were measured. The cotinine concentrations in smokers averaged 322 and 195 ng/ml for brands with yields of 0.18 and 0.10 mg nicotine, respectively. The cotinine values of the second brand were about 30 percent lower than the typical smoker population value of 300 mg/ml. Smokers of the first ultra-low brand had cotinine concentrations similar to the smoker population average. These findings were similar to those of a short-term experimental study, by Benowitz and associates, in which smokers were switched from regular to ultra-low-yield cigarettes (Benowitz *et al.*, 1986b). In that study, the intake of nicotine fell by about 30 percent when switching to ultra-low-yield cigarettes compared to the usual brand.

In summary, most studies of nicotine intake in populations smoking self-selected brands of cigarettes showed some differences in nicotine exposure when high- and low-yield brands were compared. However, the differences were quite small and not nearly quantitatively proportional to the changes in nominal yield. Thus, nicotine ratings of cigarettes are poor predictors of actual nicotine intake and of the intake of other toxins as well. The FTC method generally underestimates human exposure to nicotine, particularly in smokers who are smoking low-yield cigarettes.

**Studies of Carbon Monoxide Exposure**    Studies on CO exposure in populations of self-determined brand smokers are summarized in Table 3-2. An example of CO data from a large group of smokers recruited from shopping centers is shown in Figure 3-3 (Gori and Lynch, 1985). Similar data were reported by Woodward and Tunstall-Pedoe (1992) in the Scottish Heart Health Study (see Figure 3-2). Most other studies likewise found no relationship between machine-determined CO yield and CO exposure, although a few studies did report weak correlations. The conclusions for CO were similar to those discussed above for nicotine; that is, machine-determined yields are poor predictors of human exposure to CO, and presumably to other gaseous components of tobacco smoke as well.

**Studies of Other Tobacco Smoke Biomarkers**    Several studies have measured plasma or saliva thiocyanate concentrations, and one study measured urinary mutagenic activity. In most studies, thiocyanate concentrations were no different in smokers of cigarettes with different nominal yields. The Woodward and Tunstall-Pedoe study (1993) found a weak relationship between serum thiocyanate and cigarette yield. Benowitz and colleagues (1986b) found that smokers of ultra-low-yield cigarettes had about 25 percent lower thiocyanate levels compared to other brands, but Maron and Fortmann (1987) found no difference in thiocyanate concentration comparing smokers of ultra-low and other brands.

Hee and coworkers (1995) measured urinary mutagenicity in 108 smokers of different yield cigarettes. They found a weak relationship between urinary mutagenicity and nicotine yield (r = 0.22, P > 0.05).

Table 3-2
**Studies of Carbon Monoxide Intake Compared with Machine Yield**

| Study | Population | Machine Yields (mg) | Results |
|---|---|---|---|
| Jaffe *et al.*, 1981 | 200 recruited from urban workplaces | 0.2 - >1.0 mg nicotine | ECO vs. FTC-N $r = 0.028$ |
| Rickert and Robinson, 1981 | 159 during routine medical exams | 4-22 mg CO | COHb vs. Mach-CO $r = 0.10$ |
| Sutton *et al.*, 1982 | 55 volunteers | 11-20 mg CO | COHb vs. Mach-CO $r = 0.03$ |
| Ebert *et al.*, 1983 | 76; mix of smoking cessation, hospital employees, and ambulatory patients | 1-22 mg CO | ECO vs. Mach-CO $r = 0.03$ |
| Wald *et al.*, 1984 | 2,455 males during health screening exams in London | 0.8-28.1 mg CO | CO remained relatively constant regardless of cigarette yield |
| Gori and Lynch, 1985 | 865 recruited from shopping malls; 10 or more cigarettes per day | 2-18 mg CO | ECO vs. FTC-CO; virtually no correlation |
| Maron and Fortmann, 1987 | 713 in a community-based survey | <0.2 - >1.0 mg NIC | ECO vs. FTC-N Analysis of variance revealed NSD |
| Woodward and Tunstall-Pedoe, 1992 | 2,754 from Scottish Heart Health Study (1984–1986) | 1-19 mg CO | ECO vs. Mach Tar, N, and CO and gender (multiple regression) accounted for 19% of variance |
| Coultas *et al.*, 1993 | 298 in a population survey, primarily Hispanic | — | ECO vs. FTC-CO $r = 0.03$ |
| Hee *et al.*, 1995 | 108 volunteers, 5 or more cigarettes per day | 1.1-15.0 mg | COHb vs. Mach $r = 0.24$ |

*Key: CO = carbon monoxide; FTC-N = machine yield of nicotine by Federal Trade Commission method; ECO = expired CO; COHb = blood carboxyhemoglobin; Mach-CO = smoking-machine-measured CO.*

Figure 3-3
**Expired Cabon Monoxide Concentrations in Smokers According to FTC CO Yields of Cigarettes Smoked**

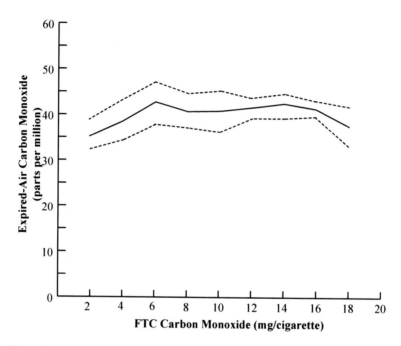

*Note: Solid line indicates mean; dashed line indicates 95% confidence intervals (from Gori and Lynch, 1985).*

Thus, the data on other biomarkers support the overall conclusions of studies that measured nicotine and CO—that there is very little difference in tobacco smoke exposure in people smoking cigarettes of different machine-determined yields. For the general population of smokers who select their own brand of cigarettes, the extent of nicotine compensation appears to be almost complete.

**SPONTANEOUS BRAND SWITCHING**  Smokers in their natural environment have chosen the brand of cigarettes they smoke. A smoker's choice of cigarette brand is influenced by a variety of factors, including the brand smoked by peers, the influence of advertising and promotional materials, a desire to reduce the health risks of smoking (which is, in turn, influenced by advertising and promotion), and the characteristics of the cigarette (*i.e.*, adequacy of nicotine dose, taste, etc.). Experimental studies of brand switching are, to some extent, artificial in that the researchers select the brand. Spontaneous brand switching studies are more informative of smokers' exposures in the real world when they switch to lower yield cigarettes.

Two studies of spontaneous brand switching were reviewed for this chapter. Lynch and Benowitz (1987) reported on 197 smokers who had measurements of plasma cotinine and COHb while smoking self-selected brands on 2 occasions, 6 years apart. Of these smokers, 104 were smoking cigarettes of the same or similar machine-determined yields as before, 62 had switched to a lower yield (0.2 mg or more reduction in nicotine delivery), and 31 had switched to higher yields (0.2 mg or more increase in nicotine delivery). Plasma samples and expired CO were measured on approximately the same day at baseline and on retesting. Smokers who did not change the nicotine yield showed a slight decrease in the numbers of cigarettes smoked per day, but there was no change in cotinine or CO levels (see Figure 3-4). Smokers who switched to lower yield cigarettes initially smoked cigarettes with higher nicotine yields (average 1.09 mg) and then switched to cigarettes with an average yield of 0.68 mg, a 38 percent reduction. Brand switching was associated with a reduction in cotinine and expired CO of about 20 percent. However, these smokers had also decreased their cigarette consumption by about 20 percent. Analysis of cotinine concentration or CO per cigarette showed no change despite reduction in yield. Thus, the smokers obtained the same dose of nicotine and CO from each cigarette even though the yield was lower. This observation is consistent with findings described previously showing that when switching from high- to low-yield cigarettes, full compensation from each cigarette is easily achieved. Reduction in daily exposure to tobacco smoke occurred primarily because certain smokers who switched to low-yield cigarettes smoked fewer cigarettes. Possibly, switching was part of an attempt by these individuals to reduce their health risks by smoking both lower yields and fewer cigarettes per day.

Switchers to high-yield cigarettes had smoked a low-yield cigarette at the initial study (average, 0.42 mg nicotine) and switched to cigarettes with an average yield of 0.85 mg, a 102 percent increase. After switching, cotinine levels increased by 23 percent and expired CO by 5 percent (see Figure 3-5). In this case, smokers did take in more nicotine and CO per cigarette, although much less than predicted by the relative increase in machine yield. Because these subjects were smoking lower yield cigarettes and had lower cotinine levels at baseline compared to subjects who switched to cigarettes of similar or lower yields, it is likely that this group was composed of smokers in an escalating phase of developing tobacco dependence. This idea was supported by the observation that, after switching, cotinine levels rose to levels similar to those of the other two groups at baseline.

Peach and coworkers studied 599 males over 13 years (from 1971 to 1984) in a study of the effects of brand switching on phlegm production on pulmonary function tests (Peach *et al.*, 1986a). Average cigarette consumption decreased in all smokers, but less so in those smokers who switched to lower yield cigarettes. Nicotine intake was estimated by a colorimetric assay of total nicotine plus metabolite excretion in the urine. At the 1984 assessment, no difference in nicotine metabolite excretion was observed in individuals who had or had not switched from higher to lower yield cigarettes. This suggests full compensation when switching to lower yield cigarettes.

Figure 3-4

**Spontaneous Brand Switching Study: Plasma Concentrations of Cotinine and Cotinine Concentration Normalized for Cigarettes Smoked per Day**

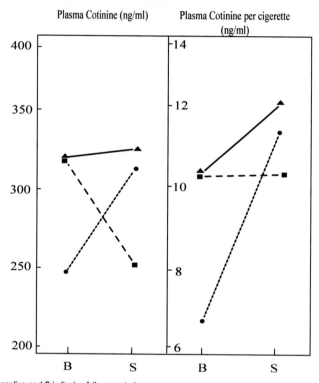

Note: B indicates baseline and S indicates follow-up study.
Symbols: Triangles=subjects who did not switch brands (n=109); solid squares=decreasers (n=62); solid circles=increasers (n=32); asteriks indicate significant change from baseline to follow-up study (from Lynch and Benowitz, 1987).

In summary, these two spontaneous brand-switching studies indicated that when smokers choose to switch to low-yield cigarettes, their intake of nicotine and CO (and presumably other smoke constituents) per cigarette does not significantly change. Thus, for spontaneous brand switchers, there appears to be a complete compensation for each cigarette smoked, reflecting more intensive smoking. These observations suggest, at least when considering modern cigarettes, that switching from higher to lower yield cigarettes per se is not likely to reduce disease risk.

**SUMMARY** Studies of subjects who smoked cigarettes with lower machine-determined yields support the idea that smokers regulate their intake of nicotine to take in the amount of nicotine that they need to sustain their addiction. Experimental switching studies show varying degrees of compensation. Variability from study to study probably reflects the characteristics of the smokers and the types of cigarettes to which they were switched. Experimental studies in which smokers were switched from regular to ultra-

Figure 3-5
**Spontaneous Brand Switching Study: Expired Air CO Concentration and CO Concentration Normalized for Cigarettes Smoked per Day**

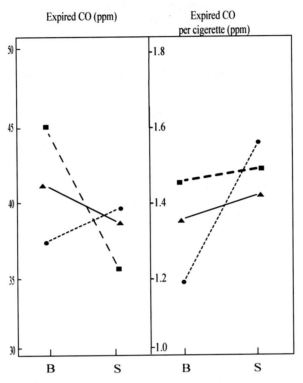

Note: B indicates baseline and S indicates follow-up study.
Symbols: Triangles=subjects who did not switch brands (n=109); solid squares=decreasers (n=62); solid circles=increasers (n=32); asteriks indicate significant change from baseline to follow-up study (from Lynch and Benowitz, 1987).

low-yield cigarettes suggest a significant but modest reduction in nicotine exposure. Spontaneous brand-switching studies suggest that there is no reduction in smoke intake per cigarette, and that any reductions that were seen in brand switchers depended upon whether or not those individuals also cut down their cigarette consumption.

Studies of smokers smoking self-selected brands assessed exposure in individuals who smoked as many of their cigarettes as they wish. These studies convincingly showed a weak relationship between nicotine yield and nicotine, CO, or thiocyanate exposure. An exception may be smokers of ultra-low-yield cigarettes, for whom in some studies there was an approximately 30 percent reduction of cotinine levels. However, the market share for ultra-low-yield cigarettes is extremely small.

Considering the overall exposure data in individuals selecting their own brands, there is little reason to expect that smokers of low-yield cigarettes will have a lower risk of disease than those smoking higher yield cigarettes. Lower tar-to-nicotine ratios could result in reduced risk, in theory, even if there is full compensation for nicotine, but the few human exposure data available to date suggest that exposure to tar compared to nicotine is not different in smokers smoking low-yield cigarettes.

The majority of smokers appear to compensate by smoking their cigarettes more intensively and/or by blocking ventilation holes. Some studies show that smokers of low-yield cigarettes smoke more cigarettes per day. Other studies indicate that occasional smokers are more likely to be in the low-yield category, which may result in estimates of smoking similar or even fewer cigarettes in the low-yield group compared to higher yield groups. Recent data from California suggest that if one looks at addicted smokers who have been smoking at a stable level for some time, smokers of low-yield cigarettes do smoke more cigarettes. This type of analysis has not been performed on other data sets, where cigarette consumption was simply taken for all smokers of a particular yield regardless of level of dependence or the stability of smoking behavior.

## CONCLUSIONS

1. Smokers regulate their intake of nicotine to obtain the amount of nicotine that they need to sustain their addiction.

2. Spontaneous brand-switching studies suggest that there is no reduction in smoke intake per cigarette, and that any reductions that are seen in brand switchers depend upon whether or not those individuals also reduce their cigarette consumption.

3. Studies of smokers smoking self-selected brands showed a weak relationship between machine-measured nicotine yield and a smoker's nicotine, CO, or thiocyanate exposure.

4. Considering the overall exposure data for individuals selecting their own brands, there is little reason to expect that smokers of low-yield cigarettes will have a lower risk of disease than those who smoke higher yield cigarettes.

## REFERENCES

Adlkofer, F., Scherer, G., Heller, W.D. Hydroxyproline excretion in urine of smokers and passive smokers. *Preventive Medicine* 13(6):670-679, 1984.

Alison, S., Frost, C., Thompson, S., Wald, N. Estimating the extent of compensatory smoking. *Nicotine, Smoking and the Low Tar Programme.* Wald, N., Fruggatt, P. (Editors). London, Oxford Medical Publishing, pp. 100-115, 1989.

Bartsch, H., Caporaso, N., Coda, M., Kadlubar, F., Malaveille, C., Skipper, P., Talaska, G., Tannenbaum, S.R., Vineis, P. Carcinogen hemoglobin adducts, urinary mutagenicity, and metabolic phenotype in active and passive cigarette smokers. *Journal of the National Cancer Institute* 82(23):1826-1831, 1990.

Benowitz, N.L. Pharmacologic aspects of cigarette smoking and nicotine addiction. *The New England Journal of Medicine* 319:1318-1330, 1988.

Benowitz, N.L. Dosimetric studies of compensatory cigarette smoking. *Nicotine, Smoking and the Low Tar Programme.* Wald, N., Froggatt, P. (Editors.). London, Oxford Medical Publishing, 1989.

Benowitz, N.L. Cotinine as a biomarker of environmental tobacco smoke exposure. *Epidemiologic Reviews* 18(2):188-204, 1996.

Benowitz, N.L. Biomarkers of environmental tobacco smoke exposure. *Environmental Health Perspectives* 107(Suppl 2):349-355, 1999a.

Benowitz, N.L. Nicotine addiction. *Primary Care* 26(3):611-631, 1999b.

Benowitz, N.L., Hall, S.M., Herning, R.I., Jacob, P., III, Jones, R.T., Osman, A.L. Smokers of low yield cigarettes do not consume less nicotine. *The New England Journal of Medicine* 309(3):139-142, 1983.

Benowitz, N.L., Jacob, P., III. Daily intake of nicotine during cigarette smoking. *Clinical Pharmacology and Therapeutics* 35(4):499-504, 1984a.

Benowitz, N.L., Jacob, P., III. Nicotine and carbon monoxide intake from high- and low-yield cigarettes. *Clinical Pharmacology and Therapeutics* 36(2):265-270, 1984b.

Benowitz, N.L., Jacob, P., III. Nicotine renal excretion rate influences nicotine intake during cigarette smoking. *The Journal of Pharmacology and Experimental Therapeutic* 234(1):153-155, 1985.

Benowitz, N.L., Jacob, P., III. Intravenous nicotine replacement suppresses nicotine intake from cigarette smoking. *The Journal of Pharmacology and Experimental Therapeutics* 254(3):1000-1005, 1990.

Benowitz, N.L., Jacob, P., III. Metabolism of nicotine to cotinine studied by a dual stable isotope method. *Clinical Pharmacology and Therapeutics* 56(5):483-493, 1994.

Benowitz, N.L., Jacob, P., III, Denaro, C. and Jenkins, R. Stable isotope studies of nicotine kinetics and bioavailability. *Clinical Pharmacology and Therapeutics* 49(3):270-277, 1991.

Benowitz, N.L., Jacob, P., III, Fong, I. and Gupta, S. Nicotine metabolic profile in man: Comparison of cigarette smoking and transdermal nicotine. *The Journal of Pharmacology and Experimental Therapeutics* 268(1):296-303, 1994.

Benowitz, N.L., Jacob, P., III, Kozlowski, L. and Yu, L. Influence of smoking fewer cigarettes on exposure to tar, nicotine, and carbon monoxide exposure. *The New England Journal of Medicine* 315(21):1310-1313, 1986.

Benowitz, N.L., Jacob, P., III, Yu, L., Talcott, R., Hall, S. and Jones, R.T. Reduced tar, nicotine, and carbon monoxide exposure while smoking ultralow- but not low-yield cigarettes. *Journal of the American Medical Association* 256(2):241-246, 1986.

Benowitz, N.L., Zevin, S., Jacob, P., III. Suppression of nicotine intake during ad libitum cigarette smoking by high dose transdermal nicotine. *The Journal of Pharmacology and Experimental Therapeutics* 287(3):958-962, 1998.

Breese, C.R., Marks, M.J., Logel, J., Adams, C.E., Sullivan, B., Collins, A.C., Leonard, S. Effect of smoking history on [3H]nicotine binding in human postmortem brain. *The Journal of Pharmacology and Experimental Therapeutics* 282(1):7-13, 1997.

Byrd, G.D., Davis, R.A., Caldwell, W.S., Robinson, J.H., deBethizy, J.D. A further study of FTC yield and nicotine absorption in smokers. *Psychopharmacology (Berl)* 13(4):291-299, 1998.

Byrd, G.D., Robinson, J.H., Caldwell, W.S., deBethizy, J.D. Comparison of measured and FTC—Predicted nicotine uptake in smokers. *Psychopharmacology (Berl)* 122(2):95-103, 1995.

Collins, A.C., Luo, Y., Selvaag, S., Marks, M.J. Sensitivity to nicotine and brain nicotinic receptors are altered by chronic nicotine and mecamylamine infusion. *The Journal of Pharmacology and Experimental Therapeutics* 271(1):125-133, 1994.

Coultas, D.B., Stidley, C.A., Samet, J.M. Cigarette yields of tar and nicotine and markers of exposure to tobacco smoke. *American Review of Respiratory Disease* 148(2):435-440, 1993.

Ebert, R.V., McNabb, M.E., McCusker, K.T., Snow, S.L. Amount of nicotine and carbon monoxide inhaled by smokers of low-tar, low-nicotine cigarettes. *Journal of the American Medical Association* 250(20):2840-2842, 1983.

Feyerabend, C., Ings, R.M.J. and Russell, M.A.H. Nicotine pharmacokinetics and its application to intake from smoking. *British Journal of Clinical Pharmacology* 19(2):239-247, 1985.

Florin, I., Rutberg, L., Curvall, M., Enzell, C.R. Screening of tobacco smoke constituents for mutagenicity using the Ames' test. *Toxicology* 15(3):219-232, 1980.

Frost, C., Fullerton, F.M., Stephen, A.M., Stone, R., Nicolaides-Bouman, A., Densem, J., Wald, N.J., Semmence, A. The tar reduction study: Randomised trial of the effect of cigarette tar yield reduction on compensatory smoking. *Thorax* 50(10):1038-1043, 1995.

Gori, G.B., Lynch, C.J. Smoker intake from cigarettes in the 1-mg Federal Trade Commission tar class. *Regulatory Toxicology and Pharmacology* 3(2):110-120, 1983.

Gori, G.B., Lynch, C.J. Analytical cigarette yields as predictors of smoke bioavailability. *Regulatory Toxicology and Pharmacology* 5(3):314-326, 1985.

Guyatt, A.R., Kirkham, A.J.T., Mariner, D.C., Baldry, A.G., Cumming, G. Long–term effects of switching to cigarettes with lower tar and nicotine yields. *Psychopharmacology (Berl)* 99(1):80-86, 1989.

Hecht, S.S. Biochemistry, biology, and carcinogenicity of tobacco-specific N-nitrosoamines. *Chemical Research in Toxicology* 11(6):559-603, 1998.

Hecht, S.S., Carmella, S.G., Murphy, S.E., Akerkar, S., Brunneman, K.D. and Hoffmann, D. A tobacco-specific lung carcinogen in the urine of men exposed to cigarette smoke. *The New England Journal of Medicine* 329(21):1543-1546, 1993.

Hee, J., Callais, F., Momas, I., Laurent, A.M., Min, S., Molinier, P., Chastagnier, M., Claude, J.R., Festy, B. Smokers' behaviour and exposure according to cigarette yield and smoking experience. *Pharmacology, Biochemistry, and Behavior* 52(1):195-203, 1995.

Jaffe, J.H., Kanzler, M., Friedman, L., Stunkard, A.J., Vereby, K. Carbon monoxide and thiocyanate levels in low tar/nicotine smokers. *Addictive Behaviors* 6:337-343, 1981.

Jahnke, G.D., Thompson, C.L., Walker, M.P., Gallagher, J.E., Lucier, G.W., DiAugustine, R.P. Multiple DNA adducts in lymphocytes of smokers and nonsmokers determined by 32P-postlabeling analysis. *Carcinogenesis* 11(2):205-211, 1990.

Jarvis, M.J., Borham, R., Primatesta, P., Feyerabend, C., Bryant, A. Nicotine yield from machine-smoked cigarettes and nicotine intakes in smokers: Evidence from a representative population survey. *Journal of the National Cancer Institute* 93(2):134-138, 2001.

Lynch, C.J., Benowitz, N.L. Spontaneous brand switching: Consequences for nicotine and carbon monoxide exposure. *American Journal of Public Health* 77(9):1191-1194, 1987.

Maron, D.J., Fortmann, S.P. Nicotine yield and measures of cigarette smoke exposure in a large population: are lower-yield cigarettes safer? *American Journal of Public Health* 77(5):546-549, 1987.

Mooney, L.A., Santella, R.M., Covey, L., Jeffrey, A.M., Bigbee, W., Randall, M.C., Cooper, T.B., Ottman, R., Tsai, W.-Y., Wazneh, L., *et al.* Decline of DNA damage and other biomarkers in peripheral blood following smoking cessation. *Cancer Epidemiology, Biomarkers & Prevention* 4(6):627-634, 1995.

Peach, H., Ellard, G.A., Jenner, P.J., Morris, R.W. A simple, inexpensive urine test of smoking. *Thorax* 40(5):351-357, 1985.

Peach, H., Hayward, D.M., Ellard, D.R., Morris, R.W., Shah, D. Phlegm production and lung function among cigarette smokers changing tar groups during the 1970s. *Journal of Epidemiology and Community Health* 40(2):110-116, 1986a.

Peach, H., Hayward, D.M., Shah, D. A double-blind randomized controlled trial of the effect of a low- versus a middle-tar cigarette on respiratory symptoms—A feasibility study. *IARC Scientific Publications* 74:251-263, 1986b.

Picciotto, M.R., Caldarone, B.J., King, S.L., Zachariou, V. Nicotinic receptors in the brain. Links between molecular biology and behavior. *Neuropsychopharmacology* 22(2):451-465, 2000.

Rickert, W.S., Robinson, J.C. Estimating the hazards of less hazardous cigarettes. II. Study of cigarette yields of nicotine, carbon monoxide and hydrogen cyanide in relation to levels of cotinine, carboxyhemoglobin, and thiocyanate in smokers. *Journal of Toxicology and Environmental Health* 7(3-4):391-403, 1981.

Rickert, W.S., Robinson, J.C., Young, J.C., Collishaw, N.E., Bray, D.F. A comparison of the yields of tar, nicotine, and carbon monoxide of 36 brands of Canadian cigarettes tested under three conditions. *Preventive Medicine* 12(5):682-694, 1983.

Robinson, J.C., Young, J.C., Rickert, W.S., Fey, G., Kozlowski, L.T. A comparative study of the amount of smoke absorbed from low yield ('less hazardous') cigarettes. Part 2: Invasive measures. *British Journal of Addiction* 78(1):79-87, 1983.

Rosa, M., Pacifici, R., Altieri, I., Pichini, S., Ottaviani, G., Zuccaro, P. How the steady-state cotinine concentration in cigarette smokers is directly related to nicotine intake. *Clinical Pharmacology and Therapeutics* 52(3):324-329, 1992.

Russell, M.A., Wilson, C., Patel, U.A., Feyerabend, C., Cole, P.V. Plasma nicotine levels after smoking cigarettes with high, medium, and low nicotine yields. *British Medical Journal* 2(5968):414-416, 1975.

Russell, M.A., Jarvis, M., Iyer, R., Feyerabend, C. Relation of nicotine yield of cigarettes to blood nicotine concentrations in smokers. *British Medical Journal* 280(6219):972-976, 1980.

Russell, M.A., Jarvis, M.J., Feyerabend, C., Saloojee, Y. Reduction of tar, nicotine and carbon monoxide intake in low tar smokers. *Journal of Epidemiology and Community Health* 40(1):80-85, 1986.

Russell, M.A.H., Sutton, S.R., Iyer, R., Feyerabend, C., Vesey, C.J. Long–term switching to low–tar low–nicotine cigarettes. *British Journal of Addiction* 77(2):145-158, 1982.

Sorsa, M., Falck, K., Heinonen, T., Vainio, H., Norppa, H. and Rimpela, M. Detection of exposure to mutagenic compounds in low-tar and medium-tar cigarette smokers. *Environmental Research* 33(2):312-321, 1984.

Sutton, S.R., Russell, M.A., Iyer, R., Feyerabend, C., Saloojee, Y. Relationship between cigarette yields, puffing patterns, and smoke intake: Evidence for tar compensation? *British Medical Journal (Clin Res Ed)* 285(6342):600-603, 1982.

U.S. Department of Health and Human Services, Public Health Service. *The Health Consequences of Smoking—Nicotine Addiction: A Report of the Surgeon General.* U.S. Department of Health and Human Services, Public Health Service, Centers for Health Promotion and Education, Office on Smoking and Health. DHHS Publication No. 88-8406, 1988.

van Maanen, J.M.S., Maas, L.M., Hageman, G., Kleinjans, J.C.S., van Agen, B. DNA adduct and mutation analysis in white blood cells of smokers and nonsmokers. *Environmental and Molecular Mutagenesis* 24(1):46-50, 1994.

Wald, N.J., Boreham, J., Bailey, A. Relative intakes of tar, nicotine, and carbon monoxide from cigarettes of different yields. *Thorax* 39(5):361-364, 1984.

West, R.J., Russell, M.A., Jarvis, M.J., Feyerabend, C. Does switching to an ultra-low nicotine cigarette induce nicotine withdrawal effects? *Psychopharmacology (Berl)* 84(1):120-123, 1984.

Woodward, M., Tunstall-Pedoe, H. Do smokers of lower tar cigarettes consume lower amounts of smoke components? Results from the Scottish Heart Health Study. *British Journal of Addiction* 87(6):921-928, 1992.

Woodward, M., Tunstall–Pedoe, H. Self-titration of nicotine: evidence from the Scottish Heart Health Study. *Addiction* 88(6):821-830, 1993.

Yamasaki, E., Ames, B.N. Concentration of mutagens from urine by adsorption with the nonpolar resin XAD-2: Cigarette smokers have mutagenic urine. *Proceedings of the National Academy of Sciences USA* 74(8):3555-3559, 1977.

Zacny, J.P., Stitzer, M.L. Cigarette brand switching: Effects on smoke exposure and smoking behavior. *The Journal of Pharmacology and Experimental Therapeutics* 246(2):619-627, 1988.

# Smoking Lower Yield Cigarettes and Disease Risks

David M. Burns, Jacqueline M. Major, Thomas G. Shanks,
Michael J. Thun, Jonathan M. Samet

**INTRODUCTION**    This chapter examines whether the disease risks of smoking
have changed as a result of the changes in cigarette design over the last 50
years. Cigarette design and manufacture have changed substantially over
the last half century, and the relationship of these changes to altered disease risks is an important scientific and public health issue. No cigarette
currently manufactured and sold can be considered safe, and the principal
recommendation for any smoker interested in reducing future disease risks
is to quit smoking. However, approximately 47 million individuals remain
cigarette smokers in the United States (CDC, 2000a), and many of these
smokers have tried to quit and failed. If these continuing cigarette smokers
could alter their risk by choosing cigarettes that differ in machine-measured
tar and nicotine yields or other characteristics, and if this choice did not
interfere with their likelihood of cessation, then advice to switch brands
might be one component of a comprehensive strategy to reduce the disease
consequences of tobacco use. Alternatively, if these lower yield products do
not reduce risks and if smokers switch brands instead of quitting, then the
changes in cigarettes and their marketing as reduced-risk products represent
a cruel deception of current smokers. For those smokers who delay cessation, the increased duration of smoking that results from delayed cessation
is likely to be a more powerful determinant of disease risk than a small, or
nonexistent, reduction in tar exposure from use of these cigarettes.

Prior reviews (U.S. DHHS, 1981; NCI, 1996) of changes in disease risk
with switching from unfiltered or higher yield to filtered or lower yield cigarettes concluded that switching probably reduced lung cancer risk somewhat, but only if smokers did not increase the number of cigarettes that
they smoked per day when they switched to lower yield cigarettes. Ninety-
seven percent of the cigarettes sold in the United States currently have filters and the sales-weighted tar yield of cigarettes has declined by more than
60 percent since the 1950s.

Assessing the consequences of changes in cigarette design and manufacturing is made difficult by the lengthy time period over which these
changes have been made, the difficulty of tracking changes in smoking
behavior over time, and the lack of validity of the FTC yield data as indica-
tors of doses of toxic compounds of cigarette smoke. Nevertheless, epidemiological evidence has provided some insights concerning the consequences
of changes in cigarettes over the last fifty years. The data have three
sources: (1) observations of national rates of lung cancer by age in relation
to age-specific smoking patterns; (2) case-control and cohort studies that
have compared lung cancer risks in smokers of different types of products
at particular points and times; and (3) comparisons of lung cancer in smok-

ers over time, coming from either a single cohort with lengthy follow-up (the British Physicians Study) or repeated cohort observations (the two CPS studies of the American Cancer Society).

Each of these sources of data has strengths and limitations when used to assess the effect of changes in cigarette design on disease risks. Changes in age-specific national lung cancer death rates over time measure the actual population burden of disease, and these rates must change if there has been any substantive benefit resulting from changes in cigarette design. They also offer the opportunity to examine change in disease rates over periods of time long enough to allow full expression of the cumulative effects of all of the changes in cigarette design, which have also occurred over multiple decades. One major limitation of these data is the absence of information on smoking status and type of cigarette smoked in national death registry data. This absence requires comparison of the lung cancer death rate data with information derived from population surveys on smoking behavior and market data on type of cigarette sold. It limits the examination of these data sets to ecological analyses and comparisons of trends over time in population measures of smoking behaviors and disease rates.

Epidemiological studies have the strength of being able to collect detailed information on smoking behaviors, type of cigarette smoked and other variables of interest that allow differences in these factors to be examined in detail, and controlled, in the analysis of disease risk. However, these studies are limited by confining their observations to relatively short slices of time or fixed cohorts of individuals. The cross-sectional nature of case-control studies requires extrapolation from differences observed across individuals who smoke different types of cigarettes at one slice of time, with the presumption that those cross-sectional differences in type of cigarette smoked reflect the longitudinal changes in cigarette design that preceded them. For example, the difference in dose of smoke received by a filter cigarette smoker compared to a non-filter cigarette smoker in 1980 may or may not correspond to the differences in smoke dose received by smokers in the 1950s (almost entirely non-filtered cigarette smokers) compared to the dose of smoke received by filtered cigarette smokers in the 1980s. A more important limitation of these studies of changing cigarette design is the possibility that the characteristic of the cigarette being studied (machine-measured yield) may directly influence smoking behavior, including the number of cigarettes smoked per day. This linkage between the characteristic being studied and the measures used to control for differences between populations of smokers in the dose of smoke received makes control for intensity of smoking problematic. In addition, the reasons for choosing the brand smoked may be linked to other demographic or behavioral characteristics which may also influence disease outcome (level of addiction, interest in cutting down or quitting, differences in other health related behaviors, etc.).

Examination of cohorts with long durations of follow-up (the British Physicians Study), or comparing similar cohorts separated by a long interval (the two CPS studies of the American Cancer Society), offer the strengths of long periods of observation and the availability of individual level data on smoking behaviors and other characteristics. Limitations of following a single cohort for long periods of follow-up include the fact that the cohort becomes less and less representative of the entire population over time; and, in particular, it is limited in its ability to examine the effects of changing cigarette design on smokers who initiate with those products rather than switch to them. Comparison of similar cohorts separated by more than 20 years allows inclusion of younger generations of smokers, but is limited by the possibility that the smokers in the two cohorts are likely to be of different composition in demographic characteristics and may differ in other characteristics as well. These differences may occur because the later cohort of smokers from the 1980s is composed of those who have been unable or unwilling to quit smoking; and therefore, it may not be directly comparable to the earlier cohort from the 1960s when the percentage of former smokers was lower.

Each of these sources of epidemiological data can expand our understanding of the disease burden that results from changing cigarette design, and together they complement each other to counter the limitations present when any one data source is examined in isolation. The question addressed in this chapter is whether cigarette smoking in the year 2000, with all of the changes in cigarette design and all of the compensatory changes in smoking behavior, is more or less hazardous than it was in 1950. The disease consequences of changes in cigarette design and the consequences of switching type of cigarette smoked can be approached from two perspectives. First, has the risk of disease per cigarette smoked changed; and second, has the risk of disease for smokers compared to nonsmokers changed. From the public health perspective, the latter is the more relevant question.

The body of existing published literature was examined to answer this question, and new analyses of data sets from the American Cancer Society and the California Tobacco Survey are provided to explore and clarify the differences between epidemiological evaluations and the national trends in lung cancer death rates.

The chapter begins with a discussion of the historical development of cigarettes that have produced ever lower machine-measured tar and nicotine yields using the Federal Trade Commission (FTC) protocol[1] (Pillsbury, 1996). It then discusses the complexity of epidemiological examination of the self-selected behavior of smoking lower yield cigarettes and outlines the potential sources of confounding likely to occur in epidemiological studies. Next, various epidemiological studies that have assessed the risks of low-yield cigarettes in relation to lung cancer and cardiovascular and chronic respiratory diseases are examined. The chapter considers the evidence on compensatory smoking, those changes in smoking behavior that allow smokers to maintain their customary nicotine intake when they switch to a cigarette with a lower machine-measured nicotine yield. It discusses two

---

[1]    The machine smokes the cigarette with 2-second, 35-ml puffs and a 58-second inter-puff interval until a 23-mm butt length or 3 mm from the filter overwrap is reached.

new epidemiological analyses that find higher daily cigarette consumption among smokers of lower yield cigarettes. Finally, the chapter considers cohort- and population-based studies that have examined temporal trends in lung cancer incidence or mortality in relation to changes in cigarette design and/or smoking behavior.

Greater weight was placed on evidence derived from trends in populations over time than on evidence from cross-sectional epidemiological studies since reductions in general population death rates are the ultimate outcome measure for the effect of changing cigarette design over the last 50 years. If the changes in cigarette design are of public health significance, they must impact the rates of disease actually occurring in the population of smokers who use these cigarettes. The true effect of changing cigarette design requires integration of the information from epidemiological studies and the population trends in disease rates. If a substantive reduction in disease risk is expected from the epidemiological studies, it should be evident as a change in population disease rates. If the effect is not evident in the population data, then one should reconsider the potential for self-selection and compensatory smoking to bias the epidemiological results or confuse their interpretation.

While the emphasis in the discussion and analyses presented in this chapter is on the tar and nicotine yields measured by the FTC protocol, the question being asked is really whether all of the changes in cigarette design and manufacture over the last half century have altered the disease risks of smoking cigarettes. Part of this focus on FTC yields comes from their use, appropriately, as exposure variables in epidemiological studies. Machine-made measurements of tar and nicotine are used in the discussion simply as convenient surrogates for the cumulative effect of all of the changes that have occurred. Arguments can be made to support differences in risk that might result from individual engineering changes in cigarette manufacturing using evidence based on changes in tobacco smoke chemistry or biological exposure studies, but ultimately, the issue of concern is the net effect of these cigarette design changes on the total disease burden in human smokers as the cigarettes are smoked by the general public. This chapter is focused on answering the question: "Have changes in cigarette manufacture and design over the last 50 years resulted in a meaningful public health benefit to human smokers?" This overall question has two related but distinct research questions. First, has the risk per cigarette smoked been changed by these product modifications; and second have the net adverse consequences of smoking for the population been changed by these product modifications.

Other chapters in this volume describe the marketing and behavioral issues of cigarettes with low machine-measured yields.

**HISTORICAL DEVELOPMENT OF THE LOWER YIELD CIGARETTE ISSUE** Cigarette smoking was definitively linked to increased lung cancer risk in the 1950s (Wynder and Graham, 1950; Doll and Hill, 1952, 1954; Hammond and Horn, 1958). It was almost simultaneously discovered that painting cigarette smoke condensate on the skin of animals produced tumors (Wynder *et al.*, 1953). A logical extrapolation of these observations was that reducing exposure of smokers to the total particulate matter in cigarette smoke should reduce the risk of developing lung cancer. Independent scientists and public health authorities recommended that cigarettes which reduced tobacco smoke delivery to the smoker be developed and marketed by tobacco companies (U.S. Congress, 1967). The tobacco industry initially responded by adding filters to cigarettes and then by offering cigarettes that delivered less tar (the total particulate matter in smoke minus the water and nicotine) in measurements made by machine smoking of cigarettes using a fixed pattern of smoking (U.S. DHHS, 1981; NCI, 1996; Warner, 1985). A variety of approaches to tar reduction were utilized, including 'puffing' the tobacco to reduce the weight of tobacco in a cigarette, altering the blends of tobacco used and porosity of the paper wrapper, changing the density of the tobacco rod, using tobacco stems and reconstituted tobacco sheet, and using a wide variety of filter materials. These changes are detailed more completely in Chapters 2 and 5. Ultimately, this effort to reduce machine-measured tar yields led to the introduction of cigarettes with ventilation holes around the filter. These ventilated filters reduced the tar measured by machine using the FTC method by diluting the smoke with entrained air. Ventilation is the principal method by which the very low levels of machine-measured tar yields of most current light and ultralight cigarettes are produced (see Chapter 2).

Both the smoke exposure and the disease risks resulting from smoking lower yield cigarettes depend on how these cigarettes are used by smokers. Machine-measured yields are only informative for the smoker to the extent that they reflect the smoker's exposure and disease risk either directly or in relation to other brands of cigarettes. Internal tobacco industry documents from the 1960s and 1970s, when filtered and lower yield cigarettes were first heavily marketed to assuage health concerns of smokers, recognized that these changes in cigarette design might not actually result in delivery of less tar to smokers. Since smokers were smoking to derive a sufficient dose of nicotine, they could compensate for reductions in nicotine delivery by changing the way that they smoked these cigarettes in order to preserve their nicotine intake. Tar yield is closely correlated with nicotine yield, and so compensation to preserve nicotine intake preserves tar intake as well.

A Philip Morris company memo (Wakeham, 1961) expressed concern about smokers' likely response to the new highly filtered cigarettes: "As we know, all too often the smoker who switches to a hi-fi cigarette winds up smoking more units in order to provide himself with the same delivery which he had before. In short, I don't believe the smoking pattern has changed much, even with the cancer scares and filter cigarettes."

A research planning memo by Claude Teague (Teague, 1972) was even more explicit: "Given a cigarette that delivers less nicotine than he desires, the smoker will subconsciously adjust his puff volume and frequency, and smoking frequency, so as to obtain and maintain his per hour and per day requirement for nicotine . . ." A Brown & Williamson Tobacco Company memo (Pepples, 1976) commented, "The new filter brands vying for a piece of the growing filter market made extraordinary claims . . . In most cases, however, the smoker of a filter cigarette was getting as much or more nicotine and tar as he would have gotten from a regular cigarette. He abandoned the regular cigarette, however, on the ground of reduced risk to health." Because tar is delivered in a relatively fixed ratio to nicotine for most conventional cigarettes (see Chapters 2 and 3), compensation to preserve nicotine intake would also preserve tar exposure, minimizing any reduction in a smoker's lung cancer risk from switching to these cigarettes. There has been a reduction in machine-measured tar-to-nicotine ratios in ultralow cigarettes when measured by the FTC method, but these same ratios in ultralow cigarettes increase when smoked under conditions that mimic those of human smokers (see Chapters 2 and 3).

The tobacco industry's response to health concerns about smoking raised by the public health community was to develop cigarettes with lower yields of tar and nicotine as measured by the FTC method. The reductions in tar were marketed as a surrogate for reductions in risk (see Chapter 7). There is no current evidence that the tobacco companies conducted any biological or animal testing to test this hypothesis of reduction in risk. Again, internal tobacco industry documents illuminated the goals and design directions taken by the industry in this effort. A report on a tobacco research conference (Green, 1968) noted, "Research staff should lay down guide lines against which alternative products can be chosen in everyday operations. Although there may, on occasions, be conflict between saleability and minimal biological activity, two types of products should be clearly distinguished, viz:

a) A Health-image (health reassurance) cigarette.

b) A Health-oriented (minimal biological activity) cigarette, to be kept on the market for those consumers choosing it."

Conversion of this line of thinking into cigarette design modifications was further specified in an undated British American Tobacco Company memo: "What would seem very much more sensible, is to produce a cigarette which can be machine smoked at a certain tar band, but which, in human hands, can exceed this tar banding . . ." (BATCO, undated). This concept is described as "elasticity of delivery," which has two definitions as used in this chapter and in tobacco industry documents. First, elasticity is used to describe the phenomenon of a smoker being able to derive markedly different amounts of tar and nicotine from a cigarette by changing the way that it is smoked. Inherent in this concept is the understanding that the elastic cigarette will provide whatever dose of nicotine the smoker wants if the smoker adjusts his or her pattern of smoking appropriately. A second, more technical definition was provided in an Imperial Tobacco of Canada document, which stated, "If the tar delivery increases in direct proportion to the increase in puff volume, the product is inelastic (*i.e.*, elasticity = 1), while if tar delivery increases faster than puff volume, elasticity > 1." (See Imperial Tobacco Limited, 1993.)

The importance of ventilation from perforated filters in achieving this elasticity was clarified by a 1982 Philip Morris memo that described tests on machine yields of cigarettes with ventilated filters when the holes in the filters were covered and uncovered, using different puff volumes to simulate smoker compensation (Goodman, 1982). The conclusion reached by Goodman stated, "The decrease in dilution from covering a portion of the perforated area can result in an increased delivery to the smoker of highly-diluted cigarettes even though the puff parameters decrease." Implications of the elasticity of delivery design for actual delivery to the smoker had been defined in a prior memo by the same individual (Goodman, 1975) that described a study which examined yields of Marlboro Light® and Marlboro 85® cigarettes when smoked by smokers who had been switched to these brands from their regular choice. The smoking puff profile for these smokers was recorded and then replicated to make measurements on a smoking machine. The conclusion reached by Goodman (1975) stated: "In effect, the Marlboro 85 smokers in this study did not achieve any reduction in smoke intake by smoking a cigarette (Marlboro Lights) normally considered lower in delivery."

These internal tobacco company documents suggest that the effort to develop low-yield cigarettes was conducted with a clear appreciation of the compensation to preserve nicotine intake that was likely to occur in smokers. Cigarettes were designed with elasticity of delivery in an effort to provide low machine yields, allowing marketing of the product as a "health-reassurance" cigarette while continuing to deliver high levels of nicotine to satisfy the addictive demands of the smokers of these cigarettes.

However, even though the impact of changes in cigarette design on actual smoke delivery to smokers was questionable, early studies of the disease risks among smokers of low-yield cigarettes were encouraging. They demonstrated a somewhat lower lung cancer risk among populations of individuals who used filtered and low-yield products, albeit a much smaller reduction in lung cancer risk than the extent of reduction in machine-measured tar. These studies led to considerable optimism about the likely public health benefits of changes that had occurred in cigarette design (U.S. Congress, 1967; U.S. DHEW, 1971, 1979). The early data were particularly encouraging because the reductions in lung cancer risks were demonstrable in populations observed during the mid to late 1960s when filtered cigarettes had only been available for a short period of time (Bross, 1968; Bross and Gibson, 1968; Hammond *et al.*, 1976, 1977). Widespread use of filtered and lower yield products began in the mid 1950s. Since the reduction in excess lung cancer risk with cessation continues to increase for 15-20 years following cessation (U.S. DHHS, 1990; Burns *et al.*, 1997b), it was expected that these modest changes in risk demonstrable with short-term use of reduced-tar products would have a growing impact on lung cancer death rates as more smokers used these products for longer periods of time (Wynder and Stellman, 1979).

Over the last 50 years, machine-measured, sales-weighted tar yields for U.S. cigarettes have declined by over 60 percent. Several careful reviews of the available scientific data (U.S. DHHS, 1981; NCI, 1996) have suggested that there is a reduction in lung cancer risk for populations of smokers who use lower yield cigarettes if they did not increase the number of cigarettes that they smoked as they decreased the yield of the cigarette that they smoked. These reviews did not identify reductions in heart or lung disease risks associated with reductions in tar and nicotine yield of the cigarette smoked. The lung cancer risk reductions offered the promise of a substantial reduction in U.S. lung cancer death rates.

A reduction in U.S. lung cancer death rates of the magnitude expected from the differences in risk found in epidemiological studies of lower yield cigarettes (15-40%) has not been realized. Lung cancer death rates have continued to rise among women, and the modest decline in lung cancer death rates observed among men is generally consistent with the temporal trends of reduced initiation and increased cessation among males. (Tolley *et al.*, 1991; Mannino *et al.*, 2001). In addition, two studies performed by the American Cancer Society 20 years apart (1960s vs. 1980s) have shown an increase in lung cancer risk among current smokers (Thun and Heath, 1997; Thun *et al.*, 1997a & b). In these studies, there was no evidence for any decline in lung cancer risk, even when the subjects were compared controlling for number of cigarettes smoked per day, duration of smoking, and age. This increase in lung cancer risk over time was confirmed by the results of the British Physicians Study (Doll *et al.*, 1994) which demonstrated an increase in lung cancer risk among continuing cigarette smokers during the last 20 years of the 40 years of follow-up (1951-1991) when compared to the first 20 years of follow-up, despite a substantial fall in machine-measured tar yield of British cigarettes over this same period.

The discrepancies between epidemiological studies demonstrating reductions in risk with the use of low-yield and filtered cigarettes and the absence of population-based reductions in the hazards of smoking led to a reexamination of the question: Does the use of lower yield cigarettes result in meaningful reductions in disease risks compared to use of higher yield cigarettes? The authors integrated what is known from published epidemiological studies of smokers of low-yield cigarettes with what is known about compensatory smoking behavior and the characteristics that lead smokers to choose low-yield products. In addition, a series of new analyses are presented in an effort to resolve the apparent differences between published epidemiological evaluations and the mortality experience in the United States.

## LIMITATIONS OF EPIDEMIOLOGICAL STUDIES IN EXAMINING THE RISKS OF LOW-YIELD CIGARETTE USE

Examination of changes in disease risks that result from changes in cigarette design raises a set of formidable challenges in human epidemiological studies. These changes come from the temporally dynamic nature of smoking over the last fifty years. The changes include changes in the product, changes in the age of smoking initiation, and changes in cessation. Related methodological challenges stem from the changing demographic distribution of tobacco use; the relationship of duration of smoking and age to disease risks; the cross-sectional slice of the population experience that is inherent in either retrospective or prospective epidemiological evaluations; the complexity and wide variety of changes that have occurred in cigarette design over the last 50 years; the changes in measures of smoking intensity that result from switching to lower yield cigarettes; the linkage between reasons for choosing lower yield cigarette brands and other behaviors intended to reduce risks (including cessation); and the limited availability of information on what changes were made to which cigarettes, over what periods of time, and their potential impacts on smoking behaviors. The tools used by epidemiologists for approaching these challenges are rather blunt; obtaining smoking histories that cover products smoked, age started smoking, and number of cigarettes smoked per day. FTC yield measurements have been used in some studies as a surrogate for changes in exposure, in spite of the well-recognized limitations of its use for this purpose (see Chapters 2 and 3).

Cigarette smoking prevalence varies with age, gender, education, race/ethnicity, and most other demographic characteristics relevant to population risks (U.S. DHHS, 1998). The distribution of smoking prevalence within demographic characteristic has also varied with calendar year over the last 50-100 years in ways that influence current differences in disease rates (Burns *et al.*, 1997a & b; Thun *et al.*, 1997b). For example, women first began to smoke in large numbers in the late 1930s and 1940s, but during those years, women initiated smoking across a wide age range (Burns *et al.*, 1997a). As a result, female smokers who are currently old enough to have high risks of lung cancer have, on average, shorter durations of smoking than males of the same age. This difference explains much of the male/female differences in U.S. lung cancer mortality rates (Mannino *et al.*, 2001). Demographic and temporal variation in smoking behaviors is also evident in patterns of smoking cessation (Burns *et al.*, 1997a).

Superimposed on this complex variation in smoking behaviors are an equally complex demographic and temporal variations in use of filtered and lower yield cigarettes, and these patterns do not always parallel those of smoking prevalence. For example, current survey data show that smoking prevalence declines with age among adults, but use of low-yield cigarette increases with age. In addition, older females, who have lower rates of smoking prevalence than their age-matched male contemporaries, are more likely to have used filtered and lower yield cigarettes and to have used them for much more of their smoking histories.

Some of these differences would be less important if smoking caused disease instantaneously, or if recent smoking was the principal determinant of disease risk. However, most diseases caused by smoking are the result of long periods of cumulative damage to the smoker and are heavily influenced by smoking that occurred 10, 20, or even 30 years or more in the past. Traditional measures of smoking intensity, such as number of cigarettes smoked per day, are recorded at entry into an epidemiological study. They have been useful approximations of lifetime smoking intensity in these studies because of the relative stability of this measure in smokers over their smoking lifetime. The same stability cannot be assumed when the smoker switches to a new type of cigarette, particularly when that new cigarette delivers less nicotine than the smoker is trying to obtain by smoking. What is often measured in epidemiological studies is the number of cigarettes currently smoked with the current type of cigarette. If the type of cigarette influences the number of cigarettes, then the current number of cigarettes smoked per day is not necessarily a valid measure of intensity of smoking in the past with other types of cigarettes. Similarly, it is also not a valid measure when comparing current smoking intensities among individuals who smoke different types of cigarettes. Thus, one of the most common measures used to control for smoking intensity in epidemiological studies may be linked to, and perhaps partly determined by, the characteristics of the cigarette that the epidemiological study is attempting to examine.

Epidemiological studies examine events during follow-up over defined slices of time in fixed populations. From these data, investigators attempt to separate the effects related to age, intensity and duration of smoking from differences in cigarette design on disease risks produced by smoking. Even prospective epidemiological studies start with a fixed population defined at a fixed point in time and follow that population forward in time. These populations define a temporally specific set of smoking experiences with a specific set of cigarette products, and these limitations restrict the range of product changes that can be observed. In other words, any study addresses only a specific time period and the products used by the smokers observed in the study. The generalizability of the findings to other time periods and other products is uncertain.

Extrapolating effects beyond the range for which one has observations is always problematic. Generalizability is a particular problem in examining changing cigarette designs because many design changes occurred simultaneously, and some of them may have influenced cigarette yields in ways that are contrary to that expected by investigators. For example, some of the filtered cigarettes introduced in the 1950s and 1960s actually had higher tar deliveries than their nonfiltered brands in the same brand family (see Chapter 7), making the use of filter cigarette smoking as a measure of lower tar exposure uncertain.

Smokers of low-yield cigarettes may differ from smokers of high-yield cigarettes in important characteristics other than the cigarette smoked. These differences need to be carefully considered in epidemiological studies in order to prevent these other characteristics from introducing confounding facts that may bias the results of these studies. If low-yield cigarette smokers have lower intensities of smoking, are more likely to quit smoking, or have other characteristics that lower their disease risks, then differences in disease risks demonstrated between populations of high- and low-yield cigarette smokers may not be due to the differences in the cigarette that they smoke. These differences can be considered as confounding, as they relate to differences between high- and low-yield cigarette smokers reflecting the differences between those selecting and not selecting the product.

The principal determinant of the chronic disease risks associated with smoking is the amount of tobacco smoke to which an individual is exposed as measured by the intensity and duration of smoking. Smoking intensity is correlated with nicotine levels in the blood (Benowitz *et al.*, 1983; Benowitz, 1996) and with the need to maintain those levels (U.S. DHHS, 1988). As discussed elsewhere in this monograph (see Chapters 2 and 3), clinical and pharmacological studies demonstrate that smokers who switch to cigarettes with low-nicotine yield modify their smoking behavior to maintain their accustomed nicotine intake. Compensatory behaviors may include: 1) taking more frequent puffs per cigarette; 2) taking larger puff volumes and inhaling more deeply; 3) obstructing the ventilation holes that would otherwise dilute the mainstream smoke; and 4) smoking more cigarettes per day. Thus, the FTC tar and nicotine ratings do not accurately reflect the exposure of an individual smoker to the carcinogens in tobacco smoke, as they do not take account of any of these compensatory behaviors.

The nicotine yield of the cigarette smoked may be a determinant of the measure of smoking intensity (number of cigarettes smoked per day) most commonly used as a control variable in epidemiological studies. If smokers who switch to lower yield cigarettes increase the number of cigarettes smoked per day to preserve a constant nicotine intake, then accounting for the number of cigarettes smoked per day in an analysis misrepresents the net consequences of changing cigarette type for dose of smoke exposure and risk. This widely employed strategy addresses the risk of different products conditional on the number of cigarettes smoked per day. For example, a smoker who smokes 10 high-nicotine cigarettes, and who switches to a low-nicotine variety, may compensate by smoking 20 low- nicotine cigarettes to maintain exactly the same level of nicotine intake. Measures of nicotine intake are good measures of total smoke dose; and, if smokers preserve the same nicotine intake, one would expect them to preserve their total smoke dose and disease risk as well. However, if the number of cigarettes smoked per day is used as a measure of smoke dose, then the smoker in this example would appear to have doubled his or her smoke dose on switching to the low-nicotine cigarette, when in reality the smoking intensity or total smoke dose had not changed at all.

## Comparing Populations of High- and Low-Yield Cigarette Smokers in Epidemiological Studies—Population Differences

Over the last several decades, there is substantial evidence showing that smokers of low yield cigarettes differ from smokers of high yield cigarettes. Some of these differences involve other risk factors for cigarette caused diseases, raising the possibility of confounding. Attribution of differences in risks between the populations to the less hazardous character of the cigarettes that they smoke requires examination of differences between these two populations of smokers in their use of cigarettes, extent of compensation, reasons for choosing these products, and other behaviors related to disease risks.

In the United States, the majority of adolescents begin smoking Marlboro®, Camel®, or Newport® cigarettes (CDC, 2000b), brands that are mid-range yield. Thus, it is brand shifting, and the decline in tar and nicotine yields of the same brands over time, rather than brand initiation that leads to the use of low machine-measured yield cigarettes among adults. Figure 4-1 presents data from the 1996 California Tobacco Survey for the fraction of adult smokers with different demographic characteristics who reported that the brand they smoke is low in tar and nicotine. Similar differences across type of cigarette smoked were evident in a national sample of smokers (Giovino *et al.*, 1996). The fraction of smokers reporting use of low-tar products increases dramatically with age, education, and income, and is higher among females than among males. These demographic differences might be expected from the marketing of these products as lower risk products.

Low-yield cigarettes have been marketed as delivering less tar, and this is commonly understood by smokers as resulting in less risk (see Chapters 6 and 7). It is, therefore, not surprising that a substantial fraction of those who switch from higher to lower yield cigarettes do so in an effort to reduce their disease risks (Cohen, 1996a & b; see Chapters 6 and 7). In addition, some smokers switch to these products hoping to quit or substantially reduce their smoking (Giovino *et al.*, 1996; see Chapters 6 and 7). Other smokers, after a failed cessation attempt, relapse to using low-yield products in an effort to mitigate the risk from resumption of smoking. Because of these health concerns, and an ongoing interest in cessation, these same low-yield cigarette smokers may also have higher rates of successful long-term smoking cessation or may voluntarily reduce the amount that they smoke for health reasons. Risk reductions that accompany cessation or lowered smoking intensity may appear to be related to the tar level of the cigarette smoked while actually resulting, at least in part, from other factors. Cohort studies following a population longitudinally for assessment of disease risk without repeated follow-up assessment of smoking status may be particularly vulnerable to this bias.

Hammond (1980) examined the American Cancer Society's first Cancer Prevention Study (CPS-I) data to look for this association between use of low-yield cigarettes and smoking cessation. Smokers of low-tar (17.6 mg or less) cigarettes midway through the study in 1965 were more likely to be former smokers than medium- or high-tar cigarette smokers at the last follow-up in 1972.

The higher educational and socioeconomic status of low-yield cigarette smokers are likely to be correlated with other positive health behaviors (diet, exercise, etc.) that may lower disease risks for reasons independent of choice of cigarette type. Giovino and colleagues (1996) showed that smokers of low-yield products have higher levels of formal education than persons who smoke higher yield products. Haddock and associates (1999) found that Air Force recruits who had switched in the previous year to lower tar and nicotine brands in order to reduce their health risks were also more likely to have more nutritious diets.

The rising level of health concerns that occur in middle age may lead individuals to a variety of changes in their behavior that are intended to improve their health, including smoking cessation. It would not be surprising to learn that these same individuals, should they relapse to smoking following a cessation attempt that is part of their efforts to change future disease risks, are more likely to smoke lower yield cigarettes. Any successful change in their diet, level of exercise, reductions in alcohol or tobacco, as well as the reductions in disease risks that result from these changes, would be linked to the use of lower yield cigarettes.

Figure 4-1
**Percentage of Smokers Over Age 18 Reporting That Their Brand is Low in Tar and Nicotine, 1996 California Tobacco Survey**

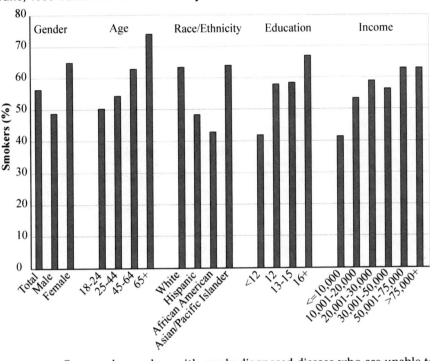

Conversely, smokers with newly diagnosed disease who are unable to quit may switch to low-yield cigarettes in the belief that there is less risk associated with their use. This would have the effect of increasing disease rates in populations of low-yield cigarette smokers.

It is also possible that less-intense and less-addicted smokers may either use, or be more likely to successfully switch to, low-yield cigarettes. Their demand for nicotine is less, and it may be more easily satisfied by cigarettes that deliver less nicotine. In contrast, heavy smokers and those who are strongly dependent may not be able to extract sufficient nicotine from these lower yield products to satisfy their addiction, so they may preferentially choose higher yield cigarettes.

These differential characteristics of smokers of different types of cigarettes may affect case-control and cohort studies in different ways. In case-control studies of lung cancer, filter or lower yield cigarette smokers are likely to be better educated, have higher incomes, and have better dietary habits than will unfiltered or higher tar cigarette smokers. The former may also be more likely to be less-intense and less-dependent smokers than the latter. These characteristics may influence the rates of lung cancer occurrence independent of any effect of cigarette type smoked; but unless they are carefully controlled in the analysis, they may bias toward finding a lower lung cancer risk among filtered or lower yield cigarette smokers.

Prospective cohort studies of lung cancer risk in relation to the type of cigarette smoked follow smokers forward in time to observe lung cancer risks. If lower yield cigarette smokers are more likely to quit successfully or adopt other healthy behaviors, and subjects are not tracked repetitively during the follow-up period, then trends toward lower risk smoking behaviors, cessation and other healthy behaviors may occur with a higher frequency in the lower yield cigarette group. A reduced rate of disease in lower yield cigarette smokers may be due to changes in their risk-related behaviors after the initial entry into the study, rather than to the type of cigarette they smoked. Many cohort studies have followed populations for a decade or more, sufficient time for differences to arise in characteristics of smokers of different types of cigarettes.

**Using Number of Cigarette Per Day to Control for Intensity of Smoking in Epidemiological Studies**

The principal method utilized to control for differences in the intensity of smoking among different populations of smokers is to use the number of cigarettes smoked per day as a measure of smoking intensity or dose of smoke received. The validity of this approach is supported by the demonstration of higher blood levels of cotinine (the major metabolite of nicotine) among smokers of larger numbers of cigarettes per day (Jarvis *et al.*, 2001; Benowitz *et al.*, 1983). Current understanding of the compensatory changes in smoking behavior that occur with the use of low yield cigarettes suggests that the bulk of compensation occurs by adjusting the topography of smoking for each individual cigarette (see Chapters 2 and 3). Smokers take larger puffs, inhale more deeply, and change their smoking pattern in other ways to extract the same amount of nicotine from cigarettes with vastly different nicotine yields by the FTC method. Smokers may also compensate by increasing the number of cigarettes smoked per day when they switch to low yield cigarettes.

Many published epidemiological studies of low-yield cigarettes have adjusted for the number of cigarettes smoked per day because it is the most readily available quantitative measure of smoke dose. It is possible for smokers who switch to lower yield cigarettes to fully preserve the daily dose of nicotine and smoke they receive from smoking (see Chapters 2 and 3). The preservation of a constant daily dose of smoke when shifting to a cigarette with a lower machine-measured yield may occur through changes in the way the cigarette is smoked, through an increase in number of cigarettes smoked per day, or through a combination of both methods. A smoker who fully compensates, and who increases the number of cigarettes smoked per day when he or she switches to a lower yield cigarette to achieve that compensation, will receive the same daily dose of smoke exposure with high and low yield cigarette smoking; but they will report different numbers of cigarettes smoked per day when smoking high and low yield cigarettes for that same daily dose of smoke. If cigarettes smoked per day is used in an epidemiological study to estimate the biologic dose of toxin or carcinogen that this smoker is receiving, then it will appear that the dose increased when the smoker switched to lower yield cigarettes; and the true dose of smoke exposure will be overestimated when smoking lower yield cigarettes as compared to higher yield cigarettes. If a substantial frac-

Figure 4-2
**Effect of Increasing the Number of Cigarettes Smoked per Day When Switching to Low-Yield Cigarettes on the Measurement of Relative Risk in Epidemiological Studies Which Control for Number of Cigarettes Smoked per Day**

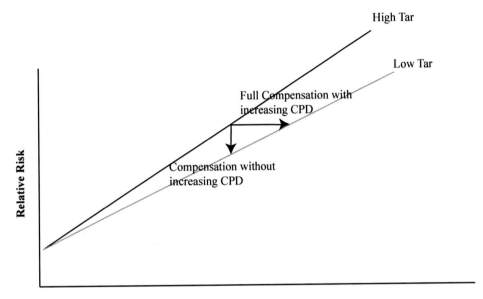

**Number of Cigarettes Smoked per Day**

*Source: Hypothetical.*

tion of lower yield cigarette smokers are compensating by increasing the number of cigarettes smoked per day, then epidemiological studies which use CPD to control for differences in daily dose will overestimate the dose received by lower yield cigarette smokers relative to higher yield cigarette smokers. This overestimation, if present, will bias the risk estimates in favor of finding lower risks among lower yield cigarette smokers when high and low yield cigarette smokers are compared in analyses that use CPD to control for daily dose of smoke received by smokers. Even slight compensation through increasing CPD can substantially bias the risk estimate.

This potential interaction between number of cigarettes smoked per day and type of cigarette smoked is illustrated in Figure 4-2 which presents theoretical relationships between disease relative risks and increasing number of cigarettes smoked per day for high and low yield cigarettes. In theory, a smoker who compensates fully could do so by either exclusively changing the pattern of smoking or by increasing the number of cigarettes smoked per day as part of that compensation. If a smoker compensates entirely by changing the pattern of smoking and does not increase the number of cigarettes smoked per day, the smoker will drop vertically from the high tar line to the low tar line. If the level of compensation is only partial, this smoker would experience a reduction in the daily smoke dose received, and one would expect a population of smokers who had this form of partial com-

79

pensation to have lower lung cancer rates. Their lung cancer risk in relation to CPD would generate a line similar to that presented as the low tar line in Figure 4-2, that is a lower risk at any given number of cigarettes smoked per day. However, if the compensation is complete, one would expect no reduction in daily dose of smoke or in lung cancer risk; and the line representing their lung cancer risk in relation to CPD would superimpose on that for high tar cigarette smokers.

However, a smoker of high-yield cigarettes may also increase the number of cigarettes smoked per day as part of the compensatory changes in smoking behavior that occur in order to preserve nicotine intake when he or she switches to low-yield cigarettes. This pattern of complete compensation is represented as a horizontal shift between the two lines in Figure 4-2; it combines the compensation that occurs due to changes in the pattern of smoking each individual cigarette with the compensation that occurs through increasing the number of cigarettes smoked per day. With complete compensation to preserve the same dose of toxic and carcinogenic intake in this pattern, no change in smoke intake or disease risk would occur; but when disease risk is plotted against number of cigarettes smoked per day, the disease risk lines would not superimpose. Instead, they would look like the two lines in Figure 4-2. The difference between these risk lines would correctly suggest that a difference in disease risk per cigarette smoked exists, when there is actually no change in disease risk for individual smokers resulting from switching to the lower yield brand of cigarettes due to the increase in number of cigarettes smoked.

Using the number of cigarettes smoked per day to control for the biological dose of smoke intake by the smoker can thus produce an artifactual difference in disease risk if the question being asked is whether risk declines when smokers switch to low yield cigarettes rather than if the risk per cigarette smoked declines. If compensatory changes include an increase in number of cigarettes smoked per day, analyses that control for intensity of smoking using CPD produce a risk estimate per cigarette smoked per day, when in reality what is needed is a risk estimate for the total smoking behavior of the smoker as he or she switches brands of cigarettes. The risk should be expressed per smoker rather than per cigarette. For example, a smoker of 20 high-tar cigarettes per day who switches to a low-tar product, and who increases his or her number of cigarettes smoked to 25 per day to fully preserve tar and nicotine intake, would also preserve the same disease risk. However, he or she would appear to have a risk on a per-cigarette-smoked basis that was 80 percent (20 divided by 25) of the risk of smoking high-tar cigarettes.

While it is possible to argue the legitimacy of expressing risk on a per-cigarette basis by suggesting that smokers should be educated not to increase the number of cigarettes smoked per day when they change brands, a public health benefit from use of low-yield cigarettes can only accrue if there is a difference in disease risks across individuals as they actually use these low-yield cigarettes. If a cigarette produces a 20-percent decrease in risk per cigarette, but its use by smokers results in 20 percent more cigarettes being smoked per day, the net result will likely be no change in disease risk for the individual or within the population.

The potential for smokers to increase the number of cigarettes that they smoke per day when they switch to lower yield cigarettes can complicate analyses of disease risks among smokers of different types of cigarettes in both case-control and prospective epidemiological evaluations. Data are presented later in this chapter to show that smokers who switched to low-yield cigarettes in the CPS-I study increased the number of cigarettes that they smoked per day, and that smokers of ultralow nicotine-yield cigarettes smoked more cigarettes per day in recent California Tobacco Surveys.

Even this limited discussion should make it apparent that epidemiological studies which simply compare the disease risks of high- and low-yield cigarette smokers must be interpreted with great caution when addressing the question of whether the cigarettes used are themselves the source of the differences in risks. Some of the published epidemiological studies have recognized this concern, and the studies cited in Tables 4-1 to 4-3 used a variety of design and statistical approaches to adjust for differences in age, duration of smoking, and intensity of smoking, as well as other characteristics of the populations.

In summary, a number of cautions are appropriate when examining epidemiological data on disease risks among those who smoke cigarettes with different machine-measured tar and nicotine yields. Comparisons of populations without controlling for differences in intensity of smoking likely to exist between high- and low-yield smokers can only define the populations as different, and these comparisons have limited ability to link the differences in risks observed to differences in the product used. However, control for intensity of smoking across populations using number of cigarettes smoked per day as the measure of dose may result in model misspecification if smokers who switch to low-yield cigarettes compensate by increasing the number of cigarettes that they smoke per day.

## PUBLISHED EPIDEMIOLOGICAL STUDIES OF HEALTH ENDPOINTS

### Lung Cancer

Tables 4-1 to 4-3 present epidemiological evaluations of smokers who used cigarettes with filters or different levels of machine-measured tar yield. An effort was made to include all of the published studies that evaluated individual smokers and presented numerical risks of disease associated with lower yield cigarettes. Studies were excluded if they used national consumption data as the measure of smoking, examined black versus blond tobacco, bidis, small cigars, hand-rolled cigarettes, cigarettes limited predominantly to other countries, clove cigarettes and other smoking products, Asian-Indian smoking behaviors, or other forms of tobacco use besides cigarettes.

Table 4-1 shows the studies that have examined lung cancer risks with low-yield products. While a few studies have not found a relationship, and several of the relationships identified were not statistically significant, the clear impression from these studies taken as a whole is that there is a lower risk of lung cancer among populations of smokers who use lower yield products. This relationship is evident in case-control studies as well as in prospective mortality studies (see Table 4-1). The vast majority of these studies controlled for intensity of smoking using the number of cigarettes

Table 4-1
**Epidemiological Studies of Low-Yield Cigarettes and Lung Cancer**

| Citation | Population | Time Period | Cigarette Type | Relative Risk | Comments |
|---|---|---|---|---|---|
| Bross, I.D., Gibson, R. Risks of lung cancer in smokers who switch to filter cigarettes. *Am. J. Public Health* 58(8):1396-1403, 1968. | Case-control study of 974 White male lung cancer patients and hospital controls. | 1960-1966 | Filter/Regular | 0.59 | Stratified by duration of smoking and number of cigarettes/day. Risk for regular is 6.48 and for filtered is 3.83. Filtered smokers were more likely to smoke more than one pack per day, 38% to 35%. Many had been smoking filtered cigarettes for leass than 3 years. |
| Bross, I.D. Effect of filter cigarettes on lung cancer risk. National Cancer Institute Monograph No. 28, *Toward a Less Harmful Cigarette.* U.S. DHEW, NCI, 1968. | Case-control study of 974 White male lung cancer patients and hospital controls. | 1960–1966 | Filter/ Regular | 0.59 | Stratified by duration of smoking and number of cigarettes/day. Risk for regular is 6.59 and for filtered is 3.9. Filtered cigarette smokers were more likely to smoke more than one pack per day, 38% to 35%. Many had been smoking filtered cigarettes for less than 3 years. |
| Hammond, E.C. *et al.* Some recent findings concerning cigarettes smoking. Cold Springs Harbor Conferences on Cell Proliferation, Volume 4. *Origins of Human Cancer,* Book A, *Incidence of Cancer in Humans.* pp. 101-112, 1977. | 12-year follow-up of CPS-I. A prospective mortality study of over 1 million men and women. | 1960-1972 | Tar yield | Male low-tar RR= 0.93 for 1960-1966, 0.82 for 1966-1972; female RR=0.81 for 1960-1966, 0.81 for 1966-1972. | |
| Hammond, E.C. *et al.* "Tar" and nicotine content of cigarette smoke in relation to death rates. *Environ. Res.* 12:263-274, 1976. | 12-year follow up of CPS-I. A prospective mortality study of over 1 million men and women. | 1960-1972 | Tar yield | Male low-tar RR= 0.93 for 1960-1966, 0.82 for 1966-1972; female RR=p.81 for 1960-1966, 0.81 for 1966-1973. | |

Table 4-1 (continued)

| Citation | Population | Time Period | Cigarette Type | Relative Risk | Comments |
|---|---|---|---|---|---|
| Lee, P.N., Garfinkel, L. Mortality and type of cigarette smoked. *J. of Epidemiol. Community Health* 35:16-22, 1981. | 12-year follow-up of CPS-I. A prospective mortality study of over 1 million men and women. | 1960-1972 | Tar yield; low/high | Male=0.82; female=0.60 | CHD risks are significantly different, but emphysema risks are not. |
| Higenbottam, T. *et al.* Cigarettes, lung cancer, and coronary heart disease: The effects of inhalation and tar yield. *J. Epidemiol. Community Health* 36:113-117, 1982. | 10-year follow-up of 17,475 male civil servants, aged 40-54, and a sample of male British residents. | 1965-1975 | Tar yield | There was a small nonsignificant difference in lung cancer mortality by tar yield that was more evident among noninhalers. | |
| Hawthorne, V.M., Fry, J.S. Smoking and health: The association between smoking behavior, total mortality, and cardiorespiratory disease in West Central Scotland. *J. Epidemiol. Community Health* 32:260-266, 1978. | Prospective follow-up of 18,786 people attending a multiphasic screening examination. | 1965-1977 | Filter/Regular | 0.83 | No significant difference in mortality rates for filter users for lung cancer or cardiovascular disease. Smokers of plain cigarettes had lower rates of respiratory symptoms than filter smokers. |
| Todd, G.F. *et al.* Four cardiorespiratory symptoms as predictors of mortality. *J. Epidemiol. Community Health* 32:267-274, 1978. | 12.4-year prospective follow-up of 10,063 subjects aged 35-69 from a random sample of the population in Great Britain. | 1965-1977 | Filter/Regular | 1.40 | The increase in lung cancer mortality with filter use was not statistically significant; there was a statistically significant decrease in all-cause mortality and male CHD mortality with filter use (standardized for number of cigarettes/day). |
| Engeland, A. *et al.* The impact of smoking habits on lung cancer risk: 28 years' observation of 26,000 | A prospective study of 26,126 Norwegian men and women drawn from a population sample. | 1966-1993 | Filter/Regular | Male=0.67; female=0.91 | Controlled for age, number of cigarettes/day, and age at initiation. |

83

Table 4-1 (continued)

| Citation | Population | Time Period | Cigarette Type | Relative Risk | Comments |
|---|---|---|---|---|---|
| Norwegian men and women. *Cancer Causes and Control* 7:366-376, 1996. | | | | | |
| Borland, C. *et al.* Carbon monoxide yield of cigarettes and its relation to cardiorespiratory disease. *BMJ* 287:1583-1586, 1983. | Prospective 10-year follow-up of the Whitehall study where 4,910 men had known CO yields of the cigarettes that they smoked. | 1967-1979 | CO yield | 0.67 | Controlled for age, grade of employment, cigarettes/day, and tar yield. Those who smoked high CO-yield cigarettes (>20 mg) tended to smoke fewer cigarettes/day. |
| Tang, J.L. *et al.* Mortality in relation to tar yield of cigarettes: a prospective study of four cohorts. *BMJ* 311:1530-1533, 1995. | Four prospective mortality studies from the United Kingdom. | 1967-1982 | Filter/Non-filter and tar level | Tar 0.94 (0.75-1.18) | Relative risks for all tobacco-related diseases combined were statistically significant. RR are adjusted for age, study, and number of cigarettes/day. |
| Wynder, E.L. *et al.* The epidemiology of lung cancer: recent trends. *JAMA* 213:2221-2228, 1970. | Case-control study of 350 lung cancer patients and approximately 700 hospital controls. | 1968-1969 | Filter for at least 10 years/Non-filter | | Decreased risk in smokers of filter cigarettes for 10 or more years controlled and stratified by number of cigarettes/day. |
| Wynder, E.L., Stellman, S.D. Impact of long-term filter cigarette usage on lung and larynx cancer risk: A case-control study. *JNCI* 62:471-477, 1979. | Case-control study of 684 lung cancer patients and 350 larynx cancer patients. | 1969-1976 | Filter for at least 10 years/Non-filter | RR for 1-10 cigarettes/day= 0.61 (M), 0.38 (F); 11-20 cigarettes/day =0.71 (M), 0.79 (F); 31-40 cigarettes/day=0.66 (M); 30+ cigarettes/day=1.03 (F); 41+ cigarettes/day=0.86 (M). | |
| Augustine, A. *et al.* Compensation as a risk factor | Case-control study of 1,242 lung cancer cases | 1969-1984 | Filter/Non-filter | | Compared to those who did not increase |

Table 4-1 (continued)

| Citation | Population | Time Period | Cigarette Type | Relative Risk | Comments |
|---|---|---|---|---|---|
| for lung cancer in smokers who switch from nonfilter to filter cigarettes. *AJPH* 79:188-191, 1989a | and 2,300 sex- and age-matched hospital controls. | | | their cigarette/day when they switched to filtered cigarettes, the odds ratios for those increased 1-10 cigarettes/day wer M=1.19, F= 1.66, for those increased 11-20 cigarettes/day, the odds ratios were M=1.75, F=2.97, and for those who increased more than 20 cigarettes/day, the odds ratios were M=2.37, F=3.89. | Mean changes in cigarettes/day after switching for cases and controls were adjusted by linear regression for age at switching and duration of non-filter smoking utilizing analysis of covariance. |
| Kabat, G.C. Aspects of the epidemiology of lung cancer in smokers and nonsmokers in the United States. *Lung Cancer* 15:1-20, 1996. | Case-control study of 7,553 lung cancer cases and 19,992 hospital controls. | 1969-1991 | Filter/Non-filter | Non-filter/filter only 0.7 (0.4-1.3);non-filter/switchers of 10+ years 0.7 (0.5-0.9). | Reduction in male filter smokers for Kreyberg I, but not Kreyberg II; effect in women not significant; odds ratios adjusted for number of cigarettes/day. |
| Rimington, J. The effect of filters on the incidence of lung cancer in cigarette smokers. *Environ. Res.* 24:162-166, 1981. | Follow-up study of 2,393 non-filter and 3,045 filter cigarette smokers from a sample of mass radio-graphy volunteers aged 40 or more in England. | 1970-1976 | Filter/Non-filter | 0.65 | Age standardized. |
| Kuller, L.H. *et al.* Cigarette smoking and mortality MRFIT Research Group. *Preventive Med.* 20:638-654, 1991. | 10.5-year follow-up of the MRFIT participants. | 1972-1985 | Tar level, nicotine level | Nicotine RR=1.0 for nicotine level≤1 mg; 0.97 (0.62-1.52) for | Adjusted for age, serum choles-terol, diastolic blood pressure, and cigarettes/day. Low-tar and low-nicotine cigarette smokers tended to smoke more cigarettes/day. |

Table 4-1 (continued)

| Citation | Population | Time Period | Cigarette Type | Relative Risk | Comments |
|---|---|---|---|---|---|
| Lubin, J.H. et al. Patterns of lung cancer risk according to type of cigarettes smoked. *Int. J. Cancer* 33:569-576, 1984. | A case-control study of 7,804 cases and 15,207 hospital-based controls in seven Western European locations. | 1976-1980 | Filter/Non-filter | Male=0.59; female=0.50 | Adjusted for years of cigarette use, number of cigarettes/day, and years since cessation. |
| Lubin, J.H. Modifying risk of developing lung cancer by changing habits of cigarette smoking. *Brit. Med. J.* 288:1953-1956, 1984a; *Brit. Med. J.* 289:921, 1984b (letter-response). | Case-control study of 7,181 lung cancer patients and 11,006 hospital controls in five Western European countries. | 1976-1980 | Filter/Non-filter | 0.54 | Risks adjusted for duration of use in years. |
| Benhamou, S. et al. Lung cancer and use of cigarettes: A French case-control study. *JNCI* 74:1169-1175, 1985. | Case-control study of 1,625 lung cancer patients and 3,091 hospital controls. | 1976-1980 | Filter/Non-filter | 0.60 | |
| Buffler, P.A. et al. Environmental associations with lung cancer in Texas coastal counties. *Annual Clinical Conference on Cancer* 28:27-34, 1986. | Case-control study of 476 cases and 466 population-based controls. | 1976-1980 | 13-14 mg/cigarette (middle) | 0.91 | No significant difference for filters. |
| Benhamou, E. et al. Lung cancer and women: Results of a French case-control study. *Brit. J. Cancer* 55:91-95, 1987. | Case-control study of 96 women with lung cancer and 192 matched hospital controls. | 1976-1980 | Filter/Non-filter | 100% non-filter; RR=0/28 (0.05-1.47) | Controlled for number of cigarettes/day duration and inhalation. |
| Benhamou, E., et al. Changes in patterns of | Case-control study of 1,057 cases and 1,503 | 1976-1980 | Filter/Non-filter | 0.7 (0.5-0.9) | Adjusted for age and duration of cigarette smoking and number of cigarettes/day. |

86

Table 4-1 (continued)

| Citation | Population | Time Period | Cigarette Type | Relative Risk | Comments |
|---|---|---|---|---|---|
| cigarette smoking and lung cancer risk: Results of a case-control study. *Br. J. Cancer* 60:601-604, 1989. | matched hospital controls in France. | | | | |
| Benhamou, S. *et al.* Differential effects of tar content, type of tobacco and use of a filter on lung cancer risk in male cigarette smokers. *Int. J. Epidemiology* 24:437-443, 1994. | Case-control study of 1,114 lung cancer patients and 1,466 hospital controls. | 1976-1980 | Filter/Non-filter | 0.63 | Risk adjusted only by age is 0.38 for filter smokers only compared to non-filtered and mixed smokers. Multivariate analysis shows slight nonsignificant increase with percentage time smoking high-tar cigarettes. |
| Vutuc, C., Kunze, M. Lung cancer risk in women in relation to tar yields of cigarettes. *Preventive Med.* 11: 713-716, 1982. | Case-control study of 297 female lung cancers and neighborhood controls from 15 lung cancer centers in Austria. | 1976-1980 | Tar level | Tar level <15, odds ratio=0.29; tar level 15-24, odds ratio= 0.49; tar level > 24, odds ratio=1.0 | Adjusted for age, duration, and number of cigarettes/day. |
| Vutuc, C., Kunze, V. Tar yields of cigarettes and male lung cancer risk. *JNCI* 71: 435-437, 1983. | Case-control study of 252 male lung cancers and hospital/neighborhood controls from 15 lung cancer centers in Austria. | 1976-1980 | Tar level | Tar level <15, odds ratio=0.30; tar 15-24, odds ratio=0.56, tar level >24, odds ratio=1.0 | Adjusted for age, duration, and number of cigarettes/day. |
| Benhamou, E., Benhamou, S. Black (air-cured) and blond (flue-cured) tobacco and cancer risk. VI: Lung cancer. *Eur. J. Cancer* 29A(12): 1778-1780, 1993. | Combination of four case-control studies in Cuba, France, Uruguay, an Italy. | 1976-1988 | Filter/Non-filter | 0.91 | Adjusted for age, duration, cigarettes/day, current smoking, and residence. |

Table 4-1 (continued)

| Citation | Population | Time Period | Cigarette Type | Relative Risk | Comments |
|---|---|---|---|---|---|
| Lange, P. *et al.* Relationship of the type of tobacco and inhalation pattern to pulmonary and total mortality. *Eur. Respir. J.* 5:1111-1117, 1992. | 6,511 men and 7,703 women selected randomly after age stratification from the general population in Copenhagen, followed for 13 years. | 1976-1989 | Filter/Non-filter | Male=0.82; Female=0.61 | |
| Gillis, C.R. *et al.* Cigarette smoking and male lung cancer in an area of very high incidence. I: Report of a case-control study in the West of Scotland. *J. Epidemiol. and Community Health* 42:38-43, 1988. | Case-control study of 656 male lung cancer patients and 1,312 age-matched hospital controls. | 1977-1981 | Low-, medium-, and high-tar yield | Relative risks did not change significantly with tar yield for smokers of 25+ cigarettes/day. For smokers of 15-24 cigarettes/day, risks fell with tar yield, but it was not statistically significant. Smokers of 1-14 cigarettes/day had a significant fall with tar yield. | |
| Alderson, M.R. *et al.* Risks of lung cancer, chronic bronchitis, ischaemic heart disease, and stroke in relation to type of cigarette smoked. *J. Epidemiol. and Community Health* 39:286-293, 1985. | Case-control study of 12,693 in-patients. | 1977-1982 | Always filter/non-filter | Male 1.48, female 0.85 | Adjusted for number of cigarettes/day. |
| Wynder, E.L., Kabat, G.C. The effect of low-yield ciga- | Case-control study of 1,278 Kreyberg I | 1977-1984 | Filter/Non-filter | Male Kreyberg I, filter-only smokers, | Adjusted for cigarettes/day, age, inhalation, and years of education. |

88

Table 4-1 (continued)

| Citation | Population | Time Period | Cigarette Type | Relative Risk | Comments |
|---|---|---|---|---|---|
| rette smoking on lung cancer risk. *Cancer* 62:1223-1230, 1988. | patients and 2,408 hospital controls and 807 Kreyberg II partients and 1,543 matched controls. | | | 0.69 (0.37-1.27); male Kreyberg II, 0.87 (0.43-1.54) | |
| Stellman, S.D. *et al.* Risk of squamous cell carcinoma and adenocarcinoma of the lung in relation to lifetime filter cigarette smoking. *Cancer* 80(3):382-388, 1997. | Case-control study of 1,442 male and 850 female lung cancers from 1977 to 1995 and hospital control. | 1977-1995 | Filter/Non-filter | Lifetime filter/non-filter: 0.4 (0.2-0.8) | Reduction in risk for squamous cell carcinoma in female lifetime filter smokers compared to lifetime non-filter smokers controlling for number of cigarettes/day, no differences for males or for adenocarcinoma. |
| Petitti, D.B., Friedman, G.D. Cardiovascular and other diseases in smokers of low yield cigarettes. *J. Chron. Dis.* 38:581-588, 1985. | 4-year prospective follow-up of 16,270 current regular smokers and 42,113 subjects who never used any form of tobacco. | 1979-1982 | Tar level and high- and low- (<15 mg tar and 1 mg nicotine) yield determined at the start of the study. | 0.87 (0.68-1.11) for a 5-mg increase in tar | Controlled for age, sex, race, and number od cigarettes/day. |
| Sidney, S. *et al.* A prospective study of cigarette tar yield and lung cancer. *Cancer Causes and Control* 4:3-10, 1993. | Prospective follow-up of 79,946 Kaiser Permanente Medical Care group members for an average of 5.6 years. | 1979-1985 | Tar yield | 1.02 (0.98-1.05) in men; 0.99 (0.96-1.03) in women | Long-term (20+ years) filter use was associated with a reduced lung cancer risk in women, RR= 0.36 (0.18-0.75), but not in men. |
| Wilcox, H.B. *et al.* Smoking and lung cancer: Risk as a function of cigarette tar content. *Preventive Med.* 17:263-272, 1988. | Case-control study of all incidence cases of lung cancer (763) in six areas of New Jersey compared to population-based controls. | 1980-1981 | Tar level | Tar level 21.1-28.0, odds ratio= 1.0; tar level 17.6-21.0, odds ratio= 1.21 (0.75-1.96); tar level | Adjusted by intensity and duration of smoking. There was an increasing intensity of smoking with decreasing level of tar among the cases when consumption in two time periods were compared. |
| Pathak, D.R. *et al.* Determinants of lung can- | Case-control study of 521 lung cancers and 769 con- | 1980-1982 | Lifelong filter/non-filter | 0.80 | Odds ratio was much lower |

89

Table 4-1 (continued)

| Citation | Population | Time Period | Cigarette Type | Relative Risk | Comments |
|---|---|---|---|---|---|
| cer risk in cigarette smokers in New Mexico. *JNCI* 76:597-604, 1986. | trols matched for age, sex, and ethnicity. | 1980-1982 | Lifelong filter/Non-filter | 0.80 | among Hispanics (0.04). |
| Kaufman, D.W. *et al.* Tar content of cigarettes in relation to lung cancer. *Am. J. Epidemiol.* 129:703-711, 1989. | Case-control study of 881 lung cancers and 2,570 hospital controls. | 1981-1986 | Tar yield: <22, 22-28, 29+ | 1, 1.9 (1.0-3.7), 3.1 (1.3-7.1) | Logistic regression controlled for age, sex, ethnicity, geographic region, years of education, year of interview, cigarettes/day, and year smoking started. |
| Khuder, S.A. *et al.* Effect of cigarettes smoking on major histological types of lung cancer in men. *Lung Cancer* 22:15-21, 1998. | Case-control study of 482 male lung cancer cases and neighborhood controls. | 1985-1987 | Filter/Non-filter | 0.46 | Adjusted for number of cigarettes/day and the confidence intervals overlap. |
| Armadans-Gil, L. *et al.* Cigarette smoking and male lung cancer risk with special regard to type of tobacco. *Int. J. Epidemiol.* 28:614-619, 1999. | Case-control study of 325 male lung cancer patients and age-matched hospital controls. | 1986-1990 | Filter/Non-filter | 0.40 | Adjusted for age and cumulative cigarette consumption. |
| Pezzotto, S.M. *et al.* Variation in smoking-related lung cancer risk factors by cell type among men in Argentina: A case-control study. *Cancer Causes and Control* 4:231-237, 1993. | Case-control study of 215 lung cancers and 433 hospital controls. | 1987-1991 | Filter/Non-filter | 0.29 | Controlled for age, hospital of admission, and intensity and duration of smoking. |

Table 4-1 (continued)

| Citation | Population | Time Period | Cigarette Type | Relative Risk | Comments |
|---|---|---|---|---|---|
| De Stefani, E. Mate drinking and risk of lung cancer in males: A case-control study from Uruguay. *Cancer Epidemiology, Biomarkers, and Prevention* 5:515-519, 1996. | Case-control study of 497 cases and 497 hospital controls. | 1988-1994 | Filter/Non-filter | 0.72 | No significant difference for filters. |
| Agudo, A. *et al.* Lung cancer and cigarette smoking in women: A case-control study in Barcelona (Spain). *Int. J. Cancer* 59:165-169, 1994. | Case-control study of 101 women with lung cancer with two matched hospital controls. | 1989-1992 | Filter/Non-filter | 0.22 | |
| Matos, E. *et al.* Lung cancer and smoking: A case-control study in Buenos Aires, Argentina. *Lung Cancer* 21: 155-163, 1998. | Case-control study of 200 male lung cancer patients and 397 hospital controls | 1994-1996 | Filter/Non-filter | Filter 0.34 (CI: 1.09-0.11) | Filter cigarettes more risky in black vs. blond comparisons and in comparisons by cell type. |
| Jockel, K.H. *et al.* Occupational and environmental hazards associated with lung cancer. *Int. J. Epidemiol.* 21:202-213, 1992. | Case-control study of 194 lung cancer patients, 194 hospital controls, and 194 population controls in five German cities. | Not stated | Filter/Non-filter | 0.41 | |

smoked per day. Measurement of cigarettes smoked per day was recorded in these studies at the same time that the brand of cigarettes smoked was recorded. As a result, the comparison in the studies is between smokers of equal numbers of different cigarettes smoked per day rather than between smokers when they are using different products. If smokers increase the number of cigarettes that they smoke per day when they switch from one type of cigarettes to another type, then comparing them on a risk per cigarette basis may result in the wrong conclusion if the question being asked is whether switching to lower yield cigarettes reduces the risk for the smoker.

One of the earliest studies (Bross and Gibson, 1968) was a case-control study of lung cancer patients diagnosed between 1960 and 1966. The study demonstrated a relative risk of 0.59 for filter smokers compared to nonfilter smokers in an analysis stratified by duration and number of cigarettes smoked per day. This analysis is of interest because it was conducted very soon following the introduction of filtered cigarettes. Figure 4-3 presents the number of filtered and nonfiltered cigarettes sold each year from 1925 to 1993, as well as their respective market shares. Essentially all cigarettes sold prior to 1955 were nonfiltered cigarettes, but the market share for filtered brands increased rapidly thereafter. Because lung cancer is often present for several years prior to its diagnosis, and 5-10 years of cessation are required to produce a 50-percent reduction in the excess risk of lung cancer, the presence of such a large reduction in relative risk following so rapidly after the introduction of filtered cigarettes raises questions concerning the biological plausibility of these results. Bross and Gibson raised these biological plausibility concerns, noting that many of the filter smokers had been using filtered cigarettes for less than 3 years. In addition, a table presented in their article demonstrated that 38 percent of the filter smokers smoked more than one pack per day in contrast to 35 percent of nonfilter smokers. This finding was in the opposite direction from the expectation that those who switched to filtered cigarettes were likely to be lighter smokers on average. It raises the likelihood that smokers who had switched to filtered cigarettes may have compensated for the decreased nicotine delivery of those cigarettes by increasing the number of cigarettes that they smoked per day, in effect biasing the analyses by moving less-intense filter smokers into strata where they were compared to more-intense nonfilter smokers.

Perhaps the most influential analyses have been those examining the 12-year follow-up of the American Cancer Society's CPS-I, which followed over 1 million men and women for up to 12 years between 1960 and 1972 (Hammond *et al.*, 1976, 1977; Lee and Garfinkel, 1981). These analyses were conducted using differences in machine-measured tar yields. Sales-weighted tar yields declined sharply during this period (see Chapter 5). Sales-weighted, machine-measured tar yields declined from 36 mg in 1954 to 19 mg in 1972. Figure 4-4 presents the market share of U.S. cigarettes by the level of machine-measured tar. Prior to 1967, most cigarettes yielded more than 20 mg of tar, but market shares of 16- to 19-mg tar cigarettes rose rapidly in the late 1960s and early 1970s.

The CPS-I compared smokers of high-tar cigarettes with more than 25.8 mg tar to smokers of mid-tar (17.6-25.8 mg) and low-tar (less than 17.6 mg)

Figure 4-3
**Market Share and Cigarette Sale of Filter and Non-Filter Cigarettes in the United States, 1925-1993**

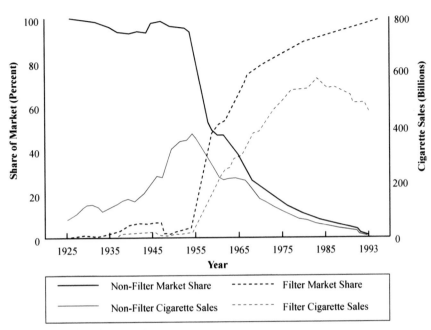

| | |
|---|---|
| —————— Non-Filter Market Share | - - - - - - Filter Market Share |
| —————— Non-Filter Cigarette Sales | - - - - - - Filter Cigarette Sales |

*Source: Maxwell Report (Maxwell, 1994).*

cigarettes. However, the 'high' group was defined as those who were in the high category from 1959 to 1960 and the high or mid category from 1965 to 1966; the low category consisted of those who were in the low category from 1959 to 1960 and either the low or medium category from 1965 to 1966. The comparison categorized smokers into groups with distinct levels of age, race, number of cigarettes smoked per day, age when smoking began, residence, occupation, education, and history of heart disease and cancer. A matched analysis of these groups was performed where the only difference between pairs was the tar level of the cigarette smoked. Measurement of the number of cigarettes smoked per day and tar levels of the cigarette smoked were at the same point in time in the follow-up, and control for number of cigarettes smoked per day was for the number smoked after switching to low-yield cigarettes. When smokers of low-yield cigarettes were compared to smokers of high-yield cigarettes in this matched analysis, the mortality ratios for lung cancer among males were 0.83 for the first 6 years of follow-up and 0.79 for the last 6 years of follow-up. Comparable ratios for females were 0.57 and 0.62, respectively. However, the researchers cautioned that the risk differences between smokers of different-yield cigarettes would disappear if smokers had increased their number of cigarettes smoked per day when they switched from high-tar to low-tar cigarettes. For example, the death rate for subjects who smoked 1-19 high-tar cigarettes per day was 75.8/100,000, but if individuals

Figure 4-4
**U.S. Market Share of Cigarettes Sold by Tar Yield of the Brand, 1967-1990 (mg of Tar by FTC Method)**

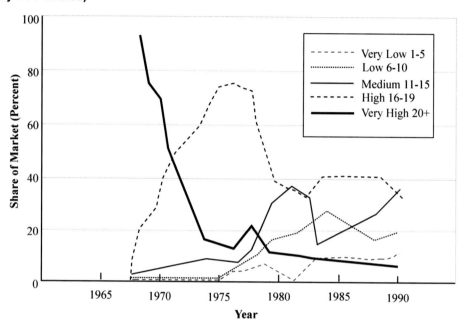

*Source: Tar levels for given years are derived from FTC Reports (for years 1967-1990). Sales data by brand are from Maxwell Report (Maxwell, 1994). Brand-specific market shares are summed by tar level of the brand in the given year to generate the market share for cigarettes with given tar yields.*

had increased to 20-39 cigarettes per day as they switched to low-yield cigarettes, the risk increased to 129.5/100,000.

This increase in lung cancer risk with compensation was examined more directly in a case-control study of lung cancer patients that examined the change in number of cigarettes smoked per day when smokers switched from nonfiltered to filtered cigarettes (Augustine *et al.*, 1989a & b). In detailed interviews with the lung cancer patients and hospital controls, the investigators constructed lifetime smoking histories by brand and number of cigarettes smoked per day for each brand. The mean number of cigarettes smoked when using nonfiltered brands was compared to the mean number of cigarettes smoked per day after switching to filtered brands. Among males, 45 percent of cases and 41 percent of controls increased the number of cigarettes that they smoked per day when they switched to filtered cigarettes. Among females, the percentages were even higher, with 59 percent of cases and 48 percent of controls increasing the number of cigarettes smoked per day. When compared to those who did not increase their cigarettes per day (CPD) when they switched to filtered cigarettes (odds ratio = 1), the lung cancer odds ratios rose with increasing compensation (the odds ratios for those who increased 1 to 10 CPD were 1.19 for males and 1.66 for females. The odds ratios for those who increased 11 to 20 CPD were 1.75

for males and 2.97 for females. The odds ratios for those who increased 21 or more CPD were 2.37 for males and 3.83 for females). The analyses were adjusted for cigarettes smoked per day with nonfiltered cigarette use (before switching), duration of nonfiltered cigarette use, age at switching, and duration of filtered cigarette use. These data demonstrated the importance of compensation with increasing number of cigarettes per day following the switch to filtered cigarettes in defining the change in lung cancer risks.

Other cohort studies have yielded mixed results. Some studies showed no significant reductions with low-yield products (Higenbottam *et al.*, 1982; Hawthorne and Fry, 1978; Todd *et al.*, 1978; Tang *et al.*, 1995; Kuller *et al.*, 1991; Petitti and Friedman, 1985; Sidney *et al.*, 1993), and others showed a decline in risk (Engeland *et al.*, 1996; Borland *et al.*, 1983; Rimington, 1981; Lange *et al.*, 1992). All of these studies controlled for intensity of smoking, using cigarettes smoked per day measured when the yield level of the brand of cigarettes smoked was entered into the analysis, and most studies controlled for a variety of other smoking (*e.g.*, duration) and demographic characteristics.

A large U.S. case-control study demonstrated significantly lower lung cancer odds ratios among filter cigarette smokers who had shifted to filtered cigarettes 10 or more years prior to diagnosis (Kabat, 1996) as well as for lifetime filter use (Stellman *et al.*, 1997). The odds ratios were adjusted for age, education, and number of cigarettes smoked per day. This study also noted that the risk decline was evident only for lung cancers in the Kreyberg I classification. Kreyberg II lung cancers showed no risk reduction with filter use. Kreyberg II lung cancers are predominantly adenocarcinoma, a form of lung cancer that has been increasing as a fraction of all lung cancers in recent decades.

Two reports from a large multicountry case-control study in Europe also reported reductions in lung cancer risk associated with lifetime filtered cigarette use (Lubin *et al.*, 1984; Lubin, 1984a & b). One study adjusted for cigarettes smoked per day at time of interview, duration of cessation, duration of smoking, and a variety of other demographic characteristics. The second study adjusted for duration of smoking, but did not adjust for CPD. There did not appear to be a systematic difference in the number of cigarettes smoked per day between filter and nonfilter smokers among the lung cancer patients. As would be expected, however, the lifetime filter smokers had substantially shorter durations of smoking. As is true of most studies of lifetime filtered cigarette users, the validity of self-reported lifetime use is in question since 63 percent of the lifetime filter smokers with lung cancer diagnoses between 1976 and 1980 in this study reported durations of filtered cigarette use of 30 or more years. Filtered cigarettes were not used in large numbers prior to the mid 1950s, making the likely maximum duration of filtered cigarette use approximately 25 years.

Epidemiological data on reduced risks of developing lung cancer among lower yield cigarette smokers are supported by a study of the histological changes in the airways of smokers (Auerbach *et al.*, 1979). The study was conducted on smokers who died of causes not associated with smoking during two time periods (1955-1960 and 1970-1977). Sales-weighted average tar yield of cigarettes declined substantially between these two periods of time. The extent and severity of histological changes in the airways were significantly and substantially less during the second calendar-year period, controlling for number of cigarettes smoked per day. The histological changes included basal cell hyperplasia, loss of cilia, occurrence of cells with atypical nuclei, and presence of advanced changes defined as carcinoma *in situ*. Comparisons were confined to examination of the airways.

In summary, most case-control and prospective mortality studies conducted in different geographic locations demonstrated differences in lung cancer risks for filter and low-tar (machine-measured) smokers compared with nonfilter and high-tar smokers when controlled for cigarettes smoked per day. The question that remains is whether differences in lung cancer experience are due to differences in machine-measured tar yield of the cigarettes smoked, due to differences in other characteristics of the smokers who use these products, or due to differences introduced by model misspecification in these studies.

**New Analyses of the American Cancer Society's Cancer Prevention Study I Data**

A reexamination of the CPS-I data set (see Appendix) was inconclusive as to whether compensatory changes in the number of cigarettes smoked per day when smokers switch to a lower nicotine cigarette introduce a bias sufficient to explain the observed increased lung cancer risk among smokers of high-yield cigarettes. If a positive gradient in lung cancer risk with tar level was present in analyses that used the tar level and number of cigarettes smoked from the most recent follow-up, and that gradient disappeared when controlling for the number of cigarettes smoked per day at the start of the study (or before smokers changed brands), then one could postulate that the compensatory shift in number of cigarettes smoked per day might be biasing the results to show an effect of tar that was not real. A survival analysis examining lung cancer risks for smokers of different-yield cigarettes using the yield of the cigarette at the most recent follow-up was performed, but it did not show a significant effect of tar for lung cancer risk with either cigarettes smoked per day at baseline or at the most recent follow-up used to control for intensity of smoking. Since there was no effect of tar on lung cancer risk to examine, it was not possible to determine whether controlling for CPD using the number of cigarettes per day prior to switching brands reduced or eliminated the effect of tar on lung cancer risk.

A survival analysis of lung cancer risk by tar level of the cigarette smoked was also conducted among those who changed the brand of cigarettes that they smoked during the CPS-I study. No significant effect was detected when using either cigarettes smoked per day measured prior to switching or at the time of the most recent follow-up to control for intensity of smoking. However, the numbers of observed lung cancer deaths were much smaller than those for the analyses of the entire smoking population.

CPS-I recorded smoking behaviors at five points during the 12-year follow-up and, therefore, some examination of the interrelationships between

Figure 4-5
**Relationship of Tar Level and Lung Cancer Risk for the American Cancer Society CPS-I Data**

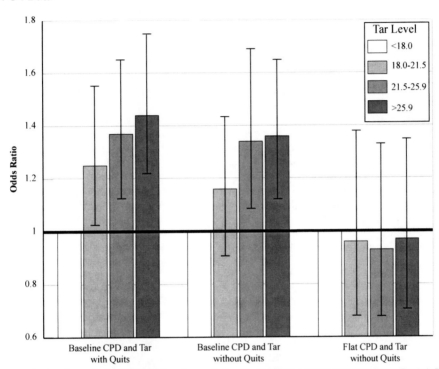

Source: American Cancer Society, CPS-I, White-male current cigarette-only smokers. Tar level interpolated from Reader's Digest (Miller & Monahan, 1959, pp.40-41) and FTC (for years 1967-1973) data by brand and year. Tar levels as indicated. Odds ratios are results of SAS lifereg survival analysis with independent variables of duration, age, CPD, and an indicator variable for first v. second 6 years of follow-up.

tar level, smoking cessation, and number of cigarettes smoked per day was possible. For the purposes of this monograph, this data set was reexamined using survival analyses that included age, number of cigarettes smoked per day, duration of smoking, and first or second 6-year period of follow-up as variables in the analyses. Three analyses of the CPS-I data set were examined in order to define the potential influences of excess cessation among low-tar smokers and the influence of shifting numbers of cigarettes smoked per day during follow-up. Figure 4-5 presents the odds ratios for four different tar levels in the three sets of survival analyses of the CPS-I data using different criteria to define which smokers are included in the analyses. The cigarettes smoked per day and tar levels of the cigarettes smoked were those recorded in the baseline survey for all of these analyses.

The first set of odds ratios was for the 12-year follow-up of smokers of cigarettes with different tar yields, with the tar level of the cigarette smoked and the number of cigarettes smoked per day derived from the baseline survey. These estimates corresponded to the approach utilized by most of the prospective mortality studies presented in Table 4-1. There was a clear and

statistically significant increase in risk with increasing tar level of the cigarette smoked, and there was a convincing dose-response relationship with
tar level. Smokers who quit were censored in the analysis at the follow-up
when they reported being former smokers. Since the last follow-up interval
was from 1965-72, this analytic approach resulted in all of the smokers who
were listed as current smokers in 1965 being considered current smokers
until the end of the study follow-up, even if they reported being former
smokers in the final follow-up survey in 1972.

The second set of analyses used the same population, but the analysis
censored those smokers who reported being former smokers in the 1972 follow-up as of the date of the next to last follow-up (1965). Because cessation
is known to influence lung cancer risk, removal of those who quit in long-
term follow-up is necessary to avoid confounding by the association of
choice of a low tar brand and subsequent cessation of smoking. Hammond
(1980) examined the CPS I data and demonstrated that smokers who were
smoking low-tar (17.6 mg or less) cigarettes in 1965 were more likely than
medium or high tar cigarette smokers to have become former smokers by
the end of the study in 1972. Removal of those who had quit by the last
follow-up did not eliminate the effect of baseline level of tar on lung cancer
risk, but the dose response relationship was less apparent.

The third set of analyses in Figure 4-5 examined only those smokers
who did not change the number of cigarettes that they reported smoking
per day over the multiple follow-up measurements. This group constituted
approximately one-third of all smokers. When using the baseline values for
tar and cigarettes smoked per day in these analyses, it was impossible to
eliminate the influence of compensatory changes in cigarettes per day that
occurred prior to the baseline measurement. However, by selecting a group
that did not change the number of cigarettes that they reported smoking
during the survey, it is possible that a group may have been identified that
also had more stable smoking practices with regard to number of cigarettes
smoked per day prior to entry into the study. When this group was examined using the baseline number of cigarettes smoked per day and tar levels,
there was no effect of tar level of the cigarette smoked on the odds ratio for
lung cancer risk. This suggested that, at least in this group with stable
smoking behavior, there was no relationship between the type of cigarette
smoked and the degree of lung cancer risk. However, it was not possible to
conclude from these analyses that the difference in lung cancer risk by type
of cigarette smoked in the larger group containing all smokers was due to
compensatory changes in the number of cigarettes smoked per day.

**Cardiovascular Disease**  Table 4-2 presents the epidemiological studies that examined cardiovascular disease risks. Relative risks of cigarette smoking for
heart disease are in the 2-4 range in contrast to the very high relative risks
for lung cancer. These lower relative risks, and the influence of the other
cardiovascular risk factors, make examination of differences in cardiovascular risks among populations who use different types of cigarettes more difficult. In contrast to the table on lung cancer risks (Table 4-1), there is no
clear consensus on coronary heart disease (CHD) risks in relation to use of
filtered or low-yield cigarettes. Some studies show increased risks and others

Table 4-2

# Epidemiological Studies of Low-Yield Cigarettes and Heart Disease

| Citation | Population | Time Period | Cigarette Type | Relative Risk | Comments |
|---|---|---|---|---|---|
| Lee, P.N., Garfinkel, L. Mortality and type of cigarette smoked. *J Epidemiol. Community Health* 35:16-22, 1981. | 12-year follow-up of CPS-I; a prospective mortality study of over 1 million men and women. | 1960-1972 | Tar yield: low/high | CHD: Male RR= 0.90; female= 0.81 | CHD risks are significantly different, but emphysema risks are not. |
| Higenbottam, T. *et al.* Cigarettes, lung cancer, and coronary heart disease: The effects of inhalation and tar yield. *J. Epidemiol. Community Health* 36:113-117, 1982. | 10-year follow-up of 17,475 male civil servants, aged 40-64, and a sample of male British residents. | 1965-1975 | Tar yield | There was a small effect of tar on CHD mortality in the inhalers | |
| Todd, G.F. *et al.* Four cardiorespiratory symptoms as predictors of mortality. *J. Epidemiol. Community Health* 32:267-274, 1978. | 12.4-year prospective follow-up of 10,063 subjects aged 35-69 from a random sample of the population in Great Britain. | 1965-1977 | Filter/Non-filter | 0.75 for males and 1.03 for females | The increase in lung cancer mortality with filter use was not statistically significant, and there was a statistically significant decrease in all-cause mortality and male CHD mortality with filter use (standardized for number of cigarettes/day). |
| Hawthorne, V.M., Fry, J.S. Smoking and health: The association between smoking behavior, total mortality, and cardiorespiratory disease in West Central Scotland. *J. Epidemiol. Community Health* 32:260-266, 1978. | Prospective follow-up of 18,786 people attending a multiphasic screening examination. | 1965-1977 | Filter/Non-filter | 1.05 for CHD mortality | No difference in mortality rates for filter users for lung cancer or cardiovascular disease. Smokers of plain cigarettes had lower rates of respiratory symptoms than filter smokers |
| Borland, C. *et al.* Carbon monoxide yield of cigarettes and its relation to cardiorespiratory disease. *BMJ* 287:1583-1586, 1983. | Prospective 10-year follow-up of the Whitehall study where 4,910 men had known CO yields of the cigarettes that they smoked. | 1967-1979 | CO yield | 1.47 for CHD mortality in those smoking cigarettes with less than 18 mg CO yield compared to those smoking 20+ mg CO yield cigarettes | Controlled for age, grade of employment, cigarettes/day, and tar yield. Those who smoked high CO-yield cigarettes (>20 mg) tended to smoke fewer cigarettes/day. |

99

Table 4-2 (continued)

| Citation | Population | Time Period | Cigarette Type | Relative Risk | Comments |
|---|---|---|---|---|---|
| Tang, J.L. *et al.* Mortality in relation to tar yield of cigarettes: a prospective study of four cohorts. *BMJ* 311:1530-1533, 1995. | Four prospective mortality studies from the United Kingdom. | 1967-1982 | Filter/Non-filter and tar yield | Tar CHD: 0.93 (0.80-1.07); stroke: 0.81 (0.59-1.12) | Relative risks for all tobacco-related diseases combined were statistically significant. Relative risks are adjusted for age, study, and number of cigarettes/day. |
| Kuller, L.H. *et al.* Cigarette smoking and mortality. MRFIT Research Group. *Preventive Med.* 20:638-654, 1991. | 10.5-year follow-up of the MRFIT participants. | 1972-1985 | Tar level, nicotine level | CHD: nicotine RR of 1.0 for nicotine level ≤1 mg. 1.04 (0.8-1.35) for 1.1-1.4 mg, and 1.27 (0.92-1.77) for 1.5+ mg; tar RR of 1.0 for tar level ≤15 mg. 1.08 (0.8-1.45) for 16-19 mg, and 1.19 (0.86-1.65) for 20+ mg. | Adjusted for age, serum cholesterol, diastolic blood pressure, and cigarettes/day. Low-tar and low-nicotine cigarette smokers tended to smoke more cigarettes/day. |
| Benhamou, E. *et al.* Lung cancer and women: Results of a French case-control study. *Br. J. Cancer* 55:91-95, 1987. | Case-control study of 96 women with lung cancer and 192 matched hospital controls. | 1976-1980 | 50+% filter/ 100% non-filter | 0.31 | Controlled for number of cigarettes/day, duration, and inhalation. |
| Alderson, M.R. *et al.* Risks of lung cancer, chronic bronchitis, ischaemic heart disease, and stroke in relation to type of cigarette smoked. *J. Epidemiol. Community Health* 39:286-293, 1985. | Case-control study of 12,693 in-patients. | 1977-1982 | Always filter/ non-filter | Age 35-54: male=1.78; female=0.24 Age 55-74: male=2.67; female=1.32 | Adjusted for number of cigarettes/day. |

Table 4-2 (continued)

| Citation | Population | Time Period | Cigarette Type | Relative Risk | Comments |
|---|---|---|---|---|---|
| Petitti, D.B., Friedman, G.D. Cardiovascular and other diseases in smokers of low yield cigarettes. *J. Chron. Dis.* 38:581-588, 1985. | 4-year prospective follow-up of 16,270 current regular smokers and 42,113 subjects who never used any form of tobacco. | 1979-1982 | Tar yield; high- and low- (less than 15 mg tar and 1 mg nicotine) yield determined at the start of the study. | 1.15 (1.03-1.28) for all cardiovascular diseases and 1.25 (0.99-1.58) for myocardial infarction for a 5-mg increase in tar. | Controlled for age, sex, race, and number of cigarettes/day. |
| Palmer, J. *et al.* Low yield cigarettes and the risk of nonfatal myocardial infarction in women. *NEJM* 320: 1569-1573, 1989. | Case-control study of 910 women with a first myocardial infarction under age 65 and 2,375 hospital controls. | 1985-1988 | Nicotine and CO levels | The estimated relative risk for women who smoked cigarettes with the lowest level of nicotine and CO was similar to that for women who smoked the brands with the highest levels of nicotine and CO. | Included in the model were terms for age, hypertension, angina, diabetes, cholesterol, family history of myocardial infarction, body mass index, type A behavior, exercise, education, residence, estrogen or oral contraceptive use, coffee consumption, alcohol consumption, and number of cigarettes/day. |
| Negri, E. Tar yield of cigarettes and risk of acute myocardial infarction. *BMJ* 306:1567-1569, 1993. | Case-control study of 916 patients with acute myocardial infarction without history of ischemic heart disease and 1,106 hospital controls in a multi-center Italian study. | 1988-1989 | Tar level | <10 mg=1, 10-15 mg=1.2 (0.7-2.1), >15-20 mg=0.8 (0.5-1.3), >20 mg= 1 (0.5-1.8). | |

Table 4-2 (continued)

| Citation | Population | Time Period | Cigarette Type | Relative Risk | Comments |
|---|---|---|---|---|---|
| Powell, J.T. *et al.* Risk factors associated with the development of peripheral arterial disease in smokers: A case-control study. *Atherosclerosis* 129:41-48, 1997. | 291 smokers with newly referred peripheral arterial disease and 828 controls without the disease from outpatient clinics. | 1988-1992 | Tar/Nicotine | Peripheral arterial disease odds ratios 1.75 for tar 14+ compared to <9 mg; 1.54 for 1.2+ mg nicotine compared to <0.8 mg; 1.62 for carboxyhemoglobin 4.5+ compared to <2.7. | Odds ratios adjusted for age, sex, and depth of inhalation. |
| Parish, S. *et al.* Cigarette smoking, tar yields, and non-fatal myocardial infarction: 14,000 cases and 32,000 controls in the United Kingdom. The International Studies of Infarct Survival (ISIS) Collaborators. *BMJ (Clin Res Ed)* 311(7003):471-477, 1995. | In the United Kingdom in the early 1990s, 14,000 cases of nonfatal myocardial infarctions and 32,000 relatives (controls) (ISIS-3 & -4) responded to questionnaires. 4,923 cases and 6,880 controls were current smokers and used in study. Unmatched case-control study assessed effects of cigarettes. | 1990 | Two groups: low-tar users (<10 mg, 7.5 mg mean) and medium-tar users (<10 mg, 13.3 mg mean) | 1.166 (1.025-1.326) for age 30-59 for medium tar compared to low tar. | Controlled for age, sex, and number of cigarettes/day. |

show decreased risks, and in many of the studies the risks are not statistically significant.

In a prospective evaluation of four cohorts from the United Kingdom
(Tang *et al.*, 1995) that included 56,255 males who were followed for an
average of 13 years, a statistically significant reduction in risk of CHD mortality (0.77; 95 percent CI, 0.61–0.97) was demonstrated with decreasing tar
yield, but the decline with filtered cigarette use was not statistically significant. These risks were adjusted for age, study, and number of cigarettes
smoked per day.

An evaluation of CHD mortality from one of these cohorts (Borland *et
al.*, 1983) revealed that CHD mortality was increased among smokers of
high carbon monoxide (CO)-yield cigarettes in an analysis that controlled
for age, employment grade, amount smoked, and tar yield of the cigarette
smoked. The differences were not statistically significant. Smokers of high
CO-yield cigarettes also tended to smoke fewer cigarettes per day. There was
little correlation between tar yield and CO yield among the different brands
of cigarettes smoked in this study, but these researchers raised the possibility that factors other than tar levels may be important in defining the exposures relevant to CHD risk.

A case-control study of nonfatal myocardial infarction in women
(Palmer *et al.*, 1989) examined disease risk in relation to nicotine yield and
CO yield of the cigarette smoked at the time of admission to the hospital.
Included in the model were terms for age, hypertension, angina, diabetes,
cholesterol, family history of myocardial infarction, body mass index, type
A behavior, exercise, education, residence, estrogen or oral contraceptive
use, coffee consumption, alcohol consumption, and number of cigarettes
smoked per day. Multivariate relative risk estimates were similar across the
categories of nicotine and CO yields from the highest to the lowest, and the
risks were not significantly different.

Parish and colleagues (1995) found that the risk ratio of nonfatal
myocardial infarction was 1.104 higher (95 percent CI, 0.998-1.222; P =
0.06) among smokers of medium-tar cigarettes compared to low-tar cigarettes in a case-control study of 14,000 survivors of myocardial infarction,
compared to 32,000 relatives who served as controls. These analyses were
controlled for age, gender, and amount smoked. When the analysis was
limited to those with no previous disease, the risk ratio declined to 1.055
(95 percent CI, 0.910-1.223, P = 0.1), raising the question of whether some
of those smokers with previously diagnosed disease might have switched to
lower yield cigarettes in an effort to reduce their risks of subsequent illness.

An analysis of the 15-year follow-up of the Multiple Risk Factor
Intervention Trial (MRFIT) participants (Kuller *et al.*, 1991) showed that
either tar or nicotine content of the cigarette smoked was only modestly,
and not statistically significantly, associated with CHD mortality in an
analysis controlled for age, serum cholesterol, diastolic blood pressure, and
cigarettes smoked per day. Petitti and Friedman (1985) found a small but
statistically significant increased risk of CHD and myocardial infarction
related to increased tar yield among 16,270 smokers compared to 42,133

never smokers who were followed for 4 years. These analyses were adjusted for age, sex, race, and number of cigarettes smoked per day as covariates. Results were similar when those with prior heart disease were removed and when the analyses were adjusted for other cardiovascular risk factors. Higenbottam and associates (1982) found a small increase in CHD mortality with lower tar yield, but the effect was evident only in the approximately 80 percent of smokers who inhaled. Todd and colleagues (1978) found a decline in CHD mortality among males, but not among females, who smoked filtered cigarettes.

In summary, while the data are not as compelling for alterations in CHD risk compared to lung cancer risk among populations who smoke low-yield cigarettes, several well-conducted epidemiological studies have demonstrated a difference in cardiovascular risk among those who smoke low-yield cigarettes when the analyses were controlled for number of cigarettes smoked per day. The complexity of examining the effect of low-yield cigarette smoking on CHD risk is exacerbated by the greater independence of the ratio of CO-to-nicotine yield among different brands of cigarettes in comparison to the ratio of tar-to-nicotine yield. CO is considered to be a major etiological agent in cardiovascular disease, and the factors that determine the CO yield of a cigarette are different from those that determine tar yield. Individual changes in cigarette design may influence tar and CO yields in different directions. These differences make interpretation of studies of cardiovascular disease risk in relation to tar yield or among filter cigarette smokers more difficult. Once again, the question that remains is whether this difference in CHD experience is due to the difference in machine-measured tar yield of the cigarettes smoked, due to the differences in other characteristics of the smokers who use these products, due to differences in other cardiovascular risk factors among smokers of different yield cigarettes, or due to differences introduced by controlling for intensity and duration of smoking in these studies.

**Chronic Respiratory Symptoms and Disease**    Table 4-3 presents the epidemiological studies that have examined respiratory disease risks. Since symptomatic chronic lung disease is commonly present for long periods prior to resulting in death, and because many smokers will quit smoking once chronic shortness of breath is manifest, it is difficult to evaluate the effect of smoking low-yield cigarettes on chronic obstructive pulmonary disease mortality. A reduced death rate from emphysema was demonstrated in the CPS-I 12-year follow-up (Lee and Garfinkel, 1981) at a point when lower yield products had not been on the market for an extended period of time. Other mortality outcome studies (Tang *et al.*, 1995; Lang *et al.*, 1992; Petitti and Friedman, 1985) have not demonstrated a similar reduction in lung disease mortality.

Sparrow and colleagues (1983) examined the relationship of tar yield to pulmonary function measurements in a group of 383 current smokers for whom pulmonary function measurements were available at two points in time 5 years apart. In a multivariate regression analysis, tar level of the cigarette smoked was not significantly associated with the forced vital capacity (FVC) or forced expiratory volume in 1 second (FEV1) in the initial exami-

Table 4-3
**Epidemiological Studies of Low-Yield Cigarettes and Respiratory Disease**

| Citation | Population | Time Period | Cigarette Type | Relative Risk | Comments |
|---|---|---|---|---|---|
| Lee P.N., Garfinkel, L. Mortality and type of cigarette smoked. *J. Epidemiol. Community Health* 35:16-22, 1981. | 12-year follow-up of CPS-I; a prospective mortality study of over 1 million men and women. | 1960-1972 | Tar yield: low/high | Emphysema: male=0.78; female=0.59 | CHD risks are significantly different, but emphysema risks are not. |
| Hawthorne, V.M., Fry, J.S. Smoking and health: The association between smoking behavior, total mortality, and cardiorespiratory disease in West Central Scotland. *J. Epidemiol. Community Health* 32:260-266, 1978. | Prospective follow-up of 18,786 people attending a multiphasic screening examination. | 1965-1977 | Filter/Non-filter | 0.61 for chronic | No difference in mortality rates for filter users for lung cancer or cardiovascular disease. Smokers of plain cigarettes had lower rates of respiratory symptoms than filter smokers. |
| Tang, J.L. *et al.* Mortality in relation to tar yield of cigarettes: a prospective study of four cohorts. *BMJ* 311:1530-1533, 1995. | Four prospective mortality studies from the United Kingdom. | 1967-1982 | Filter/Non-filter and tar yield | Tar yield chronic obstructive pulmonary disease 0.94 (0.64-1.37) | Relative risks for all tobacco-related disease combined were statistically significant. Relative risks are adjusted for age, study, and number of cigarettes/day. |
| Sparrow, D. *et al.* The relationship of tar content to decline in pulmonary function in cigarette smokers. *Am. Rev. Resp. Dis.* 127:56-58, 1983. | 383 current smokers enrolled in a longitudinal study of aging who had spirometry performed 5 years apart. | 1969-1980 | Tar level | In a multiple regression analysis, tar level did not influence FVC or FEV 1 at baseline or change in these measures at follow-up. | Controlled for age, height, and number of cigarettes/day. |
| Dean, G. *et al.* Factors related to respiratory and cardiovascular symptoms in the United Kingdom. *J. Epidemiol. Community Health* 32:86-96, 1978. | Sample of 12,736 men and women aged 37-67 living in England, Scotland, and Wales. | 1972 | Filter/Non-filter | Of eight respiratory and cardiovascular symptoms, morning cough in men and women and shortness of breath in women were lower in filter cigarette smokers. | Controlled for age, social class, number of cigarettes/day, inhalation, and occupation. |

105

Table 4-3 (continued)

| Citation | Population | Time Period | Cigarette Type | Relative Risk | Comments |
|---|---|---|---|---|---|
| Lange, P. et al. Relationships of the type of tobacco and inhalation pattern to pulmonary and total mortality. *Eur. Resp. J.* 5:1111-1117, 1992. | 6,511 men and 7,703 women selected randomly after age stratification from the general population in Copenhagen, followed for 13 years. | 1976-1989 | Filter/Non-filter | Chronic obstructive pulmonary disease: male=1.23; female=1.07 | Adjusted for number of cigarettes/day. |
| Alderson, M.R. et al. Risks of lung cancer, chronic bronchitis, ischaemic heart disease, and stroke in relation to type of cigarette smoked. *J. Epidemiol. Community Health* 39:286-293, 1985. | Case-contrl study of 12,693 in-patients. | 1977-1982 | Always filter/non-filter | Chronic bronchitis: male=0.25; female=0.75 | |
| Petitti, D.B., Friedman, G.D. Cardiovascular and other diseases in smokers of low yield cigarettes. *J. Chron. Dis.* 38:581-588, 1985. | 4-year prospective follow-up of 16,270 current regular smokers and 42,113 subjects who never used any form of tobacco. | 1979-1982 | High and low (less than 15 mg tar and 1 mg nicotine) yield determined at the start of the study | 0.97 (0.84-1.13) for all diseases of the respiratory system for a 5-mg increase in tar. | Controlled for age, sex, race, and number of cigarettes/day. |
| Krzyanowski, M. et al. Relationship of respiratory symptoms and pulmonary function to tar, nicotine, and carbon monoxide yield of cigarettes. *Am. Rev. Resp. Dis.* 143:306-311, 1991. | 690 smokers from a sample of households in Tucson, Arizona; followed to 1988. | 1981-1988 | Tar, nicotine, and CO yield | After adjustment for intensity and duration of smoking and depth of inhalation, there was no effect of tar or nicotine on chronic phlegm, cough, or dyspnea. Tar and nicotine content had no independent effect on pulmonary function. | |

Table 4-3 (continued)

| Citation | Population | Time Period | Cigarette Type | Relative Risk | Comments |
|---|---|---|---|---|---|
| Brown, C.A. *et al.* Cigarette tar content and symptoms of chronic bronchitis: Results of the Scottish Heart Health Study. *J. Epidemiol. Community Health* 45: 287-290, 1991. | 2,801 current cigarette smokers (1,154 males, 1,647 females), 40-59 years of age, from 22 districts of Scotland (Scottish Heart Health Study): cross-sectional random sample. Cigarettes smoked by subjects were assigned to one of three tar level groups: <12 mg/cig (low); 13-14 mg/cig (middle); 15+ mg/cig (high). | 1984-1986 | Tar level | Rates of chronic cough and chronic phlegm were higher for women who smoked high-tar cigarettes, but not for men. | Women in the middle-tar and high-tar group had smoked for longer and had significantly higher breath CO levels, serum thiocyanate levels, and daily cigarette consumption than women in the low-tar group. This pattern was not seen in men. |
| Withey, C.H. *et al.* Respiratory effects of lowering tar and nicotine levels of cigarettes smoked by young male middle tar smokers. II. Results of a randomised controlled trial. *J. Epidemiol. Community Health* 46(3): 281-285, 1992. | Intervention trial in 21 local authority districts in England; male middle-tar smokers aged 18-44 years; 7,029 smokers selected from 265,016 sent questionnaires; 643 controls. Assigned 1 of 3 different types of cigarettes for 6 months. | 1985-1989 | Mid-tar smokers (>12 mg/cigarette) assigned to test low-tar/ middle-nicotine, middle-tar/middle-nicotine, or low-tar/low-nicotine cigarettes for 6 months. Three cigarette groups: LM: low-tar/mid -nicotine, MM: mid-tar/mid-nicotine, LL: low-tar/low-nicotine. Per cigarette: LM: 9.5 mg tar/ 1.16 mg nicotine; MM:13.8 mg tar/ 1.24 mg nicotine; LL: 9.3 mg tar/1.04 mg nicotine. | No difference in respiratory symptoms with switching to different types of cigarettes. | Analysis of urinary nicotine metabolites showed that smokers allocated to the different cigarette type study adjusted their smoking so that throughout the trial their nicotine inhalation differed little from their pretrial intakes when they were smoking their usual cigarette for a 6-month period. |

nation, nor to change in these measures over the 5-year interval. The analyses were controlled for age, height, number of cigarettes smoked per day, and baseline lung function in the follow-up analysis.

The frequency of respiratory symptoms also has been evaluated in relation to the type of cigarette smoked. Alderson and associates (1985) demonstrated a lower risk of chronic bronchitis among those who had smoked only filtered cigarettes in an analysis adjusted for number of cigarettes smoked per day. In contrast, a smaller case-control study (Krzyzanowski *et al.*, 1991) found no difference in respiratory symptoms in relation to the tar yield of the cigarette smoked with an analysis adjusted for the duration and intensity of smoking as well as the depth of inhalation. Brown and colleagues (1991) demonstrated lower rates of chronic cough and phlegm among female smokers of lower tar cigarettes, but the effect was not evident in males. In an intervention trial (Withey *et al.*, 1992) that involved switching 7,029 smokers to one of three different types of cigarettes, no difference in respiratory symptoms after a 6-month interval was noted among those who switched to lower yield cigarettes.

In summary, there is little evidence for a substantial difference in mortality from chronic obstructive lung disease among smokers who use low-yield cigarettes. There is equivocal evidence for a reduced rate of respiratory symptoms.

**Summary of the Epidemiological Evidence**    Studies published in the epidemiological literature support a difference in lung cancer and possibly heart disease risks, but not in chronic lung disease risks, between populations of individuals who smoke filtered or lower yield cigarettes compared with individuals who smoke unfiltered or higher yield cigarettes. However, there is marked variability among the studies, with many studies finding no effect or an effect too small to be statistically significant. In some studies, the heart disease and lung cancer risks appeared to change in opposite directions with low-yield cigarette use, as did risks for male and female smokers. Most of the major studies that defined this risk used the number of cigarettes smoked per day as a measure to control for the intensity of cigarette smoking and, therefore, they may be subject to confounding due to a compensatory increase in the number of cigarettes smoked per day by some smokers when they shifted to lower yield cigarettes. Given the variability of these results, the potential for confounding and in the analyses, and the difficulty of examining the continually changing cigarette product, it is difficult to conclude from these data that there is a clearly demonstrable harm reduction that is due to the use of filtered or lower yield cigarettes in comparison to unfiltered or higher yield cigarettes.

These epidemiological data were also recently reviewed by the Tobacco Advisory Group of the Royal College of Physicians (2000) in conjunction with the evidence for compensation in smoking behavior with use of low-yield brands. They concluded, "There are therefore reasonable grounds for concern that low tar cigarettes offer smokers an apparently healthier option while providing little if any true benefit."

## BIOLOGIC IMPLICATIONS OF COMPENSATION FOR CHANGES IN CIGARETTE DESIGN

The biological significance of compensatory smoking may be more complex than is portrayed by measures of nicotine absorption or CO levels. Addition of a filter to a cigarette lowers the particulate mass passing into the smoker's mouth, and that reduction in particulate mass is usually measured as a reduction in milligrams of tar. The effects of filters and other changes in cigarette design on the particle-size distribution of the smoke are complex and somewhat dependent on the compensatory behavior of the smoker.

Filtration of cigarette smoke with a cellulose acetate filter alters the distribution of particle size in the smoke, preferentially reducing particles 0.5-micron mass median diameter (MMD) and larger as well as those particles below 0.1 micron MMD (Kieth and Derrick, 1960; Keith, 1982). The net result is a lowering of the MMD of filtered tobacco smoke. The MMD of the smoke reaching the smoker is concentrated in that range where deposition in the lung is most efficient and where there is relatively less deposition in the mouth and throat compared to the lung (International Committee on Radiation Protection, 1966; Committee on Health Risks of Exposure to Radon [BEIR VI], 1999).

Morie and colleagues (1973) examined the fibers in cigarette filters microscopically to examine the mechanism by which filters would preferentially remove both large and very small particles. They found that fibers oriented parallel to the smoke stream showed heavy deposition of particles with MMD less than 0.1 micron. Fibers oriented perpendicular to the smoke stream were coated with particles larger than 0.5 micron MMD. This finding suggests that diffusion of particles smaller than 0.1 micron MMD was the principal mechanism for deposition of these small particles on filter fibers oriented parallel to the smoke stream, and that the particles larger than 0.5 micron were trapped by interception on the fibers oriented perpendicular to the smoke stream. Particle size is a principal determinant of the deposition site of particles, with particles smaller than 0.5 micron MMD depositing in the lung rather than the upper airway (International Committee on Radiation Protection, 1966; Committee on Health Risks of Exposure to Radon [BEIR VI], 1999).

An investigation of the effect of filters on particle size, conducted for Philip Morris soon after filters had been widely introduced (Holmes *et al.*, 1959; Mitchell, 1958), suggested that filters lowered the particle size of the smoke produced by cigarettes. For example, Philip Morris regular (unfiltered) cigarettes produced smoke with an MMD of 0.94 micron and Benson and Hedges® with the filter removed produced smoke with an MMD of 1.0 micron. In contrast, filtered Parliament® cigarettes produced smoke with an MMD of 0.84 micron and Benson and Hedges® with the filter in place produced smoke with an MMD of 0.82 micron. More recent investigations (McClusker *et al.*, 1983) revealed that the particle size of the smoke generated by lower yield cigarettes is the same with and without removal of the filters. This difference in results may relate to the effect of filter ventilation on particle size. Increased ventilation results in an increase in the particle size of the smoke generated (Kieth, 1982). This effect is thought to occur because the addition of dilution, particularly in the filter, slows down the rate at which the smoke passes through the cigarette, allowing more time for coagulation of the smoke particles. This increase in particle size due to coagulation may counterbalance the reduction in particle size produced by filtration. Removal of the perforated filters on low-yield cigarettes removes both the ventilation and the filtration. As discussed elsewhere in this volume (see Chapter 3), smokers of cigarettes with ventilated filters often cover the filters with their lips or fingers in order to increase the yield of the cigarette. When these ventilation holes are occluded, the result may be filtration without increased ventilation, and particle size may be reduced. However, no studies of particle size distribution with occlusion of the ventilation holes are available.

Particles with an MMD larger than 0.75 micron contain much more tar than do smaller particles because of their larger size, but they are more likely to be deposited in the mouth before reaching the respiratory track. Thus, a filtered cigarette with a smaller particle-size distribution may deliver much more of its dose of tar to the lung than will a nonfiltered cigarette with the same machine-measured tar yield. This may result in a relative preservation of the carcinogenic dose delivered to the lung when filters are used to reduce the tar delivered at the mouth.

Nicotine in smoke is absorbed from both smoke deposited in the mouth and smoke inhaled into the lung. Venous blood levels of nicotine reflect the total smoke exposure of the smoker, not where in the respiratory track the smoke particles are deposited. Large particles contain larger amounts of nicotine, but will preferentially be deposited in the mouth and throat. Selective removal of these large particles through filtration will reduce the fraction of nicotine that is deposited in the upper airway, but may have little effect on the fraction of smoke inhaled into the lung. If the smoker compensates for the reduction in total nicotine delivery by generating and inhaling more smoke to preserve total nicotine intake, then the larger mass of smaller particles delivering that dose of nicotine in filtered smoke might produce an increased deposition of tar in the lung for the same dose of nicotine delivered to the bloodstream.

Changes in pattern of deposition of smoke aerosol have been postulated (Thun *et al.,* 1997a) as one mechanism underlying the dramatic increase in adenocarcinoma (a cancer felt to arise from the more peripheral structures of the lung) seen over the last several decades (Travis *et al.,* 1995) in the United States and other countries (Russo *et al.,* 1997; Levi *et al.,* 1997). An additional concern has been increases in the levels of tobacco-specific nitrosamines in cigarettes over time, particularly NNK, which is a potent lung carcinogen for adenocarcinoma in animals (Hecht, 1998; see Chapter 5). Recently, it was suggested (Peel *et al.,* 1999) that the formation of tobacco-specific nitrosamines in flue-cured tobacco in the United States is largely the result of using propane gas heaters in the curing process. Oxides of nitrogen generated from burning the liquid propane combine with the nicotine in the tobacco leaf to form the tobacco-specific nitrosamines. These changes in curing methods were introduced in the mid 1960s and are

Table 4-4
**Percentage of Smokers of Different Ages and Durations of Smoking Who Smoke Cigarettes with Different Tar Yields (American Cancer Society's Cancer Prevention Study I)**

| Tar Level (mg) | Age (Years) | | | | | |
| --- | --- | --- | --- | --- | --- | --- |
| | <45 | 45-55 | 55-65 | 65-75 | >75 | **Total** |
| Low ≤17.6 | 12.82 | 13.14 | 14.36 | 14.36 | 13.46 | 13.72 |
| Mid 17.6-25.8 | 52.24 | 51.74 | 53.14 | 52.23 | 51.22 | 52.36 |
| High >25.8 | 34.94 | 35.12 | 32.49 | 33.41 | 35.32 | 33.93 |
| | **Duration (Years)** | | | | | |
| | <20 | 20-29 | 30-39 | 40-49 | 50+ | **Total** |
| Low ≤17.6 | 16.18 | 14.60 | 13.48 | 13.37 | 12.77 | 13.72 |
| Mid 17.6-25.8 | 53.95 | 52.25 | 52.24 | 52.70 | 51.28 | 52.36 |
| High > 25.8 | 29.87 | 33.15 | 34.28 | 33.93 | 35.95 | 33.93 |

likely to have resulted in a substantial increase in the levels of tobacco-specific nitrosamines present in cigarettes containing tobacco cured with this method. Increased levels of tobacco-specific nitrosamines have the potential to make cigarettes manufactured after the 1960s more carcinogenic and may have contributed to the rise in adenocarcinoma, which has become the most common form of lung cancer.

**CORRELATION OF CIGARETTE BRAND CHOICE WITH NUMBER OF CIGARETTES SMOKED PER DAY AND DURATION OF SMOKING**

As discussed above, examinations of disease risks produced by lower yield cigarettes commonly adjust for differences in intensity and duration of cigarette smoking. Those adjustments can be complicated if characteristics of the cigarette itself cause changes in measures of intensity of smoking, or if concerns about disease risk influence the choice of cigarette smoked. This section examines cross-sectional and cohort studies of the correlation between type of cigarette smoked and smoking intensity or duration.

Data from the CPS-I study for the type of cigarette smoked by White male smokers of different ages and smoking durations are presented in Table 4-4 for all of the baseline and follow-up surveys combined. The fraction of smokers who smoked low-yield cigarettes was relatively constant across different ages, which was in marked contrast to the pattern of increasing use of low-yield cigarettes with advancing age that was evident in the California data from 1996 (see Figure 4.1). It is worth noting, however, that the distribution of low-tar cigarette use with duration of smoking, in contrast to age, is not uniform. When the duration of any cigarette smoking (cigarettes of any tar level) is examined, those who reported smoking high tar cigarettes at the time of follow-up had been smoking for more years than smokers of lower tar cigarettes. It is unlikely that this effect is a function of older age among high tar cigarette smokers as the distribution of tar level by age is much more uniform in the table.

As part of a case-control study of lung cancer, Augustine and colleagues (1989a & b) constructed lifetime smoking histories by cigarette brand and number of cigarettes smoked per day with each brand. They compared the mean number of cigarettes smoked per day when subjects smoked nonfiltered cigarette brands to the mean number after they switched to filtered brands. The differences in cigarettes smoked per day were adjusted for non-filter cigarettes smoked per day (before switching), duration of nonfilter and filter smoking, age at diagnosis, and age at switching. Among males, 45 percent of cases and 41 percent of controls increased the number of cigarettes that they smoked per day when they switched to filtered cigarettes. The mean increase in cigarettes per day was 5.9 for the cases and 3.9 for the controls. The percentages were even higher among females, with 59 percent of cases and 48 percent of controls increasing the number of cigarettes smoked per day. The mean increase in cigarettes per day was 7.8 for the cases and 4.7 for the controls. As measured by this study, compensation by increasing the number of cigarettes smoked per day upon switching to fil-tered cigarettes was common and involved substantial increases in the number of cigarettes smoked per day.

Assessing the impact of switching to low-yield cigarettes on the number of cigarettes smoked per day from cross-sectional data is complicated by multiple factors that may influence both choice of cigarette and the num-ber smoked daily. The strength of nicotine addiction is correlated with the number of cigarettes smoked per day, and it is possible that more-addicted smokers may not be successful in switching to low-yield cigarettes. Smokers who are trying to quit, or who are interested in quitting, may smoke fewer cigarettes per day and shift to low-yield cigarettes as part of their effort to quit.

The concentration of cotinine in the blood is correlated with the num-ber of cigarettes smoked per day (Benowitz *et al.*, 1983). Higher nicotine demand per day is met by smoking more cigarettes per day, and possibly by smoking each cigarette with more puffs and deeper inhalation. Less-addict-ed smokers have lower nicotine requirements and generally smoke fewer cigarettes per day. These lower nicotine requirements may allow the less-addicted smoker to satisfy their need for nicotine even with cigarettes that deliver lower levels of nicotine. The more heavily addicted smoker may not be able to extract sufficient nicotine from a low-yield cigarette to satisfy his or her addiction, or he or she may have to work so hard to extract the nico-tine that the experience of smoking lower yield products is unpleasant. This effect would tend to concentrate more-addicted smokers who smoke more cigarettes per day in the higher yield brands. The result of such a phenome-non in cross-sectional examinations of cotinine levels among smokers of cigarettes with different machine-measured yields would be a slight slope of increasing cotinine levels with increasing machine-measured nicotine yields, even if complete compensation occurs at the level of the individual smoker.

A similar effect would be expected if smokers who tried to quit switched to low-yield brands as part of their effort to quit, or as an effort to moderate their risk upon relapsing to cigarette smoking. Efforts to cut down prior to quitting may also involve efforts to reduce the number of cigarettes smoked per day, and those who relapse may smoke fewer daily cigarettes for a peri-od of time after reinitiating smoking. These influences been reported as reasons why smokers choose low-yield brands (Giovino *et al.*, 1996), and they would also be expected to influence the cross-sectional relationship between machine-measured nicotine yields and biological measures of nicotine intake.

Even with these influences potentially biasing the results, cross-sectional evaluations of blood cotinine levels have shown little or no relationship with machine-measured nicotine yields (Benowitz *et al.*, 1983; Benowitz, 1996; see Chapter 2). Benowitz and colleagues (1983) examined cotinine levels in smokers who smoked cigarettes with different nicotine yields as measured by the FTC method, and demonstrated a nonstatistically significant positive slope of the relationship between cotinine level in the smoker and nicotine yield of the brand smoked. In a similar comparison, but on a randomly selected population sample in the United Kingdom, a small, statistically significant positive slope was demonstrated between cotinine level in the smoker and nicotine yield of the brand smoked (Jarvis *et al.*, 2001).

In summary, these data suggest that choice of cigarette brand is only a relatively minor determinant of the amount of nicotine (and tar) that the smoker will derive from smoking. This issue is examined in more depth in Chapter 2.

**Change in Number of Cigarettes Smoked per Day with Differences in Machine-Measured Nicotine Yields in the American Cancer Society's Cancer Prevention Study I**
The CPS-I recorded cigarette brand and number of cigarettes smoked per day at five points during the 12 years of follow-up. Therefore, it was possible to examine both cross-sectional relationships between the number of cigarettes smoked per day and the machine-measured yield of the cigarette smoked, as well as the changes that take place when a smoker switches brands (see Appendix).

Table 4-5 presents the observed percentages of smokers of different numbers of cigarettes per day who smoked low-, mid-, and high-tar yield cigarettes among the CPS-I population for all of the baseline and follow-up surveys combined. The relationship between cigarettes per day and tar yield of the cigarette smoked is complex, as low-tar cigarette smokers were over-represented in both the 1-9 and 40+ cigarettes per day categories. This may suggest that choice of cigarette is conditioned by multiple factors, including the possibility that smokers with greater nicotine demands are less likely to choose and be satisfied by lower yield cigarettes, and the possibility that smokers who switch to lower yield brands increase the number of cigarettes that they smoke per day.

Hammond and Garfinkel (1964) examined the first 2 years of follow-up of the CPS-I data (1959-1961). They did not demonstrate a relationship between an increased, decreased, or unchanged tar and nicotine yield of the cigarettes smoked and a change in the categorical measure of number of cigarettes smoked per day. In an analysis that examined change over the 12-year follow-up of the CPS-I data, and which examined continuous as opposed to categorical measures of numbers of cigarettes smoked per day, Garfinkel (1979, 1980) showed a modest difference between increasing tar and nicotine yield of the cigarettes smoked and decreased numbers of cigarettes smoked per day, particularly for females, but the effect was small.

113

Table 4-5

**Percentage of Smokers of Different Numbers of Cigarettes per Day Who Smoke Cigarettes with Different Machine-Measured Tar Yields (American Cancer Society's Cancer Prevention Study I)**

| Tar Level (mg) | Cigarettes Smoked per Day | | | | | | |
|---|---|---|---|---|---|---|---|
| | 1-9 | 10-19 | 20 | 21-39 | 40 | >40 | Total |
| Low ≤17.6 | 17.37 | 13.91 | 11.64 | 14.49 | 27.27 | 15.44 | 13.72 |
| Mid 17.6-25.8 | 54.64 | 53 | 52.63 | 51.22 | 54.76 | 50.7 | 52.36 |
| High >25.8 | 27.99 | 33.08 | 35.73 | 34.3 | 17.97 | 33.86 | 33.93 |

Figure 4-6

**Nicotine Level of Brand Smoked versus Mean-Adjusted CPD Reported for All White Male Smokers (*N*=169,610): ACS CPS-I Study, Followed 1960-1972**

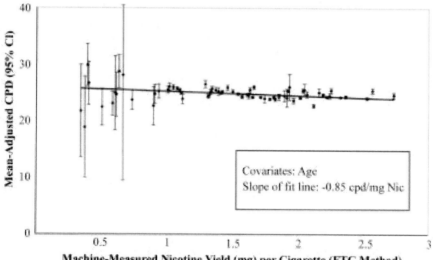

*Source: ACS CPS-I, White male current cigarette-only smokers.*
*Note: Nicotine and tar levels interpolated by year and brand from* Reader's Digest *(Miller & Monahan, 1959) and FTC (for years 1967-1973) data, mean CPD by nicotine value using the weighted mean value for each categorical level of CPD. The mean CPD values are adjusted for age and regressed on nicotine yield per cigarette. For the graph, covariate coefficients are calculated in a general regression, then points are graphed as adjusted for the covariate with the regression line shown through the adjusted points.*

The relationship between nicotine yield of the cigarette smoked and the number of cigarettes smoked per day is reexamined in this report for individual smokers among the CPS-I population of White males. Figure 4-6 presents the mean number of cigarettes smoked per day by all smokers of a given brand with the machine-measured nicotine yield of the cigarette brand. Cigarettes smoked per day were adjusted for age because of the influence of age on reported number of cigarettes smoked per day. The results were similar without the age adjustment. There was a statistically significant slope, with a 0.8 cigarette per day increase for a 1 mg decline in nicotine.

Figure 4-7

**Mean Change in Adjusted CPD Reported for Subjects Changing Brand Smoked v. Changes in Machine-Measured Nicotine Yield per Cigarettes: White Male Smokers (*N*=169,610), ACS CPS-I Study, Followed 1960-1972**

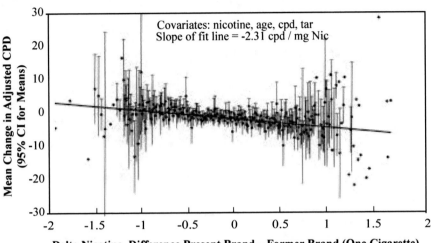

Covariates: nicotine, age, cpd, tar
Slope of fit line = -2.31 cpd / mg Nic

*Y-axis:* Mean Change in Adjusted CPD (95% CI for Means)

*X-axis:* **Delta Nicotine, Difference Present Brand—Former Brand (One Cigarette)**

*Source: ACS CPS-I, White male current cigarette-only smokers.*
*Note: Nicotine and tar levels interpolated by year and brand from* Reader's Digest *(Miller & Monahan, 1959) and FTC (for years 1967-1973) data. Each data point combines subjects with the same change in nicotine (before—after). For each CPD category, the value used in the calculations is the mean CPD value for the category as calculated across all subjects falling in the category from the final follow-up questionnaire, which has continuous CPD values available. The mean change in CPD is the average difference (after—before) in reported CPD level across subjects with the given change in nicotine. Mean change in CPD, adjusted for age, cpd, and for tar and nicotine level before changing brand, is regressed on change in nicotine yield per cigarette. For the graph, covariate coefficients are calculated in a general regression, then points are graphed as adjusted for the covariates with the regression line shown through the adjusted points.*

When the analysis was limited to those who had changed the brand of cigarettes that they reported smoking in sequential follow-up surveys, the slope of mean number of cigarettes per day in relation to change in machine-measured level of nicotine for the brand was -2.31 cigarettes/day/mg nicotine (see Figure 4-7). This analysis controlled for age, cigarettes smoked per day prior to switching brands, and tar and nicotine yields of the cigarette smoked before the switch.

The implications of these shifts in number of cigarettes smoked per day with changes in nicotine yield of the cigarette are presented in Figure 4-8. Lung cancer risks from the CPS-I study for smokers of high-tar (more than 25.8 mg) and low-tar (less than 17.6 mg) cigarettes are presented by number of cigarettes smoked per day at the baseline survey. It is possible to estimate from this figure how much compensation by number of cigarettes per day would be required to eliminate the benefit of shifting from one line to the other (*i.e.*, changing to a low-yield cigarette). In this comparison, it would require a 20-cigarette-per-day smoker who switched from a high-tar to a low-tar cigarette to smoke only 4 more cigarettes per day in order to eliminate the benefit in lung cancer risk estimated from the CPS-I data. This difference in number of cigarettes per day is that which would be predicted from a change in nicotine of 1.7 mg for individuals who switched brands in

115

Figure 4-8
**Excess Lung Cancer Death Rates for Smokers of Different Numbers of Cigarettes by Tar Level of Cigarette Smoked, American Cancer Society Cancer Prevention Study I**

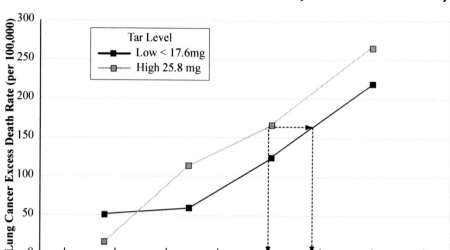

Source: ACS CPS-I White male current cigarette-only smokers.
Note: Tar levels interpolated by year and brand from Reader's Digest (Miller & Monahan, 1959) and FTC (for years 1967-1973) data. Uses base survey (1959) tar and CPD values. Restricted to subjects who smoke throughout study to personal endpoint (end of study, death, or lost-to-follow-up). The summary rates shown are age-adjusted and duration-adjusted rates for CPD and tar-level categories. For each CPD category, the value used is the mean CPD value for the category as calculated across all subjects falling in the category from the final follow-up questionnaire, which has continuous CPD values available.

the CPS-I analysis described in the previous paragraph. High tar and nicotine was defined in the CPS-I study as between 2-2.7 mg nicotine, and low tar and nicotine was below 1.2 mg nicotine. The mean nicotine level for the high-tar group in Figure 4-8 was 2.36 mg and the mean nicotine level for the low-tar group was 1.03 mg, a difference of 1.33 mg. In another context, the sales-weighted nicotine yield of U.S. cigarettes has declined from approximately 2.6 mg in the 1950s to 0.9 mg currently (see Chapter 5), a change of 1.7 mg of nicotine. The magnitude of this upward compensation, if it occurred across the entire population using lower yield cigarettes in the CPS I, is large enough to explain much of the reduction in lung cancer risks found among low yield cigarette smokers..

**Number of Cigarettes Smoked per Day among Smokers of Cigarettes with Different Machine-Measured Nicotine Yields for Current Cigarettes—California Data**

The relationship between the machine-measured nicotine yields and the number of cigarettes smoked per day was also examined for cigarettes with nicotine yields similar to those currently used in the United States. The 1990 and 1996 California Tobacco Surveys (CTS) were utilized to examine the effects of low tar and nicotine on the number of cigarettes smoked per day. This analysis was confined to a population of adult smokers who were not in the process of changing their smoking behaviors. Respondents must have smoked at least 100 cigarettes in their lifetime, smoked cigarettes daily 1 year prior to the survey, and smoked daily at the time of the survey. The analysis was further restricted to respondents who were 25-64 years old, smoked five or more cigarettes per day, and who had not tried to quit smoking in the previous 12 months. These restrictions reduced the possible influences of individuals who were starting to smoke or trying to quit, were less likely to be using cigarettes because of their dependence on nicotine as defined by smoking fewer than five cigarettes per day (Shiffman, 1989; Benowitz and Henningfield, 1994), or were switching brands based on development of an illness (those aged 65 and older).

Respondents to the 1996 CTS were asked to read the barcode number printed on the side of the cigarette package. The brand descriptions for UPC codes, versions A and E, were provided by Matthew Farrelly of the Research Triangle Institute. These brand descriptions were used to obtain the corresponding machine-measured nicotine levels provided by the FTC for the year 1996. The resulting population was 2,140.

The data were modeled using a multiple linear regression that controlled for the effects of age, gender, race/ethnicity, and level of education, variables significantly associated with number of cigarettes smoked per day in the model. This analysis was based on individual subspecies brand data and cigarettes smoked per day. Figure 4-9 shows an increase in number of cigarettes per day for smokers of low-nicotine cigarettes (slope = -2.41 cig/mg nicotine, $P < 0.005$).

This finding was supported by analyses of the CTS from 1990 and 1996 using sales-weighted nicotine as the measure of the nicotine yield of the brand smoked. Data on brand smoked were available from the 1990 CTS, but survey respondents only provided the name of the brand family and not the specific brand subspecies. An overall sales-weighted nicotine value was calculated using the 1990 and 1996 CTS for each brand using the sales and nicotine-yield data for each brand subspecies (see Appendix). The resulting populations were 2,964 in 1990 and 2,239 in 1996.

Figure 4-10 demonstrates the relationship of mean cigarettes per day to the level of nicotine in cigarettes for the 1990 and 1996 CTS. Significantly more cigarettes were smoked per day by ultralow nicotine cigarette smokers than by smokers of cigarettes with machine-measured yields of 0.75-0.90, 0.90-1.05, and 1.05+ mg nicotine in both survey years. There were no significant differences between mean cigarettes smoked per day for the 0.75-0.90, 0.90-1.05, and 1.05+ mg nicotine categories.

Data from the 1990 and 1996 CTS were modeled using a piecewise multiple linear regression that controlled for the effects of age, gender, race/ethnicity, and level of education. This model allowed for changes in the slope of the cigarettes per day versus nicotine yield line, with break points dividing the lines at defined levels of nicotine yield. The slopes of the two regression lines were compared; the left side of the piecewise regression modeled cigarettes per day for nicotine levels below 0.95 mg, while the

Figure 4-9

**Piecewise Linear Regression and Multiple Linear Regression of Cigarettes per Day, CTS, 1996, Using Individual Brand Nicotine Yield Data**

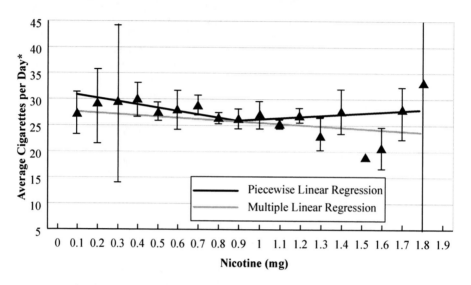

*Controlling for age, gender, race/ethnicity, and education level.*
*Note: The break point used for the piecewise regression was 0.95 mg of nicotine. FTC data for year 1996 were obtained from the FTC reports on the tar, nicotine, and carbon monoxide of domestic cigarettes (FTC, 1999). The population consisted of respondents, aged 25-64, who had smoked 100 cigarettes, smoked daily one year prior to the survey, smoked daily at the time of the survey, had not made a quit attempt in the past 12 months, and currently smoked 5+ cigarettes per day. The P-values and slopes of the piecewise regresssion are (slope$_{<0.95}$=-5.61, P$_{<0.95}$=0.0013) and (slope$_{>0.95}$=1.51, P$_{>0.95}$=0.5316).*

right side modeled cigarettes per day for nicotine levels greater than or equal to 0.95 mg. Figure 4-11 shows that there was an impact on the number of cigarettes per day for smokers of cigarettes with machine-measured nicotine yields below 0.95 mg nicotine. The slopes for the lines above 0.95 mg nicotine were not statistically different from zero. The nonstatistically significant difference in the slope of the lines from the two surveys was an artifact introduced because Marlboro® had a sales-weighted nicotine value of 0.94 in 1990 that increased slightly to 0.98 in 1996. This increase shifted the large population of Marlboro® smokers from one side of the 0.95-mg point to the other between the two analyses, and this shift resulted in a slight, nonsignificant shift in the slope of the lines above the 0.95 break point.

These analyses of the California Tobacco Surveys show a relationship between average daily cigarette consumption and the FTC nicotine yield of the cigarette smoked. More specifically, the sales-weighted analyses revealed that the average number of cigarettes smoked per day varies as a function of nicotine content below approximately 0.95 mg nicotine per cigarette. Smokers of cigarettes with ultralow nicotine levels showed a 20 percent increase in the number of cigarettes smoked per day compared to smokers of medium-nicotine cigarettes. Yet adults who smoked medium-tar and -nicotine cigarettes showed no significant difference in the mean number of

Figure 4-10
**Cigarettes Smoked per Day by Level of Sales-Weighted Nicotine Yield (California Data)**

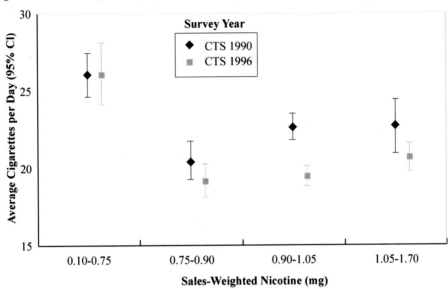

*Source: FTC data for years 1990 and 1996 were obtained from two FTC reports on the tar, nicotine, and carbon monoxide of domestic cigarettes (FTC, 1992 & 1999). Sales data for 1990 were obtained from the Maxwell Report (Maxwell, 1994). Sales data for 1996 were not available to the public. The tobacco companies, therefore, provided the 1996 sales-weighted nicotine levels using the same methodology used for the 1990 analysis. Sales-weighting for overall brand was accomplished by weighting each sub-brand nicotine level by its corresponding 1990/1996 market share. The sum of the weighted sub-brand nicotine levels provided the overall nicotine level for the brand. The population consisted of respondents, aged 25-64, who had smoked 100 cigarettes, smoked daily one year prior to the survey, smoked daily at the time of the survey, had not made a quit attempt in the past 12 months, and were currently smoking 5+ cigarettes per day.*

cigarettes per day when compared to those who smoked relatively high-tar and -nicotine cigarettes. With current cigarette designs, which depend heavily on ventilated filters to lower the machine-measured yield, smokers appear to be able to compensate within a single cigarette to maintain nicotine intake obtained from cigarettes that yield more than approximately 0.95 mg nicotine. Below that level of nicotine, compensation with increasing number of cigarettes smoked per day may also play a role. This bifurcated response of cigarettes per day with nicotine yield may be a characteristic of the engineering of cigarettes for elasticity of delivery described in the early sections of this chapter, and may not have occurred in cigarettes without ventilated filters.

**TEMPORAL TRENDS IN LUNG CANCER AND OTHER DISEASES IN MAJOR COHORT STUDIES**

Two major prospective mortality studies of smoking and disease bridged the period of greatest reduction in tar levels of cigarettes. Further examinations of these studies have revealed changes in smoking risks that have occurred as lower yield cigarettes were introduced and gained widespread acceptance.

119

Figure 4-11

**Piecewise Linear Regression of Cigarettes Smoked per Day by Sales-Weighted Nicotine Yield of the Brand Smoked (California Data)**

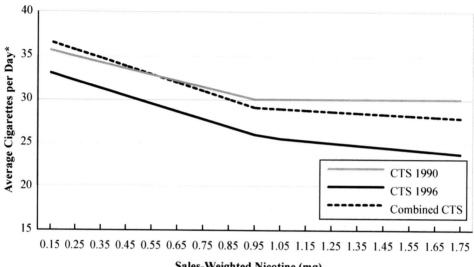

*Sales-Weighted Nicotine (mg)*

*Controlling for age, sex, race/ethnicity, and level of education.*

*Note: The break point used was 0.95 mg of nicotine for all three piecewise regressions. FTC data for years 1990 and 1996 were obtained from two FTC reports on the tar, nicotine, and carbon monoxide of domestic cigarettes (FTC, 1992 & 1999). Sales data for 1990 were obtained from the Maxwell Report (Maxwell, 1994). Sales data for 1996 were not available to the public. The tobacco companies, therefore, provided the 1996 sales-weighted nicotine levels using the same methodology used for the 1990 analysis. Sales-weighting for overall brand was accomplished by weighting each sub-brand nicotine level by its corresponding 1990/1996 market share. The sum of the weighted sub-brand nicotine levels provided the overall nicotine level for the brand. The population consisted of respondents, aged 25-64, who had smoked 100 cigarettes, had smoked daily one year prior to the survey, had not made a quit attempt in the past 12 months, and were currently smoking 5+ cigarettes per day. The p-values and slopes of the piecewise regression for CTS 1990 are (slope$_{<0.95}$=-7.12, P$_{<0.95}$<0.0001) and (slope$_{>0.95}$=-0.16, P$_{>0.95}$=0.9517). The p-values and slopes of the piecewise regression for CTS 1996 are (slope$_{<0.95}$=-9.13, P$_{<0.95}$<0.0001) and (slope$_{>0.95}$=-2.77, P$_{>0.95}$=0.5117). The P-values and slopes of the piecewise regression for the combined data are (slope$_{<0.95}$=-8.69, P$_{<0.95}$<0.0001) and (slope$_{>0.95}$=-0.80, P$_{>0.95}$=0.7171).*

The British Physicians Study examined lung cancer mortality rates (Doll *et al.*, 1994) with a follow-up period of over 40 years. The follow-up interval was divided into two 20-year periods, 1951-1971 and 1971-1991. Lung cancer death rates in male smokers, age-standardized to the same age distribution in the two follow-up intervals, increased by 19 percent to 314 per 100,000 during the second half of the study compared to 264 per 100,000 during the first 20 years of follow-up. This increase occurred during a period when the tar level of cigarettes in the United Kingdom had fallen dramatically. Lung cancer death rates for the entire U.K. population fell for males aged 35-54 and 55-74 during the 1971-1991 period (Peto *et al.*, 2000).

Differences in intensity and duration of smoking for the smokers examined in the two follow-up periods may have contributed to the increase in lung cancer death rates. Increased rates of cessation in the general population clearly contributed to the discordance of increasing lung cancer death rates among male smokers in the study as contrasted with decreasing lung cancer death rates for the male population as a whole. However, these increasing death rates among smokers also suggest that smoking may have become more hazardous over the follow-up interval. If there has been any benefit of the introduction of lower yield cigarettes in the United Kingdom for the physicians followed in the British Physicians Study, it is small enough to have been overwhelmed by the differences in intensity and duration of smoking between the first and second 20-years of the study.

Findings were similar for a comparison of the two Cancer Prevention Studies (CPS I and CPS II) which had very similar designs, but were conducted 23 years apart—CPS-I began in 1959 and CPS-II began in 1982. Comparisons of the first 6 years of follow-up in the two studies (Thun and Heath, 1997; Thun *et al.*, 1997b) demonstrated that lung cancer death rates increased between the two follow-up periods, a timeframe where substantial falls in machine-measured tar yields occurred for U.S. cigarettes. Detailed examination of the two populations studied showed that there were substantial differences in these two populations in the duration and number of cigarettes smoked per day, particularly for females (Thun *et al.*, 1997b), and these differences in smoking behaviors explained some but not all of the differences in lung cancer death rates. Figure 4-12 presents age-standardized death rates for male and female participants of CPS-I and CPS-II. There was no change in the death rates for male and female never smokers between the two studies, but the lung cancer death rates for current smokers increased dramatically between the two studies. The increase in lung cancer death rates between the two time periods was reduced, but not eliminated, when the rates were adjusted for differences in the number of cigarettes smoked per day and duration of smoking.

Nonfiltered cigarette smokers in CPS-I were compared to nonfiltered, mixed, and filtered cigarette smokers in CPS-II. Among males (see Figure 4-13), there was a dramatic increase in lung cancer risk for nonfilter smokers in CPS-II compared to CPS-I, and even the filter smokers in CPS-II had slightly higher lung cancer rates than the nonfilter smokers in CPS-I. Among females (see Figure 4-14), there were dramatically higher rates for all three categories of smokers in CPS-II compared to CPS-I. The rates in Figures 4-13 and 4-14 were age-standardized, but were not adjusted for differences in the number of cigarettes smoked per day or duration of smoking; it is likely that these differences may have contributed to the differences in lung cancer mortality between the two studies, particularly for females. However, the comparisons do not suggest that even filter smokers in CPS-II had any reduction in lung cancer risk when compared to smokers in CPS-I more than 20 years earlier. Some of this increase in lung cancer risk between the two studies may have resulted from greater availability of cigarettes and resultant heavier smoking among adolescents during the period when smokers in CPS-II were initiating their smoking behaviors. Alternatively, increased depth of inhalation with lower yield cigarettes and higher levels of tobacco-specific nitrosamines in the tobacco used in more recent cigarettes (see Chapter 5) may also have contributed to the increases. But detailed examination of the risks in these two studies separated by over 20 years does not suggest a reduction in risk resulting from lower yield cigarettes.

Figure 4-12
**Death Rates from All Lung Cancers by Smoking Status, CPS-I and CPS-II (Adjusted for Current Amount and Duration of Smoking)**

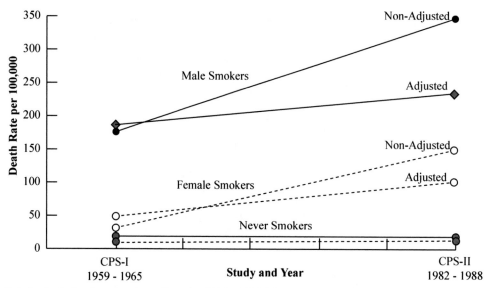

*Note: Death rates from lung cancer by smoking status, CPS-I and CPS-II (adjusted and unadjusted for current amount and duration).*

Figure 4-13
**Male Lung Cancer Death Rates by Filter Use, CPS-I and CPS-II**

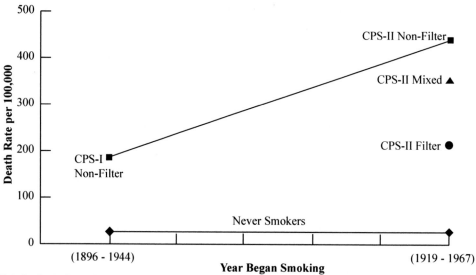

*Note: Death rates form all lung cancers among men by filter use, CPS-I and CPS-II.*

Both of these studies indicate that the lung cancer relative risks associated with smoking increased over the same time period when smokers in the U.S. and U.K. were switching to lower yield and filtered cigarettes in substantial numbers.

Figure 4-14
**Female Lung Cancer Death Rates by Filter Use, CPS-I and CPS-II**

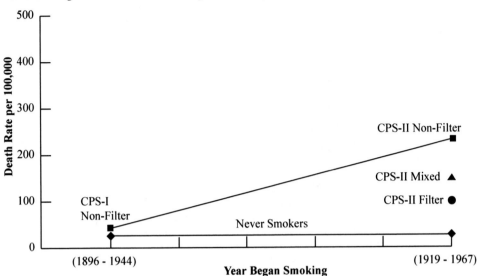

Note: Death rate from all lung cancers among women by filter use, CPS-I and CPS-II.

**TEMPORAL TRENDS IN NATIONAL LUNG CANCER DEATH RATES AND SMOKING BEHAVIORS**

The ultimate measure of a benefit from any reduction in the risk of smoking is a change in national death rates. Lung cancer death rates in both the United States and United Kingdom have declined among males in recent years. Several investigators have examined the relationships between smoking behaviors and changes in lung cancer mortality in both countries, and these analyses are now considered in relation to trends in tar yields of the cigarettes smoked in both countries.

**Published Models Using Smoking Behavior to Predict National Lung Cancer Death Rates**

In postulating the multi-stage model of carcinogenesis, Armitage and Doll (1961) suggested that multiple inheritable changes in the cell are required to cause malignant transformation. In this model, successive stages in the transformation of one cell may be separated from each other by several years, and the factors influencing early stages may be different from those influencing later stages. In its simplest form, this model implies that incidence of lung cancer at a given age is a constant times age raised to a power. Doll and Peto (1978) formulated the equation for lung cancer as Incidence = $0.273(\text{cigarettes/day} + 6)^2(\text{age} - 22.5)^{4.5}$, with the values in the formula derived from the lung cancer mortality experience of British physicians. The term (age – 22.5) was derived by assuming a uniform age of smoking uptake of 19 years and a 3.5-year latency from carcinogenic transformation of the cell to death from lung cancer. This term becomes duration of smoking prior to carcinogenic transformation for current smokers.

Variations of this model have been used by a number of investigators to match British national smoking prevalence data with British lung cancer

123

death rates. Stevens and Moolgavkar (1979, 1984) and Moolgavkar and colleagues (1989) used birth-cohort data on tobacco prevalence and birth-cohort-specific, cumulative tar-weighted cigarette consumption to construct a model that fit British birth-cohort/lung cancer death-rate data. Townsend (1978) expanded the basic multistage model to include birth-cohort-specific duration of exposure and number of cigarettes smoked per day. This model used the prevalence of smoking estimated in 5-calendar-year increments to divide each birth cohort into strata with different durations of smoking. A weighted mean of the number of cigarettes smoked per day at each age was used as the dosage term.

However, the weighting used assumed that recent smoking was more important than past smoking, decreasing the weight of duration of smoking. The number of cigarettes was also adjusted by assuming that filtered cigarettes were 40 percent less carcinogenic and that the carcinogenic risk of a cigarette was directly proportional to the machine-measured tar yield of the cigarette. The estimated lung cancer occurrence for each of the fractions with different durations of exposure was summed and added to the never-smoker risk to predict the lung cancer death rate for the birth cohort. Never-smoker death rates were taken from the American Cancer Society's prospective mortality study of 1 million males and females (Hammond, 1966).

To test this model, Townsend (1978) varied the constants in the model over a range and found the values that resulted in the best fit of the model to the British age-specific lung cancer mortality data. When the exponent for the duration of exposure term was set at 5 (the best-fit value), the model explained 98 percent of the variation in excess mortality in the male birth cohorts but only 84.8 percent of the variation in females.

Townsend's study was intended to develop a model of U.K. lung cancer mortality and was not intended to directly examine the question of risk reduction with low-yield cigarettes. The author assumed that the risk was directly proportional to the tar value of the cigarette smoked in creating their model. Adjustments for filters and tar content of the cigarettes in this study reduced the predicted risk of cigarettes by almost 40 percent from 1946 to 1966. The fit of the tar data in the model may be the result of the reduced weight given past smoking behaviors.

Brown and Kessler (1988) used a multistage model to predict U.S. lung cancer death rates to the year 2025. This model incorporated terms for calendar-year effects and a term for cohort effects and used a tar-weighted consumption measure for the number of cigarettes smoked per day. The model assumed a linear relationship between tar content and lung cancer risk and used a single cohort term to model the complex effects of differences in age of initiation and duration of exposure that occur across cohorts. These assumptions resulted in a model that predicted that lung cancer death rates in males would change very little between 1985 and 2010. The projection was not consistant with the decline in lung cancer death rates among white males that occurred following a peak in age-adjusted white male death rates in 1990 (Wingo *et al.*, 1999).

In contrast, Tolley and colleagues (1991) used a compartment model (*i.e.*, discrete state-discrete time model of health processes) to estimate lung cancer death rates using birth-cohort-specific smoking initiation, prevalence, and cessation rates for the United States and the relationship of dose and duration of smoking developed from the British Physicians Study (Peto, 1986). Without any adjustment for tar, they predicted that changes in smoking prevalence rates alone would project a decline in white male lung cancer death rates during the mid 1980s, a prediction that closely matched the actual death rate trends.

Swartz (1992) used birth-cohort-specific smoking rates estimated by Harris (1983) and a multistage carcinogenesis model developed by Whittemore (1988) to estimate U.S. lung cancer mortality. The modeled estimates predicted a 12-percent decline in lung cancer rates from 1970 to 1985, a period when lung cancer death rates increased by 26 percent. Substantial declines in tar yield of cigarettes occurred prior to and during this period, and this model suggested that risks of cigarette smoking increased rather than decreased over the period when tar yield was falling.

More recently, Mannino and colleagues (2001) examined age- and birth-cohort-specific U.S. lung cancer death rates for White males and White females, adjusting for age- and birth-cohort-specific differences in prevalence and duration of smoking. Differences between male and female lung cancer rates, and differences in lung cancer rates across birth cohorts, were eliminated by adjusting for differences in smoking prevalence and duration of smoking. These researchers noted: "Differences in lung cancer death rates across birth cohorts of U.S. men and women primarily reflect differences in the prevalence and duration of smoking. Changes in cigarette design that have greatly reduced tar yields have a relatively small effect compared with that of people's smoking status and duration of smoking."

National lung cancer death rate data in the United Kingdom were compared to two lung cancer mortality studies conducted 40 years apart (1950 and 1990) to examine the effects of changes in smoking prevalence (Peto *et al.*, 2000). The lung cancer risk produced by being a cigarette smoker increased between 1950 and 1990. This increase was attributed to the longer durations of smoking experienced by smokers as of 1990. The changes in smoking prevalence were consistent with the changes in lung cancer death rates for females and for older males, but younger males had declines in age-specific lung cancer death rates over time that were much larger than those in smoking prevalence. Reduction in lung cancer risks from smoking low-yield cigarettes was suggested as an explanation for this observation.

**Influence of Smoking Behaviors on Lung Cancer Death Rates in the United States and United Kingdom**  When considering a potential effect of changing cigarette design over time on national lung cancer death rates, it is necessary to control for changes in smoking prevalence and intensity over time because smoking intensity and duration are more powerful predictors of lung cancer risk in epidemiological studies than is tar yield of the cigarette smoked. Cigarette smoking was more widely prevalent during the early part of the twentieth century in the United Kingdom than in the United States. For example, per-capita consumption of cigarettes in the United Kingdom for the year 1905 was 380 cigarettes per adult over age 15 (Wald and Nicolaides-Bouman, 1991), whereas per-capita consumption in the United States was only 70 cigarettes per adult over age 18 for the same year (Burns *et al.*, 1997a). In contrast, filtered and low-yield cigarettes were introduced and widely accepted in the United States ahead of their use in the United Kingdom (see Figure 4-15).

Lung cancer death rates over time reached peak levels that were much higher in the United Kingdom than in the United States, particularly among males. However, male lung cancer death rates peaked earlier (around 1970) in the United Kingdom (Peto *et al.*, 2000) compared to the United States (around 1990), and they declined more steeply in the United Kingdom than in the United States. Lung cancer death rates in the United Kingdom are now lower than those in the United States for both males and females under age 70 (Peto *et al.*, 2000).

In both the United States and the United Kingdom, the prevalence of smoking among males born in the early part of the last century exceeded 70 percent, with peak smoking prevalence rates among males in the United Kingdom being somewhat higher (more than 85 percent) (Burns *et al.*, 1997a; Wald and Nicolaides-Bouman, 1991). Additionally, males among the older birth cohorts in the United Kingdom smoked hand-rolled cigarettes in high percentages (Wald and Nicolaides-Bouman, 1991). The prevalence of ever smoking has declined among male birth cohorts born after 1930 in both countries.

Lung cancer occurs predominantly at older ages due to the powerful effect of duration of smoking on lung cancer rates. However, because of the temporal trends in type of cigarettes manufactured and sold, older smokers also began smoking with much higher yield cigarettes, and they smoked these cigarettes for much more of their smoking experience than did younger smokers. As a result, changes over time in age-specific lung cancer death rates at younger ages have been suggested as a more sensitive meas-ure of the population impact of lower yield cigarettes on lung cancer rates. Younger smokers are, on average, more likely than older smokers to have begun their smoking with filtered and lower yield cigarettes and would have smoked them for a larger fraction of their smoking experience. In addition, age-specific lung cancer death rates are available from the 1950s onward allowing a long period of observation during which most of the changes in cigarette design took place.

The use of temporal changes in age-specific lung cancer death rates at younger ages as a measure of change in disease risks from low-yield ciga-rettes is somewhat limited by the observation that most younger smokers in the United Kingdom (Wald and Nicolaides-Bouman, 1991) and the United States (CDC, 2000) use cigarettes with mid-range yields of tar rather than the ultralow yield products. However, the tar values of these mid-range yield cigarettes are substantially lower than the tar yields of cigarettes sold 20-40 years earlier. In addition, use of low tar-yield cigarettes is currently

Figure 4-15
**Market Share of Filter and Non-Filter Cigarettes in the United States and United Kingdom, 1925-1990**

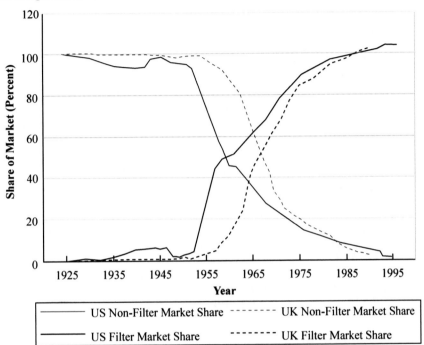

*Note: U.S. data were obtained from Maxwell Report (Maxwell, 1994). British data were obtained from UK Smoking Statistics (Wald and Nicolaides-Bouman, 1991).*

more common among older smokers than among younger smokers in both the U.S. and U.K. (see Figure 4-1 and Wald and Nicolaides-Bouman 1991), suggesting that a population effect of reduction in risk with use of these cigarettes, if present, might be larger among these older smokers. Indeed, it is among older smokers that the epidemiological data presented earlier in this chapter have suggested a decreased risk. The reduction in disease risk over time, out of proportion to declines in prevalence, is evident predominantly among younger age groups in the United Kingdom. The decline in lung cancer risk over time among older age groups is more closely matched by the decline in smoking prevalence (Peto *et al.*, 2000).

There is a difference between the United States and the United Kingdom in the rate of rise of lung cancer with age. This difference is evident across most of the birth cohorts presented in Table 4-6. Figure 4-16 presents age-specific lung cancer death rates for two separate birth cohorts. Age-specific rates in the United States start lower than in the United Kingdom but then rise more rapidly with age for both younger and older birth cohorts.

This higher rate of lung cancer at younger ages may be due to differences in the distribution of age of initiation among younger male smokers

127

in the two countries. Table 4-7 presents self-reported recall of the age of smoking initiation by smokers who were at different ages at the time of the survey. Data are presented for three surveys conducted in the United Kingdom in 1971, 1981, and 1987 (Wald and Nicolaides-Bouman, 1991) and for data from the National Health Interview Survey of the United States for the years closest to the U.K. data when the question on age of initiation was asked. For both sets of surveys, the data presented are for the entire population and age of initiation is reported for current and former smokers combined. Initiation rates prior to age 13 are similar for both countries, but there is a substantially higher rate of initiation among those 14-15 years old in the United Kingdom. This higher rate of initiation early in adolescence could contribute to the higher rate of lung cancer deaths at younger ages observed in Figure 4-16.

The reasons for the higher rate of rise with age of lung cancer death rates in the United States compared to the United Kingdom are less clear, but may relate to cessation during young adulthood in the United Kingdom occurring earlier in calendar years compared to the United States, thereby lowering the lung cancer risk as the birth cohort aged. Data are not available to make this direct comparison of cessation, but by 1984, the prevalence rates for 25- to 34-year-old males in the United Kingdom (born 1950–1959) were 39 percent (Wald and Nicolaides-Bouman, 1991), whereas the rates in comparable cohorts of White males in the United States were somewhat higher (42-43 percent) (Burns *et al.*, 1997a). This lesser cessation in the United States could contribute to the more rapid rise in lung cancer death rates with age.

The observed difference in lung cancer death rates may also relate to differences in the pattern of cigarette use at younger ages in the two countries. Differences in age of initiation, intensity of smoking during early adolescence, and rates of cessation during young adulthood all may influence lung cancer death rates at younger ages. Lung cancer death rates rise with increasing number of cigarettes smoked per day and even more powerfully with the duration of smoking (Doll and Peto, 1978), but this increase occurs with a lag of approximately 20 years from onset of exposure. That is, approximately a 20-year duration of smoking is required before lung cancer rates in smokers begin to significantly exceed those in never smokers (Burns *et al.*, 1997b). As a result, lung cancer death rates at age 35 among smokers are much more influenced by that group of smokers who began to smoke before age 15, in contrast to those smokers who first started to smoke in their mid to late 20s. The epidemiological data would suggest that it is unlikely that those smokers who began smoking after age 15 make a substantive contribution to lung cancer death rates at age 35, given the 20-year lag time demonstrated between onset of smoking and increases in the risk of lung cancer due to smoking.

Differences in the intensity of smoking at younger ages during the process of becoming a regular smoker may also play a role. To the extent that the pattern of early smoking (prior to age 15) is episodic and confined to a few cigarettes per month, which is the pattern most commonly described among adolescent smokers currently under age 15 (Johnston *et*

Table 4-6

**Age- and Birth-Cohort-Specific Lung Cancer Death Rates for the United States and United Kingdom**

| | Lung Cancer Death Rate* | | | | | | | | | | |
| | Age (Midpoint of 5-Year Age Group) | | | | | | | | | | |
| **Midpoint of** | **United Kingdom** | | | | | | | | | | |
| **Birth Cohort** | 32.5 | 37.5 | 42.5 | 47.5 | 52.5 | 57.5 | 62.5 | 67.5 | 72.5 | 77.5 | 82.5 |
|---|---|---|---|---|---|---|---|---|---|---|---|
| 1873 | | | | | | | | | | | 167.30 |
| 1878 | | | | | | | | | | 243.01 | 259.83 |
| 1883 | | | | | | | | | 305.25 | 377.48 | 391.85 |
| 1888 | | | | | | | | 329.25 | 431.62 | 506.16 | 509.23 |
| 1893 | | | | | | | 289.47 | 428.10 | 538.81 | 650.73 | 679.95 |
| 1898 | | | | | | 219.13 | 353.38 | 512.62 | 662.33 | 764.63 | 812.65 |
| 1903 | | | | | 126.17 | 232.18 | 374.27 | 528.11 | 682.74 | 796.69 | 832.76 |
| 1908 | | | | 59.72 | 125.16 | 228.23 | 369.44 | 514.73 | 655.69 | 756.35 | 767.28 |
| 1913 | | | 24.87 | 57.76 | 120.75 | 215.69 | 344.15 | 479.32 | 616.24 | 678.27 | 669.39 |
| 1918 | | 9.78 | 25.00 | 55.08 | 111.60 | 202.32 | 316.22 | 437.96 | 553.20 | 592.54 | |
| 1923 | 3.76 | 9.47 | 22.38 | 53.96 | 106.37 | 184.94 | 294.74 | 402.30 | 475.24 | | |
| 1928 | 3.53 | 9.06 | 21.01 | 46.80 | 92.11 | 158.66 | 245.40 | 326.52 | | | |
| 1933 | 2.80 | 6.29 | 16.30 | 36.15 | 69.26 | 122.78 | 184.53 | | | | |
| 1938 | 2.49 | 5.90 | 12.96 | 29.62 | 59.51 | 102.18 | | | | | |
| 1943 | 2.24 | 4.97 | 11.24 | 26.26 | 49.74 | | | | | | |
| 1948 | 1.56 | 4.07 | 9.72 | 20.74 | | | | | | | |
| 1953 | 1.09 | 3.13 | 8.02 | | | | | | | | |
| 1958 | 0.77 | 2.13 | | | | | | | | | |
| 1963 | 0.65 | | | | | | | | | | |
| | **United States** | | | | | | | | | | |
| 1873 | | | | | | | | | | | 116.80 |
| 1878 | | | | | | | | | | 138.60 | 176.30 |
| 1883 | | | | | | | | | 148.90 | 199.60 | 222.60 |
| 1888 | | | | | | | | 157.80 | 232.20 | 268.30 | 325.40 |
| 1893 | | | | | | | 135.50 | 219.70 | 302.60 | 380.60 | 431.60 |
| 1898 | | | | | | 95.90 | 180.70 | 277.30 | 371.00 | 464.00 | 477.70 |
| 1903 | | | | | 58.20 | 114.92 | 199.88 | 306.95 | 418.93 | 502.80 | 543.33 |
| 1908 | | | | 30.40 | 68.71 | 127.55 | 228.01 | 329.42 | 458.80 | 546.20 | 584.96 |
| 1913 | | | 11.60 | 31.79 | 76.79 | 152.13 | 244.30 | 359.11 | 470.70 | 565.40 | 580.60 |
| 1918 | | 4.90 | 13.99 | 38.61 | 84.32 | 150.01 | 255.74 | 367.06 | 485.89 | 529.90 | |
| 1923 | 1.70 | 5.73 | 17.26 | 44.03 | 90.91 | 162.93 | 262.46 | 374.07 | 470.90 | | |
| 1928 | 1.97 | 7.05 | 21.54 | 47.86 | 95.28 | 167.41 | 268.18 | 359.60 | | | |
| 1933 | 2.00 | 7.34 | 19.30 | 45.44 | 86.59 | 159.35 | 233.60 | | | | |
| 1938 | 2.03 | 6.15 | 17.43 | 40.26 | 80.52 | 132.70 | | | | | |
| 1943 | 1.80 | 5.29 | 15.19 | 34.64 | 66.10 | | | | | | |
| 1948 | 1.12 | 4.32 | 11.63 | 26.20 | | | | | | | |
| 1953 | 0.98 | 3.85 | 9.50 | | | | | | | | |
| 1958 | 1.16 | 3.30 | | | | | | | | | |
| 1963 | 1.20 | | | | | | | | | | |

*Deaths per 100,000

*al.*, 2000), the exposure would not be expected to contribute substantively to lung cancer death rates at age 35. To the extent that the pattern of early smoking is regular smoking of one-half pack or more per day, it would be expected to contribute relatively more to lung cancer death rates at younger ages. There are few data available to assess changes over time in the intensi-

Figure 4-16
**Birth-Cohort-Specific Male Lung Cancer Death Rates by Age**

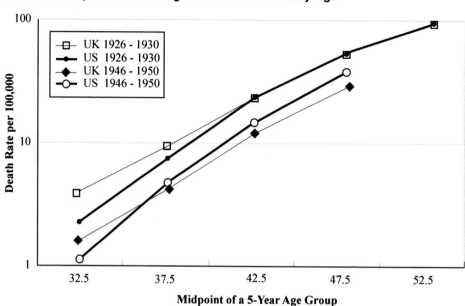

*Note: U.S. lung cancer death rates were provided for the years 1960-1994 by D.M. Mannino (personal communication, 2000).*

ty of smoking during early adolescence in either the United States or United Kingdom, but it might be expected that the intensity of smoking during early adolescence may have changed in the direction of reduced intensity due to the tobacco education and control efforts implemented in both countries. Data from the Monitoring the Future Study (Johnston *et al.*, 2000) for high school seniors in the United States showed a decline from the late 1970s to the present in the percentage of those adolescents who had smoked within 30 days of the survey who were either daily smokers or smokers of one-half pack of cigarettes per day or more. These data demonstrate a decline in intensity of smoking among high school seniors over the last 25 years, and a similar decline may have occurred among all adolescents from the mid 1950s when concerns about the disease risks of smoking were first widely publicized.

Patterns of cessation can also influence rates of lung cancer at early ages. Among birth cohorts born before 1900, the pattern of smoking behavior with age did not include substantial rates of cessation under age 60 (Burns *et al.*, 1997a). However, beginning with the widespread publication of the disease risks associated with smoking in the mid 1950s, smokers began to quit at younger ages, so more recent birth cohorts have substantial fractions of smokers who have quit prior to age 30. These smokers who quit early would not accumulate a substantial duration of smoking, and therefore would have very low risks.

Table 4-7

**Percentage of Men Starting to Smoke Any Tobacco in the United States and the United Kingdom at Different Ages (by Age at time of Survey)**

| Age at Time of Survey | Age at Initiation | Year of Survey: | United States 1970 | 1980 | 1987 | United Kingdom 1971 | 1981 | 1987 |
|---|---|---|---|---|---|---|---|---|
| 20-24 | 13 and less | | 6.9 | 8.4 | 9.7 | 31 | 9 | 10 |
| | 14-15 | | 8.3 | 11.6 | 6.8 | | 15 | 17 |
| | 16-17 | | 19.6 | 18.2 | 10.0 | 21 | 19 | 17 |
| | 18-19 | | 18.9 | 8.7 | 9.0 | 11 | 5 | 6 |
| | 20-24 | | 6.9 | 6.2 | 3.5 | 2 | 2 | 1 |
| | Don't know | | 2.5 | 1.8 | 0 | 2 | 3 | 3 |
| | Never smoked | | 36.9 | 45.1 | 61.0 | 34 | 47 | 47 |
| | | | 100 | 100 | 100 | 100 | 100 | 100 |
| | | | | | | | | |
| 25-34 | 13 and less | | 8.6 | 7.6 | 8.8 | 29 | . | . |
| | 14-15 | | 11.8 | 11.5 | 10.8 | | . | . |
| | 16-17 | | 16.6 | 14.6 | 12.1 | 24 | . | . |
| | 18-19 | | 17.9 | 17.1 | 9.9 | 13 | . | . |
| | 20-24 | | 12.5 | 10.7 | 7.3 | 8 | . | . |
| | 25-29 | | 1.6 | 0.8 | 1.1 | 1 | . | . |
| | 30-34 | | 0.2 | 0 | 0 | 0 | . | . |
| | Don't know | | 2.8 | 1.7 | 0 | 2 | . | . |
| | Never Smoked | | 28.0 | 36.0 | 49.9 | 22 | . | . |
| | | | 100 | 100 | 99.9 | 100 | | |
| | | | | | | | | |
| 25-29 | 13 and less | | 9.4 | 8.3 | 9.1 | . | 8 | 9 |
| | 14-15 | | 11.7 | 10.1 | 10.6 | . | 19 | 16 |
| | 16-17 | | 15.9 | 14.8 | 12.7 | . | 21 | 15 |
| | 18-19 | | 18.3 | 16.6 | 8.8 | . | 7 | 6 |
| | 20-24 | | 11.0 | 8.3 | 6.7 | . | 5 | 5 |
| | 25-29 | | 0.8 | 1.1 | 1.3 | . | 1 | 1 |
| | Don't know | | 2.4 | 1.4 | 0.0 | . | 5 | 3 |
| | Never Smoked | | 30.5 | 39.4 | 50.8 | . | 34 | 46 |
| | | | 100 | 100 | 100 | | 100 | 100 |
| | | | | | | | | |
| 30-34 | 13 and less | | 7.5 | 6.8 | 8.6 | . | 9 | 12 |
| | 14-15 | | 11.9 | 13.1 | 10.9 | . | 17 | 14 |
| | 16-17 | | 17.4 | 14.4 | 11.6 | . | 19 | 13 |
| | 18-19 | | 17.3 | 17.7 | 11.2 | . | 8 | 9 |
| | 20-24 | | 14.6 | 13.5 | 7.8 | . | 6 | 4 |
| | 25-29 | | 2.8 | 0.4 | 0.9 | . | 2 | 2 |
| | 30+ | | 0.4 | 0 | 0 | . | 0 | 0 |
| | Don't know | | 3.5 | 2.1 | 0 | . | 4 | 5 |
| | Never Smoked | | 24.5 | 32.1 | 49.0 | . | 36 | 42 |
| | | | 99.9 | 100.1 | 100 | | 100 | 100 |

Note: The British data were obtained from UK Smoking Statistics (Wald and Nicolaides-Bouman, 1991). The U.S. data were obtained from NHIS 1970, 1980, and 1987. The population consisted of United States White males, aged 20+, who were self-respondents for the above-mentioned NHIS years.

In the United States, most first use of cigarettes occurs before age 18 (U.S.DHHS, 1994). Changes in smoking prevalence after reaching adulthood reflect rates of cessation almost exclusively. However, data from Table 4-8 suggests that, at least for the period after 1976 and perhaps during the 1950s, the prevalence of smoking among 20-24 year old males in the

United Kingdom was substantially higher than the prevalence reported four years earlier for 16-19 year old males. This suggests that a substantial fraction of initiation in the U.K. may have occurred after age 20. These smokers will not have accumulated twenty years of smoking until they are at least 40-44 years old and are unlikely to meaningfully contribute to the lung cancer death rate for ages under age forty.

In summary, a variety of changes in the patterns of cigarette smoking have occurred in both the United States and the United Kingdom, including changes in smoking initiation as well as smoking cessation. These changes may be responsible for many of the differences across time and between the countries in national lung cancer mortality rates.

**Examination of Trends Over Time in Age-Specific Lung Cancer Death Rates in the United States and United Kingdom**
Age-specific lung cancer death rates in the United Kingdom have declined dramatically in the last several decades, and these reductions have exceeded the declines in smoking prevalence among the same age groups for those under age 45 (Peto *et al.*, 2000). One possible explanation for the more rapid decline over time in lung cancer death rates compared to trends in smoking prevalence is decreased risk from smoking lower yield cigarettes. A reduced risk from smoking lower yield products might be first evident among those who are younger because they would have had a larger proportion of their smoking experience with these lower yield cigarettes. However, as discussed in the previous section, it is important to examine other aspects of smoking behavior that could also account for changes in lung cancer rates before attributing the differences in lung cancer death rates to changes in cigarette yield.

Age- and birth-cohort-specific lung cancer death rates for the United States and United Kingdom are presented in Table 4-6. The data for the United Kingdom are those provided by Peto and associates (2000) as the mean lung cancer death rates for sequential groups of 5 calendar years presented as 5-year age-specific death rates. These rates were converted to birth-cohort rates by subtracting the mid point of the age group from the 5-year-calendar period over which the death rates were averaged to approximate the years of birth for that age group. Rates for the United States are actual birth-cohort- and age-specific lung cancer death rates provided by Mannino and colleagues (2001).

It is evident that there have been very dramatic percentage declines in male lung cancer death rates in the United Kingdom among those under age 50, with particularly dramatic percentage declines under age 40. Rates for those aged 40-49 declined by about two-thirds, with rates in the youngest age group declining by approximately 85 percent. These declines exceed the approximately 50 percent decline in smoking prevalence over time at these same ages (see Table 4-8). Among those over age 50 in the United Kingdom, declines in smoking prevalence and lung cancer death rates approximate each other more closely.

In the United States, there have been much less dramatic declines in lung cancer death rates among white males under age 50, and they more closely match changes in smoking prevalence. Data on smoking prevalence and lung cancer death rate by birth cohort and age are available for the United States and are presented in Table 4-9 for White males. At ages 30-34, the fall in lung cancer death rates across sequential birth cohorts is similar in magnitude to that observed for the fall in smoking prevalence, particularly for the fall in smoking prevalence for the same birth cohort when the cohort was age 12. At ages 35-39, lung cancer death rates fall approximately 48 percent from their peak in the 1931-1935 birth cohort to the 1951-1955 cohort, whereas smoking prevalence falls only 39 percent. However, there is also a 48 percent fall in the prevalence of smoking at age 12 across the same cohorts. Similarly, there is a 46 percent decline in lung cancer death rates at ages 40-44 from a peak in the 1926-1930 birth cohort to the last birth cohort where smoking prevalence data are available, with a decline in smoking prevalence of 36 percent, but the decline in smoking prevalence at age 12 is also 36 percent. Given the limited precision of these estimates and the difficulty in defining the exact measure of smoking behavior that should be compared (*e.g.*, no measures of intensity of smoking at younger ages are available), the changes in smoking behaviors across birth cohorts may well explain the changes in lung cancer death rates in the United States A more detailed examination of this relationship for all birth cohorts born after 1910 is presented later in this chapter.

Examination of the changes in lung cancer death rates at ages 30-34 and 35-39 with sequential birth cohorts in the United Kingdom (see Table 4-6) reveals that rates have fallen dramatically, particularly for those born after 1945. Lung cancer death rates currently occurring in those age groups in the United Kingdom approximate rates estimated for nonsmokers in these age groups by extrapolating retrogressively the rates observed among older nonsmokers in the CPS-I study to include these age groups. The rates for never smokers estimated are 1.2 at ages 30-34 and 1.9 at ages 35-39. These dramatic changes in lung cancer death rates at these younger ages in the United Kingdom are consistent with the essential elimination of a smoking effect at ages 30-34 and a near elimination of the effect at ages 35-39.

It is theoretically possible that this reduction in age-specific lung cancer death rates is due to a reduction in the carcinogenicity of the cigarettes smoked to almost zero in this younger age population, who would have initiated smoking cigarettes with substantially lower tar yields when compared with older birth cohorts, but this explanation is unlikely. In the United Kingdom (Wald and Nicolaides-Bouman, 1991), as is true in the United States, approximately 90 percent of young smokers smoke cigarettes with 10 mg or more tar yields, and approximately one-half smoke cigarettes with yields of 15 mg tar or higher. This distribution of cigarettes smoked, as well as the very modest risk reductions demonstrated in epidemiological studies and the current understanding of compensation (see Chapter 2), make it biologically implausible that smoking low-yield cigarettes would have almost no risk. An alternate, explanation is that prevalence of intense smoking at very young ages has declined dramatically, following demonstration in the 1950s of increased disease risks due to smoking and the

Table 4-8

**Prevalence of Cigarette Smoking among British Males Aged 16 and Over, by Age: ONS General Household Survey, 1976-1996**

| Year | 16-19 | 20-24 | 25-34 | 35-59 | | 60+ |
|------|-------|-------|-------|-------|---|-----|
| 1948 | 61 | 74 | 76 | 70 | | 39 |
| 1949 | 54 | 73 | 71 | 68 | | 38 |
| 1950 | 51 | 68 | 70 | 66 | | 38 |
| 1951 | 51 | 68 | 70 | 66 | | 42 |
| 1952 | 47 | 62 | 67 | 64 | | 40 |
| 1953 | 47 | 61 | 67 | 64 | | 42 |
| 1954 | 46 | 63 | 66 | 63 | | 42 |
| 1955 | 47 | 59 | 67 | 62 | | 39 |
| 1956 | 52 | 65 | 67 | 65 | | 45 |
| 1957 | 59 | 61 | 66 | 63 | | 45 |
| 1958 | 54 | 63 | 65 | 63 | | 42 |
| 1959 | 60 | 62 | 65 | 63 | | 48 |
| 1960 | 65 | 67 | 64 | 64 | | 46 |
| 1961 | 61 | 67 | 60 | 61 | | 46 |
| 1962 | 61 | 62 | 59 | 60 | | 44 |
| 1963 | 56 | 65 | 60 | 54 | | 42 |
| 1964 | 56 | 61 | 55 | 57 | | 45 |
| 1965 | 50 | 63 | 56 | 56 | | 44 |
| 1966 | 54 | 60 | 59 | 56 | | 44 |
| 1967 | 52 | 61 | 56 | 56 | | 45 |
| 1968 | 57 | 69 | 57 | 57 | | 46 |
| 1969 | 53 | 62 | 60 | 54 | | 44 |
| 1970 | 55 | 58 | 60 | 55 | | 46 |
| 1971 | 53 | 57 | 55 | 50 | | 43 |
| 1972 | 51 | 60 | 54 | 51 | | 42 |
| 1973 | 49 | 62 | 53 | 49 | | 41 |
| 1974 | 48 | 55 | 55 | 51 | | 40 |
| 1975 | 49 | 53 | 46 | 49 | | 41 |

| | 16-19 | 20-24 | 25-34 | 35-49 | 50-59 | 60+ |
|------|-------|-------|-------|-------|-------|-----|
| 1976 | 38 | 46 | 48 | 49 | 49 | 40 |
| 1978 | 35 | 46 | 49 | 47 | 47 | 38 |
| 1980 | 33 | 44 | 47 | 45 | 45 | 34 |
| 1982 | 31 | 39 | 40 | 39 | 41 | 32 |
| 1984 | 28 | 39 | 39 | 38 | 38 | 29 |
| 1986 | 30 | 41 | 37 | 37 | 34 | 28 |
| 1988 | 28 | 37 | 37 | 36 | 32 | 25 |
| 1990 | 28 | 39 | 37 | 34 | 27 | 24 |
| 1992 | 29 | 39 | 35 | 31 | 27 | 20 |
| 1994 | 28 | 42 | 34 | 31 | 26 | 17 |
| 1996 | 25 | 43 | 38 | 30 | 27 | 17 |

*Note: The prevalence of smoking for years 1976 to 1996 was obtained from the Office for National Statistics General Household Survey, 1976 to 1996 (ONS, 1998).*

social policy changes that followed the publication of the Royal College of Physicians' report on smoking (Royal College of Physicians, 1962).

Lung cancer death rates for males in the United Kingdom have also declined for ages 40-44 and ages 45-49 with each age group declining to one-third of its peak value, a proportionate reduction that exceeds the

Table 4-9

**Comparison of Birth-Cohort-Specific Current Smoking Prevalence at Different Ages with Birth-Cohort- and Age-Specific Lung Cancer Death Rates for White Males in the United States**

| | Birth-Cohort-Specific Current Smoking Prevalence | | | | | Age (Years) | | | | | | |
| BirthCohort | 12 | 17 | 22 | 27 | 30 | Lung Cancer Death Rate 30-34 | Smoking Prevalence 35 | Lung Cancer Death Rate 35-39 | Smoking Prevalence 40 | Lung Cancer Death Rate 40-44 | Smoking Prevalence 45 | Lung Cancer Death Rate 45-49 |
|---|---|---|---|---|---|---|---|---|---|---|---|---|
| 1906-1910 | 10.89 | 41.60 | 71.20 | 76.46 | 77.59 | — | 76.89 | — | 72.12 | — | 69.73 | 30.40 |
| 1911-1915 | 8.87 | 42.42 | 73.15 | 78.26 | 79.31 | — | 77.57 | — | 74.43 | 11.60 | 70.01 | 31.79 |
| 1916-1920 | 9.74 | 43.11 | 72.32 | 78.15 | 78.45 | — | 75.65 | 4.90 | 71.66 | 13.99 | 65.83 | 38.61 |
| 1921-1925 | 8.27 | 40.61 | 75.36 | 78.55 | 77.90 | 1.70 | 73.92 | 5.73 | 68.20 | 17.26 | 60.74 | 44.03 |
| 1926-1930 | 7.59 | 44.64 | 74.39 | 75.81 | 75.06 | 1.97 | 70.63 | 7.05 | 63.68 | 21.54 | 55.76 | 47.86 |
| 1931-1935 | 7.55 | 43.69 | 71.89 | 72.75 | 70.75 | 2.00 | 64.61 | 7.34 | 56.59 | 19.30 | 49.96 | 45.44 |
| 1936-1940 | 6.66 | 40.80 | 68.38 | 68.19 | 65.10 | 2.03 | 58.05 | 6.15 | 51.72 | 17.43 | 45.09 | 40.26 |
| 1941-1945 | 6.04 | 41.40 | 66.09 | 62.85 | 59.67 | 1.80 | 53.69 | 5.29 | 46.98 | 15.19 | 40.14 | 36.64 |
| 1946-1950 | 4.85 | 34.85 | 58.57 | 54.81 | 51.47 | 1.12 | 45.78 | 4.32 | 40.46 | 11.63 | — | 26.20 |
| 1951-1955 | 3.90 | 32.48 | 50.26 | 47.01 | 43.91 | 0.98 | 39.50 | 3.85 | — | 9.50 | — | — |
| 1956-1960 | 3.85 | 33.06 | 44.38 | 41.59 | 39.69 | 1.16 | — | 3.30 | — | — | — | — |
| 1961-1965 | 4.54 | 28.90 | 39.36 | — | — | 1.20 | — | — | — | — | — | — |

*Note: U.S. smoking prevalence was obtained from NCI Smoking and Tobacco Control Monograph No. 8 (Burns et al., 1997a). U.S. lung cancer death rates were obtained for years 1955 to 1995. The death rate for 1955 came from the NCI Monograph 59 (NCI, 1982). Death rates for the years 1960-1994 were provided by D.M. Mannino (personal communication, 2000). The death rate for 1995 was obtained from NCHS data.*

change in smoking prevalence within these age groups. Declines in lung cancer death rates among older age groups are more modest and are consistent with changes in smoking prevalence.

Unfortunately, birth cohort analyses of smoking behavior using the U.K. data are not available to generate a table similar to that provided for the United States (see Table 4-9). However, data are available on the prevalence of smoking by males of different ages for the calendar years 1948-1996 (see Table 4-8). These data offer some insight into the changes in age of smoking initiation and rates of cessation that have occurred among males in the United Kingdom over the time periods that relate to changes in lung cancer death rates among sequential birth cohorts of males 40-44 and 45-49 years old, as seen in Table 4-6.

The smoking prevalence rates estimated prior to 1976 in Table 4-8 for the United Kingdom are from the Tobacco Research Council/Tobacco Advisory Council surveys as reported by Wald and Nicolaides-Bouman (1991). Data after that point are from the General Household Survey (ONS, 1998), which began in 1976. The smoking prevalence estimates for males 16-19 years old prior to 1976 vary substantially from year to year, and they are too unstable to define year-to-year-to-year changes with precision. The data for males 20-24 and 25-34 years old are more stable.

In 1950, the birth cohort born between 1926 and 1930 would have been 20-24 years old, and that age group had a smoking prevalence of 68 percent in 1950 (see Table 4-8). In 1975, the 1951-1955 birth cohort would have been 20-24 years old, and that age group had a smoking prevalence of 53 percent in 1975. The decline in smoking prevalence was 22 percent in contrast to a decline of 62 percent in lung cancer rates at ages 40-44 across the same cohorts.

The birth cohort born between 1926 and 1930 had a smoking prevalence of 68 percent in 1950, and 20 years later, when they would have been ages 40-44, they had a prevalence of approximately 55 percent (as represented by the 35- to 59-year-old age group in Table 4-8). The 1951-1955 birth cohort had a prevalence of 53 percent at ages 20-24; 20 years later in 1996, their smoking prevalence would be approximately 30 percent. These changes in prevalence rates suggest that at least 19 percent of smokers in the 1926-1930 cohort had quit smoking by ages 40-44, whereas at least 43 percent of smokers in the 1951-1955 cohort had quit. These estimates are conservative because any individuals who initiated smoking after age 24 would reduce the estimated rates of cessation prior to age 40 among those smokers who initiated smoking prior to age 24. This increase in cessation during young adulthood would be expected to add to the decline in lung cancer risk produced by the fall in smoking prevalence at ages 20-24 because it would reduce the number of smokers with duration of smoking sufficient to increase their lung cancer risk.

A second characteristic of smoking behavior that differs across these birth cohorts in the United Kingdom is age of smoking initiation, particularly initiation prior to or early in adolescence. Comparison of the smoking prevalence rates in Table 4-8 at ages 20-24 in a given calendar year to those of 16- to 19-year-old smokers from 4 calendar years earlier offers some insight into the fraction of 20- to 24-year-old smokers who initiated after age 19 and who would, therefore, have had shorter durations of smoking by ages 40-44. Some caution needs to be exercised in interpreting these prevalence ratios because of the previously mentioned variability in prevalence rates for the 16- to 19-year-old smokers, but it is generally true that the fraction of 20- to 24-year-old smokers who are likely to have initiated after age 19 increased from the early 1950s, peaked in the late 1950s at approximately 25 percent of the smokers at ages 20-24, and then declined to the mid 1970s. Data from the General Household Survey have more stable rates for the 16- to 19-year-old group. These data reveal a steady fall in the ratio of 16- to 19-year-old smoking prevalence compared with the 20- to 24-year-old prevalence 4 years later. The data in Table 4-8 suggest that as of 1980, 14 percent of 20- to 24-year-old smokers began smoking after age 19. By 1996, approximately one-third of the 20- to 24-year-old smokers had begun to smoke after age 19. As described above, these late-initiating smokers will add to the smoking prevalence at age 40, but they are unlikely to contribute to an increased lung cancer risk at that age due to their short duration of smoking. They may, however, mask the reduction in smoking prevalence through cessation for those who have been smoking long enough to be at increased risk of lung cancer (those who began smoking before age 20). This masking effect might result in a greater decline in lung cancer risk at ages 40-44 than would be expected from the decline in smoking prevalence at the same age.

In summary, a combination of the decline in smoking prevalence and the increase in late initiation of smoking could explain the excess decline in lung cancer death rates observed in the United Kingdom. These considerations should be part of an examination of the dramatic decline over time in lung cancer death rates at younger ages among males in the U.K. The changes in lung cancer death rates in the United States appear to be consistent with changes in smoking prevalence.

**Matching U.S. Smoking Rates to U.S. Lung Cancer Death Rates** The question of whether U.S. lung cancer death rates have declined in a way consistent with a lowering of the lung cancer risk of smoking due to the use of lower yield cigarettes can be also examined by modeling the lung cancer death rate trends expected over time from the smoking behaviors of the U.S. population (see Appendix). The lung cancer risks that result from varying smoking intensity and duration can be defined using data from the CPS-I study. These risks can be fit to a model of lung cancer risk developed by Doll and Peto (1978) and the best fit of the CPS-I data to this model can be estimated. National birth cohort specific smoking behavior data can be used to predict national lung cancer death rates by utilizing the model of lung cancer risk derived from the CPS-I data to estimate the lung cancer rates for current, former and never smokers. Trends in these predicted estimates can be compared to the trends in actual observed lung cancer death rates. If the trends in predicted and observed rates are similar, there is no need to postulate an effect produced by changing cigarette design. If the trends are discordant, a term for changes in the tar yield of the cigarette smoked over time can be added to the model to determine whether adjusting for the changing tar yield of the cigarette improves the fit of the model.

Population data on smoking behavior over time in the United States provide the smoking intensity and duration estimates that allow the model to predict the national lung cancer death rates expected from those smoking behaviors. These predicted national rates can be compared with the actual observed U.S. mortality rates over time to evaluate whether the risks of smoking measured during the period 1960-1972 (CPS-I) continue to predict current lung cancer death rates, overestimate lung cancer rates over time suggesting a decline in the risk of smoking as the cigarettes smoked had lower machine-measured yields, or underestimate lung cancer rates over time as suggested by the comparison of the risks of smoking in CPS-I and CPS-II. The purpose of this analysis is not to develop a model of lung cancer risk, but rather to examine whether lung cancer risks, measured in a population smoking higher yield cigarettes, overestimates or underestimates current lung cancer mortality rates in a population smoking cigarettes with much lower machine-measured tar and nicotine yields than those smoked by the participants in CPS-I. If the risk is overestimated, it would suggest that cigarette smoking has become less hazardous over time. If the risk is underestimated, it suggests that smoking has not become less hazardous over time and may have become more hazardous.

Smoking prevalence estimates were based on the National Health Interview Survey data from 1965 to 1994 (Burns *et al.*, 1997a) and were adjusted for the differential mortality that occurs in smokers compared with never smokers. The smoking behaviors were estimated for each 5-year birth cohort (individuals born within the same 5 calendar years) from 1910 through 1960. Lung cancer risk estimates were derived by fitting the CPS-I data to a published model of lung cancer risk (Doll and Peto, 1978) that relates lung cancer death rates to the intensity and duration of smoking. The formulation of this model is lung cancer death rate = K(cigarettes/day + 6)$^x$(duration – 3.5)$^y$. The best-fit estimate for this equation using the CPS-I data yields values of K = 0.00000000017196, x = 0.85, and y = 3.71. Lung cancer death rates were calculated for each single year of age of initiation (which, when subtracted from age, yields duration of smoking) within each birth cohort for current smokers. The mean value for cigarettes smoked per day for all white male smokers in the National Health Interview Survey (16.45) was used as the term for cigarettes per day. The weighted sum of all the rates for individual ages of initiation yields the rate for the smokers in the cohort.

Rates in former smokers were estimated by modeling the fractional change in excess lung cancer death rates with duration of cessation using the CPS-I data (Burns, 1998). The fraction of the excess lung cancer death rate that remained with each increasing year of smoking duration was then multiplied by the excess death rate between smokers of that duration and nonsmokers of the same age. The fraction of the population who quit smoking in each year was estimated from the National Health Interview Survey data, and it was assumed that the distribution of smoking duration for those who quit was the same as that for current smokers in that year.

This generated individual cells of fractions of each cohort that had duration of smoking and duration of cessation specified by single years. Lung cancer death rates were calculated for each of these cells by subtracting the risk in never smokers from that of continuing smokers of the same age of initiation, multiplying the result by the fraction of excess mortality remaining at the appropriate duration of cessation, and adding back the rate in never smokers. The prevalence-weighted sum of all of these cells is the lung cancer death rate in former smokers for that birth cohort in that calendar year. Lung cancer death rates for never smokers were those estimated from CPS-I data (Burns *et al.*, 1997b).

Lung cancer death rates for each cohort in each calendar year were generated by summing the rates for current smokers, former smokers, and never smokers, weighted by their respective prevalence in that year. Figure 4-17 presents an example of these estimates for the cohort born between 1910 and 1914. Rates are presented by calendar year; but because the rates are for a population born during a fixed set of years, the calendar year axis also reflects increasing age of the birth cohort. This explains the increasing never smoker lung cancer death rates with calendar year in the figure, when age-specific lung cancer death rates in never smokers have not changed over time (Thun and Heath, 1997; Thun *et al.*, 1997a).

Actual observed lung cancer mortality rates by birth cohort were obtained from the U.S. mortality data and are those presented by Mannino and colleagues (2001). The birth cohorts for smoking and lung cancer are 1-year discordant, but it is unlikely that this difference contributes substantively to the results. Lung cancer death rates estimated from smoking behaviors and CPS-I risk data were scaled to the actual U.S. mortality rates to derive a single exponential scaling factor for all of the cohorts. The value for this scaling factor was 1.25. Differences between the predicted and actual lung cancer death rates were examined across calendar years for each birth cohort. A term proportional to the sales-weighted tar yield of U.S. cigarettes for each calendar year was applied to the predicted rates as $c$ times the tar value, and the optimum value for $c$ was calculated. The resultant tar-adjusted rates were tested to determine whether the addition of the term for tar to the predicted rates improved the goodness of fit of the predicted data to the observed U.S. lung cancer mortality rates by cohort. These three sets of rates (U.S. mortality, CPS-I predicted, and tar-adjusted CPS-I predicted) are presented in Figures 4-18a to 4-18i, with one graph for each 5-year birth cohort.

The fit of the CPS-I predicted rates was improved by the addition of the tar term, but the improved fit was in the direction of declining tar values increasing the risk. There was excellent agreement between the CPS-I predicted rates and the real U.S. lung cancer death rates in each cohort until the late 1970s. However, beginning in 1979 and in later years, there was a progressive underestimation of U.S. lung cancer mortality when the dose and duration risk relationships from CPS-I and U.S. smoking prevalences by birth cohort were used to estimate lung cancer death rates. In order to account for the difference in timing between transformation of a cell into a cancer and death from the growth of that cancer, the analysis was repeated

Figure 4-17
**Contribution to White Male Lung Cancer Rates by Smoking Status: Birth Cohort 1910-1914**

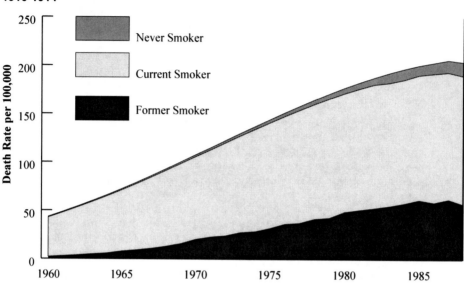

Note: Prevalence rates of cigarette smoking, initiation, and cessation by year for U.S. White males were obtained from NCI Smoking and Tobacco Control Monograph No. 8 (Burns et al., 1997a). U.S. population estimates stratified by age, sex, and race were obtained from CDC and U.S. Bureau of the Census web sites (CDC, 2000c; USBC, 2000). U.S. lung cancer mortality of White males were provided by D.M. Mannino (personal communication). These risk data were stratified by 5-year birth cohorts for each calendar year, 1960-1994. The 5-year birth cohorts began with 1901-1905 and ended with 1961-1965. See Appendix for details.

with the tar values lagged by 4 years, and the results were not substantively nor significantly different. These analyses suggest that, if anything, there has been an increase rather than a decrease in the carcinogenicity of smoking over the last several decades in the United States.

In order to address the question of changes in age-specific lung cancer death rates at younger ages, the difference was examined between the observed lung cancer death rates and the death rates predicted using the CPS-I risk data (without a term for tar) at fixed ages across multiple birth cohorts. If the most recent birth cohorts have lung cancer death rates that are declining more rapidly than would be predicted from differences in their smoking prevalence (*i.e.*, an effect suggesting a reduction in risk of smoking with lower yield cigarettes), then the difference between actual and predicted lung cancer death rates at fixed ages should have a slope when plotted across sequential cohorts. When sequential birth cohorts are examined in this manner for age-specific lung cancer death rates at ages under 50, there is no discernible slope for cohorts born after 1930, and the slope for older cohorts and for older ages is in the direction of increasing risk with the younger cohorts. Therefore, even when the model is examined in an age-specific format and confined to younger ages, there is no evidence to suggest that there is a decline in risk for smokers who would have had higher proportions of their smoking experience using filtered or low-yield cigarettes.

Figure 4-18a
**Lung Cancer Death Rates: White Males, Birth Cohort 1910-1914**

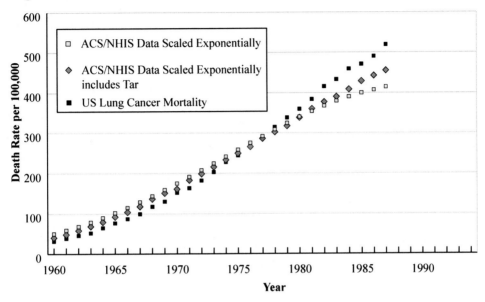

Figure 4-18b
**Lung Cancer Death Rates: White Males, Birth Cohort 1915-1919**

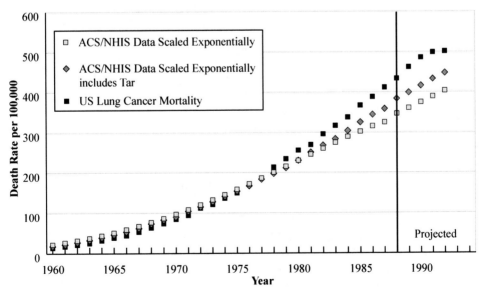

Figure 4-18c
**Lung Cancer Death Rates: White Males, Birth Cohort 1920-1924**

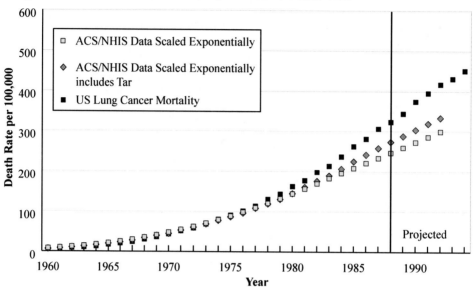

Figure 4-18d
**Lung Cancer Death Rates: White Males, Birth Cohort 1925-1929**

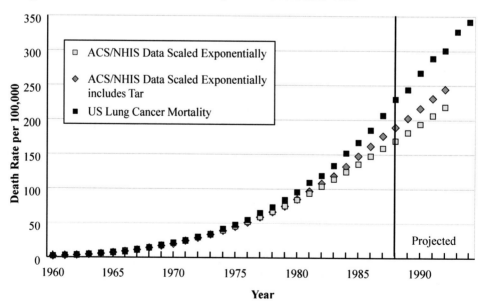

Figure 4-18e
**Lung Cancer Death Rates: White Males, Birth Cohort 1930-1934**

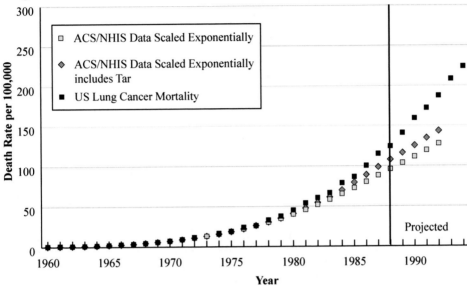

Figure 4-18f
**Lung Cancer Death Rates: White Males, Birth Cohort 1935-1939**

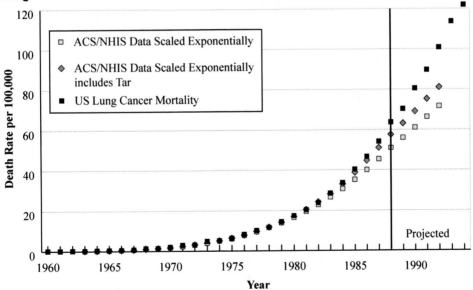

Figure 4-18g
**Lung Cancer Death Rates: White Males, Birth Cohort 1940-1944**

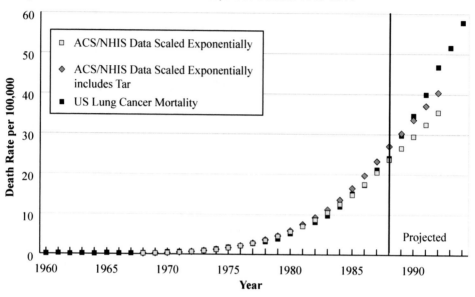

Figure 4-18h
**Lung Cancer Death Rates: White Males, Birth Cohort 1945-1949**

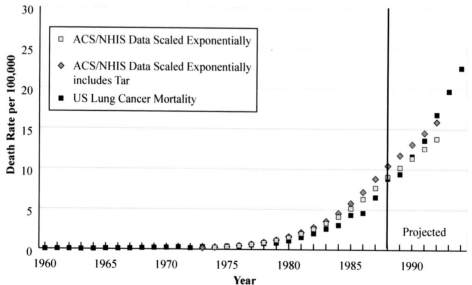

Figure 4-18i
**Lung Cancer Death Rates: White Males, Birth Cohort 1950-1954**

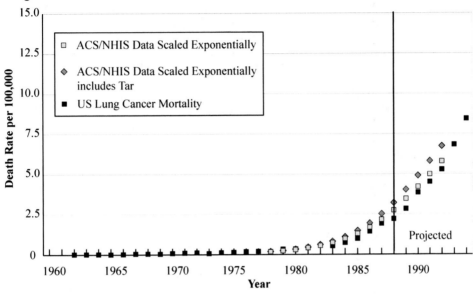

Note for Figures 18a-18i: Estimated lung cancer death rates were obtained by using a model developed by Peto (Doll and Peto, 1978). U.S. lung cancer death rates were provided for the years 1960-1995 by D.M. Mannino (personal communication, 2000). See Appendix for further details.

In these analyses, tar is a surrogate for the overall changes in cigarette design and manufacture over the last five decades, rather than a specific measure of the actual tar intake by the smoker. This analytical approach is an attempt to answer the question of whether the sum total of the changes occurring in cigarette design and composition over the last 45 years produced a reduction in carcinogenicity of smoking, and there appears to be little evidence for a population effect in the direction of a reduced risk. Moreover, this analysis supports the comparison of the two American Cancer Society prospective mortality studies (CPS-I and CPS-II) in suggesting that cigarette smoking may have become more, rather than less, hazardous, based on the cumulative effects of all the changes in cigarette design and manufacture that have occurred over the last half century.

**SUMMARY**

The three lines of evidence on lung cancer risk in relation to changes in cigarette design provide somewhat inconsistent findings, perhaps reflecting methodological limitations and the limited number of studies available. Detailed examination of lung cancer rates by age in the United States and the United Kingdom provide seemingly conflicting patterns from the two countries. Lesser risks for more recent cigarettes are one potential explanation for the rapid decline of lung cancer mortality at younger ages in the United Kingdom over recent years. However, the temporal pattern of lung cancer mortality at younger ages in the United States is not consistent with

145

this explanation. The temporally cross-sectional findings from several case-control and cohort studies provide some evidence of reduced risk for smokers of lower yield products at time points across the 1960s through the 1980s. These studies, however, provide only relative comparisons of risk and data analysis methods raise concern about biased findings in some. Finally, both the British Physician's Study and the CPS I and II studies provide powerful evidence that both relative and absolute risks of lung cancer in smokers have risen from the 1950s through the 1980s. The different findings across these three lines of epidemiological evidence cannot be reconciled with available information. Overall, however, they do not provide evidence that public health has benefited from changes in cigarette design and manufacture over the last fifty years.

## CONCLUSIONS

1. Changes in cigarette design and manufacturing over the last fifty years have substantially lowered the sales-weighted, machine-measured tar and nicotine yields of cigarettes smoked in the United States.

2. Cigarettes with low machine-measured yields by the FTC method are designed to allow compensatory smoking behaviors that enable a smoker to derive a wide range of tar and nicotine yields from the same brand, offsetting much of the theoretical benefit of a reduced-yield cigarette.

3. Existing disease risk data do not support making a recommendation that smokers switch cigarette brands. The recommendation that individuals who cannot stop smoking should switch to low yield cigarettes can cause harm if it misleads smokers to postpone serious efforts at cessation.

4. Widespread adoption of lower yield cigarettes by smokers in the United States has not prevented the sustained increase in lung cancer among older smokers.

5. Epidemiological studies have not consistently found lesser risk of diseases, other than lung cancer, among smokers of reduced yield cigarettes. Some studies have found lesser risks of lung cancer among smokers of reduced yield cigarettes. Some or all of this reduction in lung cancer risk may reflect differing characteristics of smokers of reduced-yield compared to higher-yield cigarettes.

6. There is no convincing evidence that changes in cigarette design between 1950 and the mid 1980s have resulted in an important decrease in the disease burden caused by cigarette use either for smokers as a group or for the whole population.

# Appendix

**Description of Cancer Prevention Study-I Data
and Methods of Analysis**

The first Cancer Prevention Study (CPS-I) was a major cohort study carried out by the American Cancer Society (ACS). Over one million individuals were followed for more than 12 years, from 1959 to 1972. The protocol included a baseline survey that covered smoking history and present use, as well as information about health history and behaviors. The major outcome variable was mortality by specific cause as indicated on the death certificate. CPS-I provided strong evidence that confirmed relationships between smoking and specific diseases, including lung cancer and coronary heart disease.

**DESCRIPTION OF THE DATA**    The focus of this analysis is the White male subset of cigarette smokers. The baseline data were gathered in 1959 and included 174,997 White male current cigarette smokers who were not using other forms of smoked or oral tobacco. These are the subjects for the present analysis. Major follow-ups were conducted in 1961, 1963, 1965, and 1972 that included questions about the brand of cigarette smoked and number of cigarettes smoked per day. This provided enough information to be able to consider the changing smoking habits during the 12-year period as well as relationships to disease outcomes.

**TAR AND NICOTINE LEVEL**    The database available from ACS did not retain the specific brand smoked from the baseline survey, but it has the brands re-coded into categories of tar and nicotine level crossed by filter/nonfilter. This simplification of the data can be understood by recalling that this was the era of data entry and analysis using punched cards. For the present study, this means that the baseline tar and nicotine levels for individuals are not known explicitly beyond a category of combined tar and nicotine levels. The subsequent follow-up efforts did retain the specific brand smoked by the individual, though the particular subspecies of the brand was not retained, such as king size or regular, low tar versus full flavor, etc.

The tar and nicotine levels for specific brands were determined in 1959 in laboratory studies commissioned and published by the *Reader's Digest* (Miller and Monahan, 1959). These values were used by the ACS for the baseline categorizations. Subsequently, brand-specific tar and nicotine assessments were carried out by the Federal Trade Commission (FTC) in 1967, 1970, and 1974 (FTC, 1967, 1970, 1974). Because these years do not correspond to the years of the CPS-I follow-up surveys, linear interpolation was used within brands to estimate tar and nicotine levels for the years of the follow-up. When multiple subspecies were tested by the FTC within brands, market share information from the Maxwell Report (Maxwell, 1994) was used to develop a market-share-weighted tar and nicotine value for each brand for each survey year. These values allowed a specific tar and nicotine estimate to be attached to each smoker at each follow-up period for which he provided a brand. When an individual showed a consistent pattern of smoking the same brand and when the tar and nicotine level for that brand was consistent with the category assigned to that individual at baseline, it was assumed that he smoked that brand at baseline and the category values were adjusted to the explicit tar and nicotine values for that brand.

**CIGARETTES PER DAY**   At baseline as well as for the follow-up surveys, smokers were asked how many cigarettes were smoked each day. Responses were categorized into levels 1-9, 10-19, 20, 21-39, 40, 40+ for all except the final follow-up, where the specific number of cigarettes smoked per day was recorded. For most analyses, the final follow-up was also converted to the categorical levels with 40 and 40+ combined. When an explicit value for a category was needed for graphing or regression, the weighted mean value for the category was used, based on the distribution of observed cigarettes per day values at the time of the final follow-up. These means were: 4.48, 11.97, 20, 29.15, and 43.52, respectively.

**CHANGES IN TAR AND NICO-TINE AND CIGARETTES PER DAY ACROSS YEARS OF STUDY**   The cross-sectional follow-up surveys provided estimates of tar and nicotine level and cigarettes per day for each smoker. By comparing responses at subsequent surveys, changes over time in the balance of tar and nicotine and cigarettes per day can be assessed. The baseline and four follow-up surveys provided four sequential measures of change for each subject who completed the five cross-sectional surveys. The cross-sectional combination of variables and changes between adjacent surveys allowed analysis of temporal changes in the interrelationships of these variables.

**ASSEMBLING DATA SET FOR ANALYSIS**   SAS and Pascal programs were used to assemble simplified data sets for analysis. For a given subject, the four periods of follow-up were assembled with the tar and nicotine levels for the beginning of the follow-up period and the reported cigarettes per day level at that time. Additional criteria were sometimes used to isolate individuals who: changed brands, did not change brands, never reported an attempt to quit, changed to a cigarette with a lower tar value, etc. For each individual, possible endpoints included death with date and international code for cause of death (WHO, 1957), lost to follow-up, or censored at end of study.

**METHODS OF ANALYSIS**   Several kinds of regression analyses were undertaken. These included survival analysis, regression analysis of log of death rates on tabular data, and regression analysis of interrelationships between factors.

**Survival Analysis**   Survival analysis was undertaken using the SAS *lifereg* procedure, using a database of individual subjects with the combinations of factors present at the beginning of the interval and an observed time period of follow-up with factors assumed at that level. Generally, the dependent variable for these analyses was the likelihood of death by a specific cause, such as lung cancer. The independent variables included combinations of tar level (continuous or stratified to 3-5 levels), cigarettes per day (continuous or stratified), age (continuous), and duration of smoking (continuous).

**Regression Analysis of Tabular Data**    Alternatively, in some instances the observations were assembled into cells of observations stratified by 5-year age groups, 5-year duration groups, cigarettes per day level, and tar level (3-5 levels), with observed death rates calculated for each cell. Typically, these cell-wise analyses were carried out in S-Plus2000, as a *glm* (generalized linear model) regression analysis of the log of the death rates or excess mortality rates (compared to never smokers), and regressed on the explanatory variables.

**Regression Analysis of Combinations of Factors**    Several analyses were also undertaken to examine the interrelationships between factors, such as the relationship between nicotine level and cigarettes smoked per day. In these analyses, the data points representing combinations reported by individuals at various points in the follow-up were analyzed. These analyses included examination of distributions of factors occurring together, and examination of relationships between changes in one factor as related to changes in another. For these analyses, the database assembled was similar to that reported for survival analyses, but sometimes also included changes in factors between consecutive follow-up surveys. Generally, these regression analyses were undertaken in SAS using the GLM procedure.

**DETAILED NOTES TO FIGURE 4-17**    This figure shows the estimated population-based lung cancer death rates for the specific birth cohort by smoking status (current, former, or never smokers). Ever and current smoking prevalence among 5-year birth cohorts of U.S. White males were obtained from Chapter 2 of the National Cancer Institute's (NCI) Monograph 8 (Burns *et al.*, 1997a). Former smoking prevalence in a given year was obtained by subtracting the current smoking from the ever smoking prevalence in the same year. The prevalence of never smokers in a given year was obtained by subtracting the prevalence of ever smokers from 100 percent, where 100 percent represents the entire population.

To determine the contribution of current and former smokers to the overall lung cancer death rate, the prevalence rates and risks of death from lung cancer were linked over time, accounting for changes in initiation and cessation rates of white males by specific 5-year birth cohorts.

**Current Smokers' Contributions**    The age-of-initiation profile for each birth cohort was estimated using the change in prevalence of ever smoking by year under age 30. The rate of initiation in a given year was estimated by taking the difference between the ever smoking prevalence for a given year and that for the previous year. This generated a distribution of age of initiation by age/calendar year for those in the cohort who started smoking under the age of 30. The percentage of the population who are current smokers of given durations for each calendar year of a birth cohort was obtained by proportioning the current smokers to the age-of-initiation profile.

Data on lung cancer death rates among smokers of different durations along with numbers of cigarettes smoked per day were used to estimate the parameters for a model of lung cancer risk in relation to smoking behaviors (Doll and Peto, 1978). These fitting parameters were applied to the data on birth-cohort-specific smoking prevalence by duration to obtain estimates of lung cancer death rates for current smokers. An average number of 16.45

149

cigarettes smoked per day was used in this calculation based on the average number of cigarettes per day reported in the National Health Interview Surveys (NHIS). These surveys were conducted between 1965 and 1999 and controlled for age and race. This model required estimation of three parameters. The maximum likelihood procedure was applied to lung cancer deaths of White male cigarette smokers using data from the ACS CPS-I to estimate the necessary parameters (a = 0.85285 the exponent on the cigarettes/day term; b = 3.70895 the exponent on the duration term; and c = $1.7196 \times 10^{-10}$, a constant).

The current smokers' contribution to the national lung cancer death rate for each calendar year equals the sum of the predicted lung cancer death rates for smokers of each given duration divided by the white male population for that year, and it is expressed per 100,000.

**Former Smokers' Contributions**   The incidence of smoking cessation in each cohort for each calendar year was estimated by subtracting the prevalence of former smokers in a given year from the prevalence of former smokers in the previous year. The fraction of the population that quit in a given year is distributed into discrete durations of smoking using the distribution of age of initiation for that cohort and the year of the estimate.

Modeled estimates were generated for given durations of smoking as described for current smokers. However, for former smokers, the estimated lung cancer death rates were reduced using length of time since quitting. The fractions of excess lung cancer risk (risk in smokers minus the risk in nonsmokers) that remained after increasing durations of cessation were estimated using data from the ACS CPS-I study (Shanks, 1999).

To determine the contribution of former smokers to the national White male lung cancer rate for each birth cohort by calendar year, the predicted death rates for each duration of smoking at each duration of cessation for each calendar year were summed and divided by that year's corresponding White male population for the birth cohort. The result was expressed per 100,000.

**Never Smokers' Contributions**   The observed lung cancer death rates for White male never smokers by 5-year age groups were obtained from NCI Monograph 8, page 303 (see Burns *et al.*, 1997b), using data from CPS-I. Using the midpoint of each 5-year age group, the observed death rates were modeled using linear regression of log rates weighted to person-years of observation to obtain the death rates for each age in 1-year increments (from ages 25 to 88), using S-Plus software (S-Plus 2000, June 1999).

To determine the contribution of never smokers to the national White male lung cancer rate for each birth cohort by calendar year, the predicted death rates were calculated as the product of the prevalence of never smokers in the year, the death rate of never smokers for that cohort in that year using the median age of the birth cohort at each calendar year, and the corresponding White male population for the birth cohort. The result was expressed per 100,000. Nine sequential birth cohorts were evaluated, the first being 1910-1914 and the last being 1950-1954.

**DETAILED NOTES TO FIGURES 4-18a TO 4-18i**    The estimated lung cancer death rates by smoking status (current, former, and never smokers) for individual birth cohorts of the U.S. White male population were summed to obtain the total death rates for each birth cohort by year. Total lung cancer death rates were then scaled to the actual national death rates for each birth cohort and year strata using a single exponential scaling factor.

To investigate the effects of tar on lung cancer death rates, a term for sales-weighted tar was added. Fit of the modeled lung cancer rate data to actual lung cancer death rates was examined before and after adding tar. The model was further enhanced by including an additional term for the mean cigarettes smoked per day for each calendar year. The GLM procedure in SAS/STAT was used to obtain mean cigarettes per day by year while controlling for age and race. Data sources for the means were the NHIS for the years 1965-1995. The mean cigarette per day rates for the years 1960-1964 were assumed to equal that of the NHIS for 1965.

To compare these estimates to the actual lung cancer death rates, the estimates were scaled exponentially and graphed against the actual national lung cancer mortality. Sales-weighted average tar deliveries of U.S. cigarettes for the years 1954-1994 were provided by The American Health Foundation (Hoffmann, 1997). The modeling procedures were performed using S-Plus 2000 software (S-Plus 2000, June 1999).

# REFERENCES

Agudo, A., Barnadas, A., Pallares, C., Martinez, I., Fabregat, X., Rosello, J., Estape, J., Planas, J., Gonzalez, CA. Lung cancer and cigarette smoking in women: a case-control study in Barcelona (Spain). *International Journal of Cancer* 59:165-169, 1994.

Alderson, M.R., Lee, P. N., Wang, R. Risks of lung cancer, chronic bronchitis, ischaemic heart disease, and stroke in relation to type of cigarette smoked. *Journal of Epidemiology & Community Health* 39:286-293, 1985.

Armadans-Gil, L. Vaque-Rafart, J., Rossello, J., Olona, M., Alseda, M. Cigarette smoking and male lung cancer risk with special regard to type of tobacco. *International Journal of Epidemiology* 28:614-619, 1999.

Armitage, P., Doll, R. Stochastic models for carcinogenesis. *Proceedings of the Fourth Berkeley Symposium on Mathematical Statistics and Probability, Vol. 4.* Berkeley, CA: University of California Press, 1961.

Auerbach, O., Hammond, E.C., Garfinkel, L. Changes in bronchial epithelium in relation to cigarette smoking, 1955–1960 vs. 1970–1977. *New England Journal of Medicine* 300:381-385, 1979.

Augustine, A. Harris R.E., Wynder E.L. Compensation as a risk factor for lung cancer in smokers who switch from nonfilter to filter cigarettes. *American Journal of Public Health* 79:188-191, 1989a.

Augustine, A. Harris R.E., Wynder E.L. Compensation as a risk factor for lung cancer in smokers who switch from nonfilter to filter cigarettes. *Progress in Clinical and Biological Research* 293:221-230, 1989b.

Benhamou, E., Benhamou, S. Black (air-cured) and blond (flue-cured) tobacco and cancer risk. VI: Lung cancer. *European Journal of Cancer* 29A(12):1778-1780, 1993.

Benhamou, E., Benhamou, S., Auquier, A., Flamant, R. Changes in patterns of cigarette smoking and lung cancer risk: Results of a case-control study. *British Journal of Cancer* 60:601-604, 1989.

Benhamou, E., Benhamou, S., Flamant, R. Lung cancer and women: Results of a French case-control study. *British Journal of Cancer* 55:91-95, 1987.

Benhamou, S., Benhamou, E., Auquier, A., Flamant, R. Differential effects of tar content, type of tobacco and use of a filter on lung cancer risk in male cigarette smokers. *International Journal of Epidemiology* 23:437-443, 1994.

Benhamou, S., Benhamou, E., Tirmarche, M., Flamant, R. Lung cancer and use of cigarettes: A French case–control study. *Journal of the National Cancer Institute* 74:1169-1175, 1985.

Benowitz, N.L. Biomarkers of cigarette smoking. *The FTC Cigarette Test Method for Determining Tar, Nicotine, and Carbon Monoxide Yields of U.S. Cigarettes. Report of the NCI Expert Committee.* Smoking and Tobacco Control Monograph No.7. U.S. Department of Health and Human Services, National Institutes of Health, National Cancer Institute, NIH Publication No. 96-4028, 1996.

Benowitz, N.L., Hall, S.M., Herning, R.I., Jacob, P., Jones, R.T., Osman, A. Smokers of low-yield cigarettes do not consume less nicotine. *New England Journal of Medicine* 309:139-42, 1983.

Benowitz, N.L., Henningfield, J.E. Establishing a nicotine threshold for addiction. *New England Journal of Medicine* 331:123-125, 1994.

Borland, C., Chamberlain, A., Higenbottam, T., Shipley, M., Rose, G. Carbon monoxide yield of cigarettes and its relation to cardiorespiratory disease. *British Medical Journal* 287:1583-1586, 1983.

British American Tobacco Company. Structured creativity group. Thoughts by C.C. Greig – R&D, Southampton, Marketing scenario. Florida AG tobacco litigation, undated. Bates No. 100515909.

Bross, I.D., Gibson, R. Risks of lung cancer in smokers who switch to filter cigarettes. *American Journal of Public Health and the Nations Health* 58(8):1396-1403, 1968.

Bross, I.D. Effect of filter cigarettes on lung cancer risk. *Toward a Less Harmful Cigarette.* NCI Monograph No. 28. Wynder, E.L., Hoffmann, D. (Editors.). U.S. Department. of Health, Education, and Welfare, National Institutes of Health, National Cancer Institute, 1968.

Brown, C., Kessler, L. Projections of lung cancer mortality in the United States: 1985–2025. *Journal of the National Cancer Institute* 80:43-51, 1988.

Brown, C.A., Crombie, I.K., Smith, W.C., Tunstall-Pedoe, H. Cigarette tar content and symptoms of chronic bronchitis: Results of the Scottish Heart Health Study. *Journal of Epidemiology and Community Health* 45:287-290, 1991.

Buffler, P.A., Contant, C.F., Pickle, L.W., Burau, K., Cooper, S.P., Mason, T.J. Environmental associations with lung cancer in Texas coastal counties. *Lung Cancer: Current Status and Prospects for the Future. Twenty-eighth Annual Clinical Conference on Cancer.* Mountain, C.F., Carr, D.T. (Editors.). Houston, Texas, USA, November 7–10, 1984. Austin, TX: University of Texas Press, 1986.

Burns, D. *Primary prevention, smoking, smoking cessation—Implications for future trends in lung cancer prevention.* Proceedings of the International Conference on Prevention and Early Diagnosis of Lung Cancer. Varese – Ville Ponti, December 9-10, 1998. Dominioni, L., Strauss, G. (Editors.), 1998.

Burns, D., Lee, L., Shen, Z., Gilpin, B., Tolley, D., Vaughn, J., Shanks, T. Cigarette smoking behavior in the United States. *Changes in Cigarette-Related Disease Risks and Their Implication for Prevention and Control.* Smoking and Tobacco Control Monograph No. 8. U.S. Department of Health and Human Services, National Institutes of Health, National Cancer Institute, NIH Publication No. 97-4213, 1997a.

Burns D., Shanks, T., Choi, W., Thun, M., Heath, C., Garfinkel L. The American Cancer Society Cancer Prevention Study I: 12-year follow-up of 1 million men and women. *Changes in Cigarette-Related Disease Risks and Their Implication for Prevention and Control.* Smoking and Tobacco Control Monograph No. 8. U.S. Department of Health and Human Services, National Institutes of Health, National Cancer Institute, NIH Publication No. 97-4213, 1997b.

Centers for Disease Control and Prevention. Cigarette smoking among adults—United States, 1998. *Morbidity and Mortality Weekly Report* 49(39):881-884, 2000a.

Centers for Disease Control and Prevention. Ahern, C.H., Batchelor, S.M., Blanton, C.J., Law, M., Loo, C.M., Pevzner, E.S., Ryan, H.A., Stolfus, S.A., Tabladillo, M., Warren, C.W., Zinner, L.R., Eriksen, M.P., Healton, C.G., Messeri, P.A., Reynolds, J.H., Stokes, C., Ross, J.G., Flint, K., Robb, W.H. Youth tobacco surveillance—United States, 1998–1999. *Morbidity and Mortality Weekly Report* 49(SS10):1-93, 2000b.

Centers for Disease Control and Prevention. *U.S. Population Estimates by Age, Sex, Race.* Centers for Disease Control and Prevention, 2000. Available from www.cdc.gov/nchs/datawh/statab/unpubd/mortabs/pop6079.html.

Cohen, J. B. Consumer/smoker perceptions of Federal Trade Commission tar ratings. *The FTC Cigarette Test Method for Determining Tar, Nicotine, and Carbon Monoxide Yields of U.S. Cigarettes. Report of the NCI Expert Committee.* Smoking and Tobacco Control Monograph No. 7. U.S. Department of Health and Human Services, National Institutes of Health, National Cancer Institute, NIH Publication No. 96-4028, 1996a.

Cohen, J. B. Smokers' knowledge and understanding of advertised tar numbers: Health policy implications. *American Journal of Public Health* 86:18-24, 1996b.

Committee on Health Risks of Exposure to Radon (BEIR VI). *Health Effects of Exposure to Radon: BEIR VI.* National Research Council. Washington, DC: National Academy Press, 1999.

Dean, G., Lee, P.N., Todd, G.F., Wicken, A.J., Sparks, D.N. Factors related to respiratory and cardiovascular symptoms in the United Kingdom. *Journal of Epidemiology and Community Health* 32:86-96, 1978.

De Stefani, E. Mate drinking and risk of lung cancer in males: A case-control study from Uruguay. *Cancer Epidemiology, Biomarkers and Prevention* 5:515-519, 1996.

Doll, R., Hill, A.B. A study of the aetiology of carcinoma of the lung. *British Medical Journal* 2:1271-1286, 1952.

Doll, R., Hill, A.B. The Mortality of doctors in relation to their smoking habits: A preliminary report. *British Medical Journal* 1(4877):1451-1455 (June 26), 1954.

Doll, R., Peto, R. Cigarette smoking and bronchial carcinoma: dose and time relationships among regular smokers and lifelong non-smokers. *Journal of Epidemiology and Community Health* 32:303-313, 1978.

Doll, R., Peto, R., Wheatley, K., Gray, R., Sutherland, I. Mortality in relation to smoking: 40 years' observations on male British doctors. *British Medical Journal* 309:901-911, 1994.

Engeland, A., Haldorsen, T., Andersen, A., Tretli, S. The impact of smoking habits on lung cancer risk: 28 years' observation of 26,000 Norwegian men and women. *Cancer Causes and Control* 7:366-376, 1996.

Federal Trade Commission. *Report of Tar and Nicotine Content of the Smoke of 59 Varieties of Cigarettes.* Federal Trade Commission, Washington, D.C., 1967.

Federal Trade Commission. *Report of Tar and Nicotine Content of the Smoke of 126 Varieties of Cigarettes [for year 1968].* Federal Trade Commission, Washington, D.C., 1969.

Federal Trade Commission. *Report of Tar and Nicotine Content of the Smoke of 118 Varieties of Cigarettes.* Federal Trade Commission, Washington, D.C., 1969.

Federal Trade Commission. *Report of "Tar" and Nicotine Content of the Smoke of 120 Varieties of Cigarettes.* Federal Trade Commission, Washington, D.C., 1970.

Federal Trade Commission. *Report of "Tar" and Nicotine Content of the Smoke of 130 Varieties of Cigarettes.* Federal Trade Commission, Washington, D.C., 1974.

Federal Trade Commission. *Report of "Tar" and Nicotine Content of the Smoke of 145 Varieties of Cigarettes [for year 1975].* Federal Trade Commission, Washington, D.C., 1976.

Federal Trade Commission. *Report of "Tar" and Nicotine Content of the Smoke of 166 Varieties of Cigarettes [for year 1976].* Federal Trade Commission, Washington, D.C., 1977.

Federal Trade Commission. *Report of "Tar" and Nicotine Content of the Smoke of 167 Varieties of Cigarettes [for year 1977].* Federal Trade Commission, Washington, D.C., 1978.

Federal Trade Commission. *Report of "Tar", Nicotine and Carbon Monoxide of the Smoke of 187 Varieties of Cigarettes [for year 1979].* Federal Trade Commission, Washington, D.C., 1981.

Federal Trade Commission. *Report of "Tar", Nicotine and Carbon Monoxide of the Smoke of 200 Varieties of Cigarettes [for year 1981].* Federal Trade Commission, Washington, D.C., 1981.

Federal Trade Commission. *Report of "Tar", Nicotine and Carbon Monoxide of the Smoke of 207 Varieties of Domestic Cigarettes [for year 1982].* Federal Trade Commission, Washington, D.C., 1984.

Federal Trade Commission. *Report of "Tar", Nicotine and Carbon Monoxide of the Smoke of 207 Varieties of Domestic Cigarettes [for year 1984].* Federal Trade Commission, Washington, D.C., 1985.

Federal Trade Commission. *Report of "Tar", Nicotine and Carbon Monoxide of the Smoke of 370 varieties of domestic cigarettes [for year 1988].* Federal Trade Commission, Washington, D.C., 1990.

Federal Trade Commission. *Report on Tar, Nicotine, and Carbon Monoxide Content of the Smoke of 534 Varieties of Domestic Cigarettes [for year 1990].* Federal Trade Commission, Washington D.C., 1992.

Federal Trade Commission. *Report on Tar, Nicotine, and Carbon Monoxide Content of the Smoke of 1262 Varieties of Domestic Cigarettes [for year 1996].* Federal Trade Commission, Washington D.C., 1999.

Garfinkel, L. Changes in the cigarette consumption of smokers in relation to changes in tar/nicotine content of cigarettes smoked. *American Journal of Public Health* 69:1274-1276, 1979.

Garfinkel, L. Changes in number of cigarettes smoked compared to changes in tar and nicotine content over a 13-year period. A Safe Cigarette? *Banbury Report 3, Proceedings of a Meeting Held at the Banbury Center, Cold Spring Harbor Laboratory, NY, Oct. 14–16, 1979.* Gori, G.B., Bock, F.G. (Editors.). Cold Spring Harbor, NY: Cold Spring Harbor Laboratory, 1980.

Gillis C.R., Hole, D.J., Boyle, P. Cigarette smoking and male lung cancer in an area of very high incidence. I: Report of a case-control study in the West of Scotland. *Journal of Epidemiology and Community Health* 42:38-43, 1988.

Giovino, G.A., Tomar, S.L., Reddy, M.N., Peddicord, J.P., Zhu, B.P., Escobedo, L.G., Eriksen, M.P. Attitudes, knowledge, and beliefs about low-yield cigarettes among adolescents and adults. *The FTC Cigarette Test Method for Determining Tar, Nicotine, and Carbon Monoxide Yields of U.S. Cigarettes. Report of the NCI Expert Committee.* Smoking and Tobacco Control Monograph No. 7. U.S. Department of Health and Human Services, National Institutes of Health, National Cancer Institute, NIH Publication No. 96-4028, 1996.

Goodman, B. to Meyer, L.F. September 17, 1975. Memo by Barboro Goodman. Marlboro-Marlboro Lights study delivery data. Bates No. 2021544486.

Goodman, B. to Meyer, L.F. October 21, 1982. Memo by Barboro Goodman. Effect of reduced dilution on tar delivery to a smoker. Phillip Morris Archive Document I.D. No. 1003415278/5280.

Green, S.J. Research conference held at Hilton Head Island S.C., September 24-30, 1968. University of California San Francisco Tobacco Archive Document I.D. 1112.01, 1968.

Haddock, CK; Talcott, GW; Klesges, RC; Lando, H. An examination of cigarette brand switching to reduce health risks. *Annals of Behavioral Medicine* 21:128-134, 1999.

Hammond, E.C., Horn, D. Smoking and Death Rates—A report on 44 months of follow-up of 187,783 men. II. Death rates by cause. *Journal of the American Medical Association* 166:1294-1308, 1958.

Hammond, E.C., Garfinkel, L. Changes in cigarette smoking. *Journal of the National Cancer Institute* 32:49, 1964.

Hammond, E.C. Smoking in relation to the death rates of one million men and women. *National Cancer Institute Monograph* 19:127-204, 1966.

Hammond, E.C. The long term benefits of reducing tar and nicotine in cigarettes. *A Safe Cigarette? Banbury Report 3, Proceedings of a Meeting Held at the Banbury Center, Cold Spring Harbor Laboratory, NY, Oct. 14–16, 1979.* Gori, G.B., Bock, F.G. (Editors.). Cold Spring Harbor, NY: Cold Spring Harbor Laboratory, 1980.

Hammond, E.C., Garfinkel L., Seidman, H., Lew, E.A. Some recent findings concerning cigarette smoking. *Origins of Human Cancer. Book A: Incidence of Cancer in Humans.* Cold Springs Harbor Conferences on Cell Proliferation, Volume 4. 1977.

Hammond, E.C., Garfinkel, L., Seideman, H., Lew, E.A. "Tar" and nicotine content of cigarette smoke in relation to death rates. *Environmental Research* 12:263-274, 1976.

Harris, J. Cigarette smoking among successive birth cohorts of men and women in the United States during 1900–1980. *Journal of the National Cancer Institute* 71:473-479, 1983.

Hawthorne, V.M., Fry, J.S. Smoking and health: The association between smoking behavior, total mortality, and cardiorespiratory disease in West Central Scotland. *Journal of Epidemiology and Community Health* 32:260-266, 1978.

Hecht, S.S. Biochemistry, biology, and carcinogenicity of tobacco-specific N-nitrosamines. *Chemical Research in Toxicology* 11:559-603, 1998.

Higenbottam, T., Shipley, M.J., Rose, G. Cigarettes, lung cancer, and coronary heart disease: The effects of inhalation and tar yield. *Journal of Epidemiology and Community Health* 36:113-117, 1982.

Hoffmann, D., Hoffmann, I. The changing cigarette, 1950–1995. *Journal of Toxicology and Environmental Health* 50:307-364, 1997.

Holmes, J.C., Hardcastle, J.E., Mitchel, R.I. Determination of particle size and electric charge distribution in cigarette smoke. *Tobacco Science* 3:148-153, 1959.

Imperial Tobacco Limited. Research & Development Division, Progress report July 1993-December 1993. Bates No. 402415194-402415196. Available at www.tobaccopapers.org/documents/psc8.pdf.

International Committee on Radiation Protection, Task Group in Lung Dynamics. Deposition and retention models for internal dosimetry of the human respiratory tract. *Health Physics* 12:173-207, 1966.

Jarvis, M.J., Boreham, R., Primatesta, P., Feyerabend, C., Bryant, A. Nicotine yield from machine-smoked cigarettes and nicotine intakes in smokers: Evidence from a representative population survey. *Journal of the National Cancer Institute* 93:134-138, 2001.

Jöckel, K.H., Ahrens, W., Wichmann, H.E., Becher, H., Bolm-Audorff, U., Jahn, I., Molik, B., Greiser, E., Timm, J. Occupational and environmental hazards associated with lung cancer. *International Journal of Epidemiology* 21:202-213, 1992.

Johnston, L.D., O'Malley, P.M., Bachman, J.G. Cigarette use and smokeless tobacco use decline substantially among teens. University of Michigan News and Information Services: Ann Arbor, MI. [On-line], 2000. Available: www.monitoringthefuture.org; accessed 1/16/01.

Kabat, G.C. Aspects of the epidemiology of lung cancer in smokers and nonsmokers in the United States. *Lung Cancer* 15:1-20, 1996.

Kaufman, D.W., Palmer, J.R., Rosenberg, L., Stolley, P; Warshauer, E., Shapiro, S. Tar content of cigarettes in relation to lung cancer. *American Journal of Epidemiology* 129:703-711, 1989.

Khuder, S.A., Dayal, H.H., Mutgi, A.B., Willey, J.C., Dayal, G. Effect of cigarette smoking on major histological types of lung cancer in men. Lung *Cancer* 22:15-21, 1998.

Kieth, C.H. Particle size studies on tobacco smoke. *Beitrage zur Tabakforschung International* 11:123-131, 1982.

Kieth, C.H., Derrick, J.C. Measurement of the particle size distribution and concentration of cigarette smoke by the "conifuge." *Journal of Colloid Science* 15:340-356, 1960.

Krzyzanowski, M., Sherrill, D.L., Paoletti, P., Lebowitz, M.D. Relationship of respiratory symptoms and pulmonary function to tar, nicotine, and carbon monoxide yield of cigarettes. *American Review of Respiratory Disease* 143:306-311, 1991.

Kuller, L.H. Ockene, J.K., Meilahn, E., Wentworth, D.N., Svendsen, KH., Neaton, J.D. Cigarette smoking and mortality. Cigarette smoking and mortality. MRFIT Research Group. *Preventive Medicine* 20:638-654, 1991.

Lange, P., Nyboe, J., Appleyard, M., Jensen, G., Schnohr, P. Relationship of the type of tobacco and inhalation pattern to pulmonary and total mortality. *European Respiratory Journal* 5:1111-1117, 1992.

Lee, P.N., Garfinkel, L. Mortality and type of cigarette smoked. *Journal of Epidemiology and Community Health* 35:16-22, 1981.

Levi, F., Franceschi, S., La Vecchia, C., Randimbson, L., Te, V. Lung carcinoma trends by histological type in Valud and Neuchatel, Switzerland, 1974–1994. *Cancer* 79:906-914, 1997.

Lubin, J.H., Blot, W.J., Berrino, F., Flamant, R., Gillis, C.R., Kunze, M., Schmahl, D., Visco, G. Patterns of lung cancer risk according to type of cigarette smoked. *International Journal of Cancer* 33:569-576, 1984.

Lubin, J.H. Modifying risk of developing lung cancer by changing habits of cigarette smoking. *British Medical Journal* 288:1953-56, 1984a.

Lubin, J.H. [letter-response] *British Medical Journal* 289:921, 1984b.

Mannino, D.M., Ford, E., Giovino, G.A, Thun, M. Lung cancer mortality rates in birth cohorts in the United States from 1960 to 1994. *Lung Cancer* 31(2-3):91-99, 2001.

Matos, E., Vilensky, M., Boffetta, P., Kogevinas, M. Lung cancer and smoking: A case-control study in Buenos Aires, Argentina. *Lung Cancer* 21:155-163, 1998.

Maxwell, J. C., Jr. *Historical Sales Trends in the Cigarette Industry, a Statistical Summary Covering 69 Years (1925-93)*. 1994. Richmond, VA, Wheat, First Securities, Inc.

McClusker, K., Hiller, F.C., Wilson, J.D., Mazumder, M.K., Bone R. Aerodynamic sizing of tobacco smoke particulate from commercial cigarettes. *Archives of Environmental Health* 38:215-218, 1983.

Miller, L.M., Monahan, J. The search for "safer" cigarettes. *The Reader's Digest* 38:37-45, 1959.

Mitchell, R.I. Second phase report on the determination of particle size in cigarette smoke. Report to Philip Morris Inc. Battelle Memorial Institute. October 30, 1958. Bates No. 1001905717.

Moolgavkar, S.H, Dewanji, A., Luebeck, G. Cigarette smoking and lung cancer: Reanalysis of the British Doctor's Data. *Journal of the National Cancer Institute* 81:415-420, 1989.

Morie, G.P., Sloan, C.H., Peck, V.G. Study of cigarette smoke filtration by means of the scanning electron microscope. *Beitrage zur Tabakforschung International* 7:99-104, 1973.

National Cancer Institute. *Cancer Mortality in the United States: 1959–1977.* NCI Monograph 59. U.S. Department of Health and Human Services, Public Health Service, National Institutes of Health, National Cancer Institute, NIH Publication No. 82-2435. 1982.

National Cancer Institute. *The FTC Cigarette Test Method for Determining Tar, Nicotine, and Carbon Monoxide Yields of U.S. Cigarettes. Report of the NCI Expert Committee.* Smoking and Tobacco Control Monograph No. 7. U.S. Department of Health and Human Services, National Institutes of Health, National Cancer Institute, NIH Publication No. 96-4028, 1996.

Negri, E., Franzosi, M.G., La Vecchia, C., Santoro, L., Nobili, A., Tognoni, G. Tar yield of cigarettes and risk of acute myocardial infarction. *British Medical Journal* 306:1567-1569, 1993.

Office for National Statistics (ONS). Statistics on Smoking: England. 1976–1996. *Statistical Bulletin* 1998/25, July 1998.

Palmer, J., Rosenberg, L., Shapiro, S. Low yield cigarettes and the risk of nonfatal myocardial infarction in women. *New England Journal of Medicine* 320:1569-1573, 1989.

Parish, S., Collins, R., Peto, R., Youngman, L., Barton, J., Jayne, K., Clarke, R., Appleby, P., Lyon, V., Cederholm-Williams, S., et al. Cigarette smoking, tar yields, and non-fatal myocardial infarction: 14,000 cases and 32,000 controls in the United Kingdom. The International Studies of Infarct Survival (ISIS) Collaborators. *British Medical Journal (Clin Res Ed)* 311[7003], 471-477, 1995.

Pathak, D.R., Samet, J.M., Humble, C.G., Skipper, B.J. Determinants of lung cancer risk in cigarette smokers in New Mexico. *Journal of the National Cancer Institute* 76:597-604, 1986.

Peel, D.M., Riddick, M.G., Edwards, M.E., Gentry, J.S., Nestor, T.B. *Formation of Tobacco Specific Nitrosamines in Flue-Cured Tobacco.* Presented at the 53rd Tobacco Science Research Conference. Montreal, Quebec, Canada. September 12–15, 1999.

Pepples, E. Industry response to cigarette/health controversy. February 4, 1976. University of California San Francisco Tobacco Archive Document I.D. 2205.01.

Petitti, D.B., Friedman, G.D. Cardiovascular and other diseases in smokers of low-yield cigarettes. *Journal of Chronic Diseases* 38:581-588, 1985.

Peto, R. Influence of dose and duration of smoking on lung cancer rates. *Tobacco: A Major International Health Hazard.* Zaridze, D.G., Peto, R. (Editors.). Lyons, France: International Agency for Research on Cancer, 1986.

Peto, R., Darby, S., Deo, H., Silcocks, P., Whitley, E., Doll, R. Smoking, smoking cessation, and lung cancer in the U.K. since 1950: Combination of national statistics with two case-control studies. *British Medical Journal* 321:323-329, 2000.

Pezzotto, S.M., Mahuad, R., Bay, M.L., Morini, J.C., Poletto, L. Variation in smoking-related lung cancer risk factors by cell type among men in Argentina: A case-control study. *Cancer Causes and Control* 4:231-237, 1993.

Pillsbury, H.C. Review of the Federal Trade Commission Method for determining cigarette tar and nicotine yield. *The FTC Cigarette Test Method for Determining Tar, Nicotine, and Carbon Monoxide Yields of U.S. Cigarettes. Report of the NCI Expert Committee.* Smoking and Tobacco Control Monograph No. 7. U.S. Department of Health and Human Services, National Institutes of Health, National Cancer Institute, NIH Publication No. 96-4028, 1996.

Powell, J.T., Edwards, R.J., Worrell, P.C., Franks, P.J., Greenhalgh, R.M., Poulter, N.R. Risk factors associated with the development of peripheral arterial disease in smokers: A case-control study. *Atherosclerosis* 129:41-48, 1997.

Rimington, J. The effect of filters on the incidence of lung cancer in cigarette smokers. *Environmental Research* 24:162-166, 1981.

Royal College of Physicians. *Smoking and Health. Summary and Report of the Royal College of Physicians of London on Smoking in Relation to Cancer of the Lung and Other Diseases.* New York: Pitman Publishing Corp, 1962.

Russo, A., Crosignani, P., Franceschi, S., Berrino, F. Changes in lung cancer histological types in Varese cancer registry, Italy 1976–1992. *European Journal of Cancer* 33:1643-1647, 1997.

S-Plus 2000. Guide to Statistics. Data Analysis Products Division, MathSoft, Inc. Seattle, WA. June, 1999.

Shanks, T.G. Reduction in disease risks after quitting smoking. Presentation APHA. Chicago, IL. November 1999.

Shiffman, S. Tobacco "chippers"—Individual differences in tobacco dependence. *Psychopharmacology (Berlin)* 97:539-547, 1989.

Sidney, S., Tekawa, I.S., Friedman, G.D. A prospective study of cigarette tar yield and lung cancer. *Cancer Causes and Control* 4:3-10, 1993.

Sparrow, D., Stefos, T., Bosse, R., Weiss, S.T. The relationship of tar content to decline in pulmonary function in cigarette smokers. *American Review of Respiratory Disease* 127:56-58, 1983.

Stellman, S.D., Muscat, J.E., Thompson, S., Hoffmann, D., Wynder, E.L. Risk of squamous cell carcinoma and adenocarcinoma of the lung in relation to lifetime filter cigarette smoking. *Cancer* 80(3):382-388, 1997.

Stevens, R., Moolgavkar, S. Estimation of relative risk from vital data: smoking and cancers of the lung and bladder. *Journal of the National Cancer Institute* 63:1351-1357, 1979.

Stevens, R., Moolgavkar, S. A cohort analysis of lung cancer and smoking in British males. *American Journal of Epidemiology* 119:624-641, 1984.

156

Swartz, J.B. Use of a multistage model to predict time trends in smoking induced lung cancer. *Journal of Epidemiology and Community Health* 46:311-315, 1992.

Tang, J.L., Morris, J.K., Wald, N.J., Hole, D., Shipley, M., Tunstall-Pedoe, H. Mortality in relation to tar yield of cigarettes: A prospective study of four cohorts. *British Medical Journal* 311:1530-1533, 1995.

Teague, C. Research planning memorandum on a new type of cigarette delivering a satisfying amount of nicotine with a reduced "tar"-to-nicotine ratio. March 28, 1972. Engle Plantiffs Exhibit No. 0111.

Thun, M.J., Heath, C.W. Changes in mortality from smoking in two American Cancer Society prospective studies since 1959. *Preventive Medicine* 26:422-426. 1997.

Thun, M.J., Lally, C.A., Flannery, J.T., Calle, E.E., Flanders, W.D., Heath, C.W. Cigarette smoking and changes in the histopathology of lung cancer. *Journal of the National Cancer Institute* 89:1580-1586, 1997a.

Thun, M., Myersm D., Day-Lallym C., Myers, D.G., Calle, E., Flanders, W.D., Zhu, B.P., Namboodiri, M., Heath, Jr, C. Trends in tobacco smoking and mortality from cigarette use in cancer prevention studies I (1959 through 1965) and II (1982 through 1988). *Changes in Cigarette-Related Disease Risks and Their Implications for Prevention and Control*. Smoking and Tobacco Control Monograph No. 8. U.S. Department of Health and Human Services, National Institutes of Health, National Cancer Institute, NIH Publication No. 97-4213, 1997b.

Tobacco Advisory Group (of the Royal College of Physicians). *Nicotine Addiction in Britain*. Royal College of Physicians of London, 2000.

Todd, G.F., Hunt, B.M., Lambert, P.M. Four cardiorespiratory symptoms as predictors of mortality. *Journal of Epidemiology and Community Health* 32:267-274, 1978.

Townsend, J. Smoking and lung cancer: A cohort study of men and women in England and Wales 1935–70. *Journal of the Royal Statistical Society* A141[pt 1]:95-107, 1978.

Tolley, H.D., Crane, L., Shipley, N. Smoking prevalence and lung cancer death rates. *Strategies to Control Tobacco Use in the United States: A Blueprint for Public Health Action in the 1990s*. Smoking and Tobacco Control Monograph No. 1. U.S. Department of Health and Human Services, National Institutes of Health, National Cancer Institute, Publication No. [PHS] 92-3316, 1991.

Travis, W.D., Travis, L.B., Devesa, S.S. Lung cancer. *Cancer* 75:191-202, 1995.

U.S. Bureau of the Census. U.S. population estimates by age, sex, race. Washington, D.C., 2000 Available from ww.census.gov/population/www/estimates/nat_80s_detail.html and nat_90s_detail.

U.S. Congress. Hearings before the Consumer Subcommittee of the Committee on Commerce. Senate, 90th Congress, August 23, 24, 1967.

U.S. Department of Health, Education, and Welfare. *The Health Consequences of Smoking: A Report to the Surgeon General*. U.S. Department of Health, Education, and Welfare, Public Health Service, Health Services and Mental Health Administration, Office on Smoking and Health. DHEW Publication No. (HSM) 71-7513, 1971.

U.S. Department of Health, Education, and Welfare. *Smoking and Health. A Report of the Surgeon General*. U.S. Department of Health, Education, and Welfare, Public Health Service, Office of the Assistant Secretary for Health, Office on Smoking and Health. DHEW Publication No. (PHS) 79-50066, 1979.

U.S. Department of Health and Human Services. *The Health Consequences of Smoking: The Changing Cigarette. A Report of the Surgeon General*. U.S. Department of Health and Human Services, Public Health Service, Office of the Assistant Secretary for Health, Office on Smoking and Health. DHHS Publication No. 81-50156, 1981.

U.S. Department of Health and Human Services. *The Health Consequences of Smoking: Nicotine Addiction. A Report of the Surgeon General*. U.S. Department of Health and Human Services, Public Health Service, Centers for Disease Control and Prevention, Center for Health Promotion and Education, Office on Smoking and Health, 1988. DHHS Publication No. (CDC) 88-8406.

U.S. Department of Health and Human Services. *The Health Benefits of Smoking Cessation. A Report of the Surgeon General*. U.S. Department of Health and Human Services, Public Health Service, Centers for Disease Control and Prevention, Center for Chronic Disease Prevention and Health Promotion, Office on Smoking and Health, DHHS Publication No. (CDC) 90-8416, 1990.

U.S. Department of Health and Human Services. *Preventing Tobacco Use Among Young People: A Report of the Surgeon General*. U.S. Department of Health and Human Services, Public Health Service, Centers for Disease Control and Prevention, National Center for Chronic Disease Prevention and Health Promotion, Office on Smoking and Health, 1994.

U.S. Department of Health and Human Services. *Tobacco Use Among U.S. Racial/Ethnic Minority Groups: A Report of the Surgeon General*. U.S. Department of Health and Human Services, Public Health Service, Centers for Disease Control and Prevention, National Center for Chronic Disease Prevention and Health Promotion, Office on Smoking and Health, 1998.

Vutuc, C., Kunze, M. Lung cancer risk in women in relation to tar yields of cigarettes. *Preventive Medicine* 11:713-716, 1982.

Vutuc, C., Kunze, M. Tar yields if cigarettes and male lung cancer risk. *Journal of the National Cancer Institute* 71:435-437, 1983.

Wakeham, H to Cullman, H. March 24, 1961. Memo by H. Wakeman. Trends in tar and nicotine deliveries over the last 5 years. Bates No. 1000861953.

Warner, KE. Tobacco industry response to public health concern: A content analysis of cigarette ads. *Health Education Quarterly* 12:115-27, 1985.

Wald, N., Nicolaides-Bouman, A. (Editors.). *UK Smoking Statistics.* 2nd Edition. Oxford, UK: Oxford University Press, 1991.

Wilcox, H.B., Schoenberg, J.B., Mason, T.J., Bill, J.S., Stemhagen, A. Smoking and lung cancer: Risk as a function of cigarette tar content. *Preventive Medicine* 17:263-272, 1988.

Wingo, P.A, Ries, L.A.G., Giovino, G.A., Miller, D.S., Rosenberg, H.M., Shopland D.R., Thun, M.J., Edwards, B.K. Annual report to the nation on the status of cancer, 1973–1996, with a special section on lung cancer and tobacco smoking. *Journal of the National Cancer Institute* 91:675-690, 1999.

Withey, C.H., Papacosta, A.O., Swan, A.V., Fitzsimons, B.A., Ellard, G.A., Burney, P.G., Colley, J.R., Holland, W.W. Respiratory effects of lowering tar and nicotine levels of cigarettes smoked by young male middle tar smokers. II. Results of a randomised controlled trial. *Journal of Epidemiology and Community Health* 46(3):281-285, 1992.

Whittemore, A.S. Effect of cigarette smoking in epidemiological studies of lung cancer. *Statistics in Medicine* 7:223-238, 1988.

World Health Organization. *Manual of the International Statistical Classification of Diseases, Injuries, and Causes of Death* (7th Ed. Rev. of the *International Lists of Diseases and Causes of Death,* adapted 1955). Vol. 1. Geneva: World Health Organization, 1957.

Wynder, E.L., Graham, E.A. Tobacco smoking as a possible etiologic factor in bronchogenic carcinoma. A study of six hundred and eighty-four proved cases. *Journal of the American Medical Association* 143:329-336, 1950.

Wynder, E.L., Graham, E.A., Croninger, A.B. Experimental production of carcinoma with cigarette tar. *Cancer Research* 13:855-864, 1953.

Wynder, E.L., Kabat, G.C. The effect of low-yield cigarette smoking on lung cancer risk. *Cancer* 62:1223-1230, 1988.

Wynder, E.L., Mabuchi, K., Beattie, E.J., Jr. The epidemiology of lung cancer: Recent trends. *Journal of the American Medical Association* 213:2221-2228, 1970.

Wynder, E.L., Stellman, S.D. Impact of long-term filter cigarette usage on lung and larynx cancer risk: A case–control study. *Journal of the National Cancer Institute* 62:471-477, 1979.

# The Changing Cigarette: Chemical Studies and Bioassays

Dietrich Hoffmann, Ilse Hoffmann

**INTRODUCTION**    In 1950, the first large-scale epidemiological studies on smoking and lung cancer conducted by Wynder and Graham, in the United States, and Doll and Hill, in the United Kingdom, strongly supported the concept of a dose response between the number of cigarettes smoked and the risk for cancer of the lung (Wynder and Graham, 1950; Doll and Hill, 1950).

In 1953, the first successful induction of cancer in a laboratory animal with a tobacco product was reported with the application of cigarette tar[a] to mouse skin (Wynder et al., 1953). The particulate matter of cigarette smoke generated by an automatic smoking machine was suspended in acetone (1:1) and painted onto the shaven backs of mice three times weekly for up to 24 months. A clear dose response was observed between the amount of tar applied to the skin of the mice and the percentage of skin papilloma- and carcinoma-bearing animals in the test group (Wynder et al., 1957). Since then, mouse skin has been widely used as the primary bioassay method for estimating the carcinogenic potency of tobacco tar and its fractions, as well as of particulate matters of other combustion products (Wynder and Hoffmann, 1962, 1967; NCI, 1977a, 1977b, 1977c, 1980; Hoffmann and Wynder, 1977; IARC, 1986a). Intratracheal instillation in rats of the PAH-containing neutral subfraction of cigarette tar led to squamous cell carcinoma of the trachea and lung (Davis et al., 1975). A cigarette tar suspension in acetone painted onto the inner ear of rabbits led to carcinoma with metastasis in thoracic organs (Graham et al., 1957).

Dontenwill and colleagues (1973) developed a method that involved placing Syrian golden hamsters individually into plastic tubes and exposing them to cigarette smoke diluted with air (1:15) twice daily, 5 days a week, for up to 24 months (Dontenwill et al., 1973). The method led to lesions primarily in the epithelial tissue of the outer larynx. Using an inbred strain of Syrian golden hamsters with increased susceptibility of the respiratory tract to carcinogens, long-term exposure to cigarette smoke produced a high tumor yield in the larynx (Bernfeld et al., 1974). A dose response was recorded between the degree of smoke exposure and the induction of benign and malignant tumors in the larynges of the hamsters.

In general, inhalation studies have not found that tobacco smoke leads to squamous cell carcinoma of the lung (Wynder and Hoffmann, 1967; Mohr and Reznik, 1978; IARC, 1986a & b). Dalbey and associates from the National Laboratory in Oak Ridge, Tennessee, exposed female F344 rats to diluted smoke of up to 7 cigarettes daily, 5 times a week for up to 2.5 years. A high percentage of the smoke-exposed rats developed hyperplasia and

---

[a]    Throughout the article, the term "tar" is only used as descriptive noun.

159

metaplasia in the epithelium of the nasal turbinates and in the larynx, and also some hyperplasia in the trachea. The sham-treated rats developed a small number of lesions in nasal and laryngeal epithelia but none in the trachea. Ten tumors of the respiratory system were observed in 7 out of 80 smoke-exposed rats. These were 1 adenocarcinoma, 1 squamous cell carcinoma in the nasal cavity, 5 adenomas of the lung, 2 alveologenic carcinomas, and 1 squamous cell carcinoma of the lung (Dalbey *et al.*, 1980). In the control group of 93 sham-smoked rats, 1 developed an alveologenic carcinoma (Dalbey *et al.*, 1980). In 1952, Essenberg reported that cigarette smoke induces an excessive number of pulmonary adenomas; whereas, the sham-exposed mice, as well as the untreated mice, developed significantly lower rates of pulmonary tumors (Essenberg, 1952). In the following years, the Leuchtenbergers repeatedly confirmed the findings by Essenberg. They also demonstrated that even the gas phase increased the occurrence of pulmonary tumors in mice (Leuchtenberger *et al.*, 1958; Leuchtenberger and Leuchtenberger, 1970). Several additional studies demonstrated the induction of pulmonary tumors in several strains of mice exposed to diluted cigarette smoke (Mühlbock, 1958; Wynder and Hoffmann, 1967; Mohr and Reznik, 1978; IARC, 1986a & b). Otto exposed mice to diluted cigarette smoke for 60 minutes daily for up to 24 months. Of 30 mice, 4 developed lung adenomas and 1 an epidermoid carcinoma of the lung. In the untreated control group, 3 of 60 mice developed lung adenomas (Otto, 1963).

## IDENTIFICATION OF CARCINOGENS, TUMOR PROMOTERS, AND CARCINOGENS IN TOBACCO SMOKE

Green and Rodgman (1996) estimated that there were about 4,800 compounds in tobacco smoke. In addition, additives out of a list of 599 compounds disclosed by tobacco companies (Doull *et al.*, 1994) may be added to cigarette tobacco in the process of manufacturing a cigarette in the United States (Green and Rodgman, 1996; Doull *et al.*, 1994). Tables 5-1 and 5-2 list the major constituents of the vapor phase (Table 5-1) and the particulate phase (Table 5-2) and their concentrations in the mainstream smoke (MS) of non-filter cigarettes (Hoffmann and Hecht, 1990; Ishiguro and Sugawara, 1980). The agricultural chemicals and pesticides, as well as their specific thermic degradation products, are omitted from the two tables because of the many variations in the nature and amount of these agents in tobacco from country to country and from year to year (Wittekindt, 1985). Table 5-3 lists the major toxic components in the MS of cigarettes (Hoffmann *et al.*, 1995).

Development of highly sensitive analytical methods, as well as reproducible short-term and long-term assays, has led to the identification of 69 carcinogens (Table 5-4). Of these, 11 are known human carcinogens (Group I), 7 are probably carcinogenic in humans (Group 2A), and 49 of the animal carcinogens are possibly also carcinogenic to humans (Group 2B). This classification of the carcinogens is according to the International Agency for Research on Cancer (IARC, 1983, 1984, 1986b, 1987, 1988, 1991, 1992, 1994a–e, 1995a & b, 1996, 1999a & b). Two suspected carcinogens have yet to be evaluated by the IARC.

Table 5-1
**Major Constituents of the Vapor Phase of the Mainstream Smoke of Non-Filter Cigarettes**

| Compound[a] | Concentration/Cigarette (% of Total Effluent) |
|---|---|
| Nitrogen | 280-320 mg (56-64%) |
| Oxygen | 50-70 mg (11-14%) |
| Carbon dioxide | 45-65 mg (9-13%) |
| Carbon monoxide | 14-23 mg (2.8-4.6%) |
| Water | 7-12 mg (1.4-2.4%) |
| Argon | 5 mg (1.0%) |
| Hydrogen | 0.5-1.0 mg |
| Ammonia | 10-130 µg |
| Nitrogen oxides ($NO_x$) | 100-600 µg |
| Hydrogen cyanide | 400-500 µg |
| Hydrogen sulfide | 20-90 µg |
| Methane | 1.0-2.0 mg |
| Other volatile aromatic alkanes (20) | 1.0-1.6 mg[b] |
| Volatile alkenes (16) | 0.4-0.5 mg |
| Isoprene | 0.2-0.4 mg |
| Butadiene | 25-40 µg |
| Acetylene | 20-35 µg |
| Benzene | 12-50 µg |
| Toluene | 20-60 µg |
| Styrene | 10 µg |
| Other volatile hydrocarbons (29) | 15-30 µg |
| Formic acid | 200-600 µg |
| Acetic acid | 300-1,700 µg |
| Propionic acid | 100-300 µg |
| Methyl formate | 20-30 µg |
| Other volatile acids (6) | 5-10 µg |
| Formaldehyde | 20-100 µg |
| Acetaldehyde | 400-1400 µg |
| Acrolein | 60-140 µg |
| Other volatile aldehydes (6) | 80-140 µg |
| Acetone | 100-650 µg |
| Other volatile ketones (3) | 50-100 µg |
| Methanol | 80-180 µg |
| Other volatile alcohols (7) | 10-30 µg |
| Acetonitrile | 100-150 µg |
| Other volatile nitriles (10) | 50-80 µg[b] |
| Furan | 20-40 µg |
| Other volatile furans (4) | 45-125 µg[b] |
| Pyndine | 20-200 µg |
| Pyridine (3) | 15-80 µg |
| 3-Vinylpyridine | 10-30 µg |
| Other volatile pyridines (25) | 20-50 µg[b] |
| Pyrrole | 0.1-10 µg |
| Pyrrolidine | 10-18 µg |
| N-Methylpyrrolidine | 2.0-3.0 µg |
| Volatile pyrazines (18) | 3.0-8.0 µg |
| Methylamine | 4-10 µg |
| Other aliphatic amines (32) | 3-10 µg |

[a]*Numbers in parentheses represent the individual compounds identified in a given group*
[b]*Estimate*

161

Table 5-2

## Major Constituents of the Particulate Matter of the Mainstream Smoke of Non-Filter Cigarettes

| Compound[a] | µg/Cigarette[b] |
|---|---|
| Nicotine | 1.000-3.000 |
| Nornicotine | 50-150 |
| Anatabine | 5-15 |
| Anabasine | 5-12 |
| Other tobacco alkaloids (17) | NA |
| Bipyridyls (4) | 10-30 |
| $n$-Hentriacontane ($n$-C$_{31}$H$_{64}$)[c] | 100 |
| Total nonvolatile hydrocarbons (45)[c] | 300-400[c] |
| Naphthalene | 2-4 |
| Naphthalenes (23) | 3-6[c] |
| Phenanthrenes (7) | 0.2-0.4[c] |
| Anthracenes (5) | 0.05-0.1[c] |
| Fluorenes (7) | 0.6-1.0[c] |
| Pyrenes (6) | 0.3-0.5[c] |
| Fluoranthenes | 0.3-0.45[c] |
| Carcinogenic polynuclear aromatic hydrocarbons (11)[b] | 0.1-0.25 |
| Phenol | 80-160 |
| Other phenols (45)[c] | 60-180[c] |
| Catechol | 200-400 |
| Other catechols (4) | 100-200[c] |
| Other dihydroxybenzenes (10) | 200-400[c] |
| Scopoletin | 15-30 |
| Other polyphenols (8)[c] | NA |
| Cyclotenes (10)[c] | 40-70[c] |
| Quinones (7) | 0.50 |
| Solanesol | 600-1,000 |
| Neophytadienes (4) | 200-350 |
| Limonene | 30-60 |
| Other terpenes (200-250)[c] | NA |
| Palmitic acid | 100-150 |
| Stearic acid | 50-75 |
| Oleic acid | 40-110 |
| Linoleic acid | 150-250 |
| Linolenic acid | 150-250 |
| Lactic acid | 60-80 |
| Indole | 10-15 |
| Skatole | 12-16 |
| Other indoles (13) | NA |
| Quinolines (7) | 2-4 |
| Other aza-arenes (55) | NA |
| Benzofurans (4) | 200-300 |
| Other 0-heterocyclic compounds (42) | NA |
| Stigmasterol | 40-70 |
| Sitosterol | 30-40 |
| Campesterol | 20-30 |
| Cholesterol | 10-20 |
| Aniline | 0.36 |
| Toluidines | 0.23 |
| Other aromatic amines (12) | 0.25 |
| Tobacco-specific $N$-nitrosamines (6) | 0.34-2.7 |
| Glycerol | 120 |

[a]*Numbers in parentheses represent individual compounds identified.*
[b]*For details, See Table 5-4*
[c]*Estimate. NA=Not available.*

Table 5-3
**Major Toxic Agents in Cigarette Smoke[a]**

| Agent | Concentration/ Non-Filter Cigarette | Toxicity |
|---|---|---|
| Carbon monoxide | 10-23 mg | Binds to hemoglobin, inhibits respiration |
| Ammonia | 10-130 µg | Irritation of respiratory tract |
| Nitrogen oxide (NO$_x$) | 100-600 µg | Inflamation of the lung |
| Hydrogen cyanide | 400-500 µg | Highly ciliatoxic, inhibits lung clearance |
| Hydrogen sulfide | 10-90 µg | Irritation of respiratory tract |
| Acrolein | 60-140 µg | Ciliatoxic, inhibits lung clearance |
| Methanol | 100-250 µg | Toxic upon inhalation and ingestion |
| Pyridine | 16-40 µg | Irritates respiratory tract |
| Nicotine[b] | 1.0-3.0 mg | Induces dependence, affects cardiovascular and endocrine systems |
| Phenol | 80-160 µg | Tumor promoter in laboratory animals |
| Catechol | 200-400 µg | Cocarcinogen in laboratory animals |
| Aniline | 360-655 µg | Forms methemoglobin, and this affects respiration |
| Maleic hydrazide | 1.16 µg | Mutagenic agent |

[a]This is an incomplete list.
[b]Toxicity: oral/rat, $LD_{50}$ free nicotine 50 mg/kg, nicotine bitartrate 65 mg/kg.
*Source: Hoffmann et al., 1998.*

Table 5-4
**Carcinogens in Cigarette Smoke**

| Agent | Conc./Non-filter Cigarette | IARC Evaluation Evidence of Carcinogenicity in Lab Animals | in Humans | Group[a] |
|---|---|---|---|---|
| **PAH** | | | | |
| Benz(*a*)anthracene | 20-70 ng | Sufficient | | 2A |
| Benzo(*b*)fluoranthene | 4-22 ng | Sufficient | | 2B |
| Benzo(*j*)fluoranthene | 6-21 ng | Sufficient | | 2B |
| Benzo(*k*)fluoranthene | 6-12 ng | Sufficient | | 2B |
| Benzo(*a*)pyrene | 20-40 ng | Sufficient | Probable | 2A |
| Dibenz(*a,h*)anthracene | 4 ng | Sufficient | | 2A |
| Dibenzo(*a,l*)pyrene | 1.7-3.2 ng | Sufficient | | 2B |
| Dibenzo(*a,e*)pyrene | Present | Sufficient | | 2B |
| Indeno(1,2,3-*cd*)pyrene | 4-20 ng | Sufficient | | 2B |
| 5-Methylchrysene | 0.6 ng | Sufficient | | 2B |
| **Heterocyclic Compounds** | | | | |
| Quinoline[b] | 1-2 ng | | | |
| Dibenz(*a,h*)acridine | 0.1 ng | Sufficient | | 2B |
| Dibenz(*a,j*)acridine | 3-10 ng | Sufficient | | 2B |
| Dibenzo(*c,g*)carbazole | 0.7 ng | Sufficient | | 2B |
| Benzo(*b*)furan | Present | Sufficient | | 2B |
| Furan | 18-37 ng | Sufficient | | 2B |

Table 5-4 (continued)

| Agent | Conc./Non-filter Cigarette | IARC Evaluation Evidence of Carcinogenicity in Lab Animals | in Humans | Group[a] |
|---|---|---|---|---|
| ***N*-Nitrosamines** | | | | |
| *N*-Nitrosodimethylamine | 2-180 ng | Sufficient | | 2A |
| *N*-Nitrosoethylmethylamine | 3-13 ng | Sufficient | | 2B |
| *N*-Nitrosodiethylamine | ND-2.8 ng | Sufficient | | 2A |
| *N*-Nitrosodi-*n*-propylamine | ND-1.0 ng | Sufficient | | 2B |
| *N*-Nitroso-di-*n*-butylamine | ND-30 ng | Sufficient | | 2B |
| *N*-Nitrosopyrrolidine | 3-110 ng | Sufficient | | 2B |
| *N*-Nitrosopiperidine | ND-9 ng | Sufficient | | 2B |
| *N*-Nitrosodiethanolamine | ND-68 ng | Sufficient | | 2B |
| *N*-Nitrosonornicotine | 120-3,700 ng | Sufficient | | 2B |
| 4-(Methylnitrosamino)-1-(3-pyridyl)-1-butanone | 80-770 ng | Sufficient | | 2B |
| | | | | |
| **Aromatic Amines** | | | | |
| 2-Toluidine | 30-337 ng | Sufficient | | 2B |
| 2,6-Dimethylaniline | 4-50 µg | Sufficient | | 2B |
| 2-Naphthylamine | 1-334 ng | Sufficient | Sufficient | 1 |
| 4-Aminobiphenyl | 2-5.6 ng | Sufficient | Sufficient | 1 |
| | | | | |
| ***N*-Heterocyclic Amines** | | | | |
| AaC | 25-260 ng | Sufficient | | 2B |
| IQ | 0.3 ng | Sufficient | | 2B |
| Trp-P-1 | 0.3-0.5 ng | Sufficient | | 2B |
| Trp-P-2 | 0.8-1.1 ng | Sufficient | | 2B |
| Glu-P-1 | 0.37-0.89 ng | Sufficient | | 2B |
| Glu-P-2 | 0.25-0.88 ng | Sufficient | | 2B |
| PhIP | 11-23 ng | Sufficient | Possible | 2A |
| | | | | |
| **Aldehydes** | | | | |
| Formaldehyde | 70-100 µg | Sufficient | Limited | 2A |
| Acetaldehyde | 500-1,400 µg | Sufficient | Insufficient | 2B |
| | | | | |
| **Volatile Hydrocarbons** | | | | |
| 1,3-Butadiene | 20-75 µg | Sufficient | Insufficient | 2B |
| Isoprene | 450-1,000 µg | Sufficient | | 2B |
| Benzene | 20-70 µg | Sufficient | Sufficient | 1 |
| Styrene | 10 µg | Limited | | 2B |
| | | | | |
| **Misc. Organic Compounds[c]** | | | | |
| Acetamide | 38-56 µg | Sufficient | | 2B |
| Acrylamide | Present | Sufficient | | 2B |
| Acrylonitrile | 3-15 µg | Sufficient | Limited | 2A |
| Vinyl chloride | 11-15 ng | Sufficient | Sufficient | 1 |
| DDT | 800-1,200 µg | Sufficient | Probable | 2B |
| DDE | 200-370 µg | Sufficient | | 2B |
| Catechol | 100-360 µg | Sufficient | | 2B |
| Caffeic acid | < 3 µg | Sufficient | | 2B |
| 1,1-Dimethylhydrazine | Present | Sufficient | | 2B |
| Nitromethane | 0.3-0.6 µg | Sufficient | | 2B |

Table 5-4 (continued)

| Agent | Conc./Non-filter Cigarette | IARC Evaluation Evidence of Carcinogenicity in Lab Animals | in Humans | Group[a] |
|---|---|---|---|---|
| 2-Nitropropane | 0.7-1.2 µg | Sufficient | | 2B |
| Nitrobenzene | 25 µg | Sufficient | | 2B |
| Ethyl carbamate | 20-38 µg | Sufficient | | 2B |
| Ethylene oxide | 7 µg | Sufficient | Sufficient | 1 |
| Propylene oxide | 12-100 ng | Sufficient | | 2B |
| Methyleugenol | 20 ng | | | |
| **Inorganic Compounds** | | | | |
| Hydrazine | 24-43 ng | Sufficient | Inadequate | 2B |
| Arsenic | 40-120 µg | Inadequate | Sufficient | 1 |
| Beryllium | 0.5 ng | Sufficient | Sufficient | 1 |
| Nickel | ND-600 ng | Sufficient | Sufficient | 1 |
| Chromium (only hexavalent) | 4-70 ng | Sufficient | Sufficient | 1 |
| Cadmium | 7-350 ng | Sufficient | Sufficient | 1 |
| Cobalt | 0.13-0.2 ng | Sufficient | Inadequate | 2B |
| Lead | 34-85 ng | Sufficient | Inadequate | 2B |
| Polonium-210 | 0.03-1.0 pCi | Sufficient | Sufficient | 1 |

*Abbreviations: ND, not detected; PAH, polynuclar aromatic hydrocarbons; AaC, 2-amino-9H-pyrido[2,3-b]indole; IQ, 2-amino-3-methylimidazo[4,5-b]quinoline; Trp-P-1, 3-amino-1,4-dimethyl-5H-pyrido[4,3-b]indole; Trp-2, 3-amino-1-methyl-5H-pyrido[4,3-b]indole; Glue-P-1, 2-amino-6-methyl[1,2-a:3',2"-d] imidazole; Glu-P-2, 2-aminodipyrido[1,2-a:3'2"-d]imidazole; PhIP, 2-amino-1-methyl-6-phenylimidazo [4,5-b]pyridine.*
[a]*IARC Monographs on the Evaluation of Carcinogenic Risks. Volume 1 and Supplements 1-8, 1972-1999. (1) Human carcinogens; (2A) Probably carcinogenic in humans; (2B) Possibly carcinogenic to humans; (3) Not classifiable as to their carcinogenicity to humans.*
[b]*Unassigned carcinogenicity status by IARC at this time*
[c]*In 1982, the IARC assigned di(2-ethylhexyl)phthalate as sufficient to Group 2B. However, in 2000, re-evaluation of the carcinogenicity was classified as not carcinogenic (IARC 1982, 2000). We cited di(2-ethylhexyl)phthalate as a 2B carcinogen (Hoffmann and Hoffmann, 1997) and in this article, it is deleted from Table 5-4, "Carcinogenicity in Cigarette Smoke."*
*Sources: International Agency for Research on Cancer, 1982, 2000.*

**SMOKING CONDITIONS**      In 1936, the American Tobacco Company began using standard machine smoking conditions, which, to some extent, reflected the smoking habits of cigarette smokers at that time. The estimated sales-weighted average nicotine yields of the cigarettes smoked at that time were around 2.8 mg (Bradford *et al.*, 1936). In agreement with the U.S. tobacco industry, the Federal Trade Commission (FTC) adapted the 1936 standard method in 1969 with only slight modifications. Since then, machine-smoking conditions are one puff/minute with a volume of 35 ml drawn during 2 seconds, leaving a butt length of 23 mm for a non-filter (plain) cigarette, and length of the filter and overwrap plus 3 mm for a filter cigarette (Pillsbury *et al.*, 1969). In Canada and the United Kingdom, the standard smoking conditions of the International Standards Organization (ISO) have been accepted since 1991 (ISO, 1991). In other European countries, the standard smoking conditions for cigarettes are those developed by CORESTA (Centre De Cooperation Pour Les Recherches Scientifiques Relative Au Tabac), which are similar to the FTC standard smoking conditions (CORESTA, 1991). In Japan, the FTC standard smoking conditions are employed for the machine smoking of cigarettes (Pillsbury *et al.*, 1969). The FTC method defines tar as smoke particulates minus water and nicotine, whereas CORESTA defines tar as total particulates minus water (Pillsbury *et al.*, 1969; ISO, 1991; CORESTA, 1991). The standard conditions for machine smoking of tobacco products used by the different testing protocols are presented in Table 5-5. Using the FTC method, the sales-weighted average tar and nicotine yields of U. S. cigarettes decreased from about 37 mg and 2.7 mg in 1954 to 12 mg and 0.85 mg in 1993 (Figure 5-1).

More than 20 years ago, M.A.H. Russell in the United Kingdom and N.L. Benowitz in the United States reported that long-term smokers of cigarettes with lower nicotine yields took more than one puff per minute, drew puff volumes exceeding 35 ml, and inhaled the smoke more deeply than smokers of higher yield cigarettes (Russell, 1976, 1980; Benowitz *et al.*, 1983).

Table 5-6 presents the smoking characteristics of 56 volunteer smokers who regularly consumed low-yield cigarettes ($\leq$ 0.8 mg nicotine/cigarette according to the FTC smoking machine method) and of 77 volunteer smokers regularly consuming medium-nicotine cigarettes (FTC, 0.9–1.2 mg/cigarette). These two ranges of nicotine yield constituted more than 73.4 percent of all cigarettes smoked in the U.S. in 1993 (FTC, 1995). The results of this study clearly indicated that the majority of U.S. smokers smoked their cigarettes much more intensely to satisfy their acquired need for nicotine. Comparing the yields of the same cigarettes smoked under FTC standard machine smoking conditions with the smoke inhaled by the consumers of cigarettes with low- and medium-nicotine content revealed that smokers inhaled 2.5 and 2.2 times more nicotine/cigarette, 2.6 and 1.9 times more tar, 1.8 and 1.5 times more carbon monoxide, 1.8 and 1.6 times more BaP, and 1.7 and 1.7 times more NNK than is generated by the FTC machine-smoking method (Table 5-6; Djordjevic *et al.*, 2000).

The discrepancy in exposure assessment between recent measurements and former interpretations of machine-smoking data has led to criticism of the FTC standard machine smoking method for consumer guidance. The suggestion that there is a meaningful quantitative relationship between the FTC-measured yields and actual intake (by the cigarette smoker) is misleading (Benowitz, 1996). In view of these concerns, it appears "that the time has come for meaningful information on the yields of cigarettes" (Wilkenfeld *et al.*, 2000a & b). The FTC agrees, in principle, that a better and more comprehensive test program for cigarettes is needed (Peeler and Butters, 2000).

**CHANGES IN CIGARETTE SMOKE COMPOSITION WITH VARIOUS DESIGN CHANGES**

**Filter Tips**

In 1959, Haag *et al.* reported the selective reduction of volatile smoke constituents by filtration through charcoal filter tips (Haag *et al.*, 1959). Several of the compounds that are selectively removed from mainstream smoke (MS) in this fashion are major ciliatoxic agents, such as hydrogen cyanide, formaldehyde, acrolein, and acetaldehyde. Charcoal filters reduce the MS levels of these agents by up to 66 percent (Kensler and Battista, 1966; Tiggelbeck, 1976; Battista, 1976). However, for tar reduction, charcoal filters are less efficient than cellulose acetate filters. Several types of combination filters are in use. The early charcoal-activated dual and triple filter tips were cellulose acetate filters with embedded charcoal powder or granulated char-

Table 5-5
**Standard Conditions for Machine Smoking of Tobacco Product**

| Parameters | Cigarettes | | Bidis | Little Cigars | Small Cigars | Cigars | Premium | Pipes |
|---|---|---|---|---|---|---|---|---|
| | FTC | CORESTA | | FTC | CORESTA | CORESTA | CORESTA | CORESTA |
| **Weight** (g) | 0.8-1.1 | 0.8-1.1 | 0.55-0.80 | 0.9-1.3 | 1.3-2.5 | 5-17 | 6-20 | * |
| **Puff** | | | | | | | | |
| Frequency (sec) | 60.0 | 60.0 | 30.0 | 60.0 | 40.0 | 40.0 | 40.0 | 20.0 |
| Duration (sec) | 2.0 | 2.0 | 2.0 | 2.0 | 1.5 | 1.5 | 1.5 | 2.0 |
| Volume (ml) | 35.0 | 35.0 | 35.0 | 35.0 | 40.0 | 40.0 | 40.0 | 50.0 |
| **Butt length (mm)** | | | | | | | | |
| Non-filter | 23.0 | 23.0 | 23.0 | 23.0 | 33.0 | 33.0 | 33.0 | |
| Filter | | F&OW+3F+8 | F&OW+3 | | | | | |

*Abbreviations: FTC = Federal Trade Commission method; CORESTA = Centre de Cooperation Pour Les Reherches Scientifiques Relative au Tabac Method; F = filter tip; OW = overwrap.*
*One gram of pipe tobacco smoked.*
*Sources: Hoffmann et al., 1974; International Committee for Cigar Smoking, 1974; Miller, 1963.*

Figure 5-1
**Sales-Weighted Tar and Nicotine Values for U.S. Cigarettes as Measured by Machine Using the FTC Method, 1954*-1998**

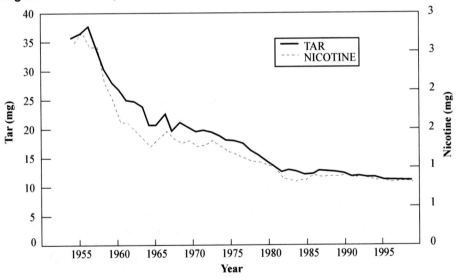

*Values before 1968 are estimated from available data.*

coal sandwiched between cellulose acetate segments. These filters have been improved by innovative filter designs, incorporating cellulose acetate, charcoal, and cigarette filter paper (Shepherd, 1994). In the United States, however, cigarettes with charcoal filters have accounted for only about 1 percent of all cigarette sales over the past 15 years. In most developed coun-

Table 5-6

**A Comparison of Smoke Data for Two Low-Yield U.S. Filter Cigarettes Smoked According to the FTC-Method and by Smokers**

| Parameters | FTC Machine Smoking | Cigarette Smokers | |
|---|---|---|---|
| | | FTC 0.6-0.8 Nicotine | FTC 0.9-1.2 Nicotine |
| **Puff** | | | |
| Volume (ml) | 35.0 | 48.6 (45.2-52.3)[a] | 44.1 (40.8-46.8)[b] |
| Interval (sec) | 58.0 | 21.3 (19.0-23.8)[a] | 18.5 (16.5-20.6)[b] |
| Duration (sec) | 2.0 | 1.5 (1.4-1.7)[a] | 1.5 (1.4-1.6)[b] |
| **Nicotine** (mg/cig) | 0.7 (0.6-0.8) | 1.74 (1.54-1.98)[c] | |
| | 0.1 (1.09-1.13) | | 2.39 (2.20-2.60)[d] |
| **Tar** (mg/cig) | 8.5 (7.7-9.5) | 22.3 (18.8-26.5)[e] | |
| | 15.4 (14.2-14.9) | | 29.0 (25.8-32.5)[f] |
| **CO** (mg/cig) | 9.7 (9.0-10.4) | 17.3 (15.0-20.1)[g] | |
| | 14.6 (14.2-14.9) | | 22.5 (20.3-25.0)[h] |
| **Ba P** (ng/cig) | 10 (8.2-12.3) | 17.9 (15.3-20.9)[i] | |
| | 14 (10.1-19.4) | | 21.4 (19.2-23.7)[j] |
| **NNK** (ng/cig) | 112.9 (96.6-113.0) | 186.5 (158.3-219.7)[i] | |
| | 146.2 (132.5-165.5) | | 250.9 (222.7-282.7)[j] |

*Test Groups:* [a]*56 smokers;* [b]*71 smokers;* [c]*30 smokers;* [d]*42 smokers;* [e]*18 smokers;* [f]*19 smokers;* [g]*15 smokers;* [h]*16 smokers;* [i]*6 smokers;* [j]*3 smokers.*

*Source: Djordjevic et al., 2000.*

tries, charcoal filter cigarettes have accounted for, at most, a small percentage of the open cigarette market, exceptions are Japan, South Korea, Venezuela and Hungary, where at least 90 percent of the cigarettes have charcoal filter tips (John, 1996; Fisher, 2000).

Cellulose acetate filter cigarettes first became popular in Switzerland, during the early 1950s, and soon thereafter in Germany. Their popularity spread to the U.S., the UK and Japan, and finally to France. In 1956, the market share of filter cigarettes in Switzerland was 57.2 percent, in Germany 16.7 percent, and in the USA 29.6 percent, with only a few percent in Japan, England, and France. By 1965, the filter cigarette market share in these countries had risen to about 82 percent, 80 percent, 63 percent, 50 percent , 52 percent , and 21 percent, respectively. At this time, cellulose acetate filter cigarettes accounted for at least 95 percent of the cigarette markets in all of the developed countries, except France, where filter cigarettes remained at 85 percent of all cigarette sales (Wynder and Hoffmann, 1994; Waltz and Häusermann, 1963; Hoffmann and Hoffmann, 1997).

In the early 1960s, investigators found that cellulose acetate filter tips retained up to 80 percent of the volatile phenols from the smoke. Reduction of the emissions of volatile phenols from cigarettes was desirable because their tumor promoting activity had been demonstrated in carcinogenesis assays (Roe *et al.*, 1959; Wynder and Hoffmann, 1961; Hoffmann and Wynder, 1971). When tested on a gram-to-gram basis, the tar from cellulose acetate-filtered smoke is somewhat more toxic, but less carcinogenic, than tars obtained from charcoal-filtered smoke or from the smoke of non-filter cigarettes (Hoffmann and Wynder, 1963; Spears, 1963; Wynder and Mann, 1957; Bock *et al.*, 1962; NCI, 1977c). Cellulose acetate filter tips also selectively remove up to 75 percent of the carcinogenic volatile *N*-nitrosamines (VNA), whereas charcoal-filter tips are much less effective in removing VNA (Brunnemann *et al.*, 1977). Exposure of Syrian golden hamsters twice daily, 5 days per week, for over 60 weeks to the diluted smoke from two different cellulose acetate filter cigarettes elicited a significantly lower incidence of carcinoma of the larynx than exposure to the diluted smoke from the non-filter cigarette ($p<0.01$). In contrast, the incidence rate of carcinoma of the larynx of hamsters exposed to diluted smoke from charcoal-filter cigarettes did not differ significantly from that of larynx carcinoma in hamsters exposed to diluted smoke from the non-filter cigarette (Dontenwill *et al.*, 1973).

Filter perforation allows air dilution of smoke during puff drawing. The velocity of airflow through the burning cone of cigarettes with perforated filters is slowed down because the negative pressure generated by drawing a puff is reduced by drawing air through the filter perforations, and the pressure drop across the tobacco rod is reduced, thus slowing the flow of smoke through the rod. This results in more complete combustion of the tobacco and a higher retention of particulate matter by cellulose acetate in the filter tip (Hoffmann and Hoffmann, 1997; Norman *et al.*, 1984; Durocher, 1984; Baker, 1984). Presently, more than 50 percent of all cigarettes have perforated filter tips. Table 5-7 compares smoke yields of cigarettes without filter tips, cigarettes with cellulose acetate filter tips, and cigarettes with cellulose acetate filter tips that are perforated. The filling tobaccos of these experimental cigarettes were made of an identical blend. The conventional filter tip of cellulose acetate retains more tar, nicotine, and phenol, but releases more CO and ciliatoxic agents, hydrogen cyanide, acetaldehyde, and acrolein than does the cigarette with the perforated filter tip (NCI, 1977c). In mouse skin assays, the tars from both types of filter cigarettes have comparable tumorigenic activity. However, one needs to bear in mind that (a) these comparative data are generated with tars obtained by the standardized machine smoking method, with a 35-ml puff, taken once a minute over 2 seconds; (b) more than 60 percent of today's smokers in the United States and in many developed countries smoke cigarettes with nicotine yields of only 1.2 mg or less (according to FTC standards of smoking); and (c) most of these smokers compensate for the low nicotine delivery.

Compensation and greater smoke intake is governed by the smoker's acquired need for nicotine and, in essence, negates the intended benefits of reducing smoke yields by technical means (Russell, 1976, 1980; Benowitz *et al.*, 1983; Benowitz and Henningfield, 1994; Schultz and Seehofer, 1978; Moody, 1980; Herning *et al.*, 1981; Gritz *et al.*, 1983; Nil *et al.*, 1986; Djordjevic *et al.*, 1995, 2000; see Chapter 2).

**Paper Porosity**     Since about 1960, higher cigarette paper porosity and treatment of paper with citrate have significantly contributed to the reduction of smoke yields of several smoke components. During and in between puff drawing, porous paper enhances the outward diffusion through the paper of hydrogen, NO, CO, $CO_2$, methane, ethane, and ethylene. On the other hand, it

Table 5-7
**Comparison of Experimental Cigarettes (Yield/Cigarette)[a,b]**

| SmokeComponents | Unit of Measurement | Non-FilterCelluloseAcetate Cigarette | CelluloseAcetate FilterCigarette | CelluloseAcetate Filter w/Perforation | CelluloseAcetate Filter w/Perforation & Highly Porous Paper |
|---|---|---|---|---|---|
| Carbon monoxide | ml | 16.2 | 19.2 | 8.62 | 6.66 |
| Hydrogen cyanide | µg | 368 | 296 | 201 | 109 |
| Nitrogen oxides-NOx | µg | 406 | 438 | 364 | 224 |
| Formaldehyde | µg | 36.0 | 20.9 | 31.7 | 21.4 |
| Acetaldehyde | µg | 1,040 | 1,290 | 608 | 550 |
| Acrolein | µg | 105 | 104 | 58.6 | 48.6 |
| Tar | mg | 27.0 | 14.7 | 19.2 | 19.5 |
| Nicotine | mg | 1.8 | 0.94 | 1.31 | 1.5 |
| Phenol | µg | 161 | 61.7 | 122 | 129 |
| Benz(a)anthracene | µg | 40.6 [1.40] | 35.3 [2.25] | 38.5 [1.88] | 40.1 [1.91] |
| Benzo(a)pyrene | ng | 29.9 [1.09] | 19.6 [1.25] | 29.2 [1.13] | 23.9 [1.14] |

[a]*The composition of the cigarette tobacco is identical in all four experimentsal cigarettes*
[b]*Numbers in square brackets = µg/dry tar*
*Source: National Cancer Institute, 1977c.*

accelerates the diffusion of $O_2$ and $N_2$ into the tobacco column; this, in turn, causes more rapid smoldering during puff intervals (Hoffmann and Hoffmann, 1997; Owens, 1998). Porous cigarette paper causes a significant decrease of CO, hydrogen cyanide, nitrogen oxides, volatile aldehydes; yet, it hardly changes the yields of tar, nicotine, benz(a)anthracene (BaA), and BaP. Importantly, the significant reduction of nitrogen oxides in the smoke of these cigarettes reduces the formation and, thus, significantly lowers the yields of volatile and tobacco-specific *N*-nitrosamines (TSNA) (Owens, 1998; Brunnemann *et al.*, 1994).

**Cigarette Construction** Smoke yields of cigarettes are also dependent on physical parameters, such as length and circumference of the cigarette, and the width of the cut (number of cuts per inch) of the tobacco filler. Extending the cigarette length from 50 mm to 130 mm produces an increase in the level of oxygen in the mainstream smoke, while the absolute levels of hydrogen, carbon monoxide, methane, ethane, and ethylene decrease. The major reason for this lies in the diffusion of oxygen through the paper into the smoke stream (Terrell and Schmeltz, 1970). This phenomenon is also reflected in an increased CO delivery with ascending number of puffs because the available surface area of the paper diminishes as the cigarette is smoked. With increasing length of the cigarette, the overall yields of tar, nicotine, PAH, and other particulate components increase (DeBardeleben *et al.*, 1978). A circumference of cigarettes smaller than the regular 24.8–25.5 mm (*e.g.*, 23 mm or less) translates into less tobacco being burned and a greater volume of oxygen available during combustion. Thus, the smoke yields of tar, nicotine, and other particulate components are lowered (DeBardeleben *et al.*, 1978; Lewis, 1992; Brunnemann *et al.*, 1994; Hoffmann and Hoffmann, 1997). Cigarettes with small circumference also have a lower ignition propensity toward inflammable materials than cigarettes that have a 24.8- to 25.5-mm circumference. It has been estimated that in all fire deaths in the U.S. in 1997, 30% were caused by smoking, and worldwide, 10% (Lecstikoo *et al.*, 2000).

The number of cuts per inch (width of tobacco strands) applied to the filler tobacco of cigarettes has an impact on smoke yields and/or on the carcinogenicity of the tars. The first investigation on the importance of tobacco cuts per inch, with regard to smoke yields and tumorigenicity of the resulting tars, was published in 1965 (Wynder and Hoffmann, 1965). It compared the smoke yields of tar and BaP when 8, 30, 50, and 60 cuts per inch of tobacco were applied. Tar yields per cigarette decreased from 29.1 to 23.0 mg and Ba P from 37 to 21 ng. The tumorigenicities of tars derived from cigarettes made with 8, 30, or 50 cuts per inch of tobacco declined from 27 percent to 16 percent and 13 percent of tumor-bearing mice. In a large-scale study of cigarettes filled with an identical blend, cut 20 and 60 times per inch, the smoke yields per cigarette of tar, nicotine, volatile aldehydes, BaA, and BaP were significantly reduced for the fine-cut. However, hydrogen cyanide was insignificantly increased. Gram-to-gram comparison of tumorigenicities of both tars on mouse skin revealed statistically insignificant differences (NCI, 1977a). As the large-scale bioassay was repeated twice, one has to conclude that, in terms of mouse skin carcinogenicity, activities of tars obtained from coarse-cut and fine-cut tobaccos are comparable.

**Tobacco Types**     The botanical genus *Nicotiana* has two major subgenera: *N. rustica* and *N. tabacum*. *Nicotiana rustica* is primarily grown in Russia, the Ukraine, and other East European countries, including Georgia, Moldavia, and Poland. It is also grown in South America and, to a limited extent, in India. In the rest of the world, *Nicotiana tabacum* is grown as the major tobacco crop; it is classified into flue-cured type (often called bright, blond, Virginia or Maryland tobacco), air-cured type (often called burley tobacco; light air-cured tobacco grown in Kentucky, and dark air-cured type grown in parts of Tennessee and Kentucky, South America, Italy, and France) and sun-cured type (often called oriental tobacco; primarily grown in Greece and Turkey). In addition, there are special classes of air-cured tobaccos for cigars, chewing tobacco, and snuff (Tso, 1990).

Prior to the last two decades, flue-cured tobaccos were used exclusively for cigarettes in the United Kingdom and in Finland; they were also the predominate type used in Canada, Japan, China, and Australia. Air-cured tobaccos are preferred for cigarettes in France, southern Italy, some parts of Switzerland and Germany, and South America. Cigarettes made exclusively from sun-cured tobaccos are popular in Greece and Turkey. In the rest of Western Europe and in the United States, cigarettes contain blends of flue-cured and air-cured tobaccos as major components. Today, in many countries, such as the United Kingdom, France, and other developed nations, the U.S. blended cigarette is gaining market share. In the United States, the composition of the cigarette blend has undergone gradual changes. In the 1960s and early 1970s, 45–50 percent of the cigarette blend were flue-cured (Virginia) tobaccos, 35 percent were air-cured (burley) tobaccos, and a few percent were Maryland air-cured and oriental tobaccos. By 1980, the average blend was composed of 38 percent flue-cured, 33 percent air-cured, and a few percent each of Maryland and oriental tobaccos. In the early 1990s, these proportions were about 35 percent, 30 percent, and, again, a few percent of Maryland and oriental tobaccos (Hoffmann and Hoffmann, 1997; Spears and Jones, 1981). The blended cigarette is preferred in many countries, in part because each of the three major *N. tabacum* types adds a certain aroma to the smoke. Some isoprenoids, and a relatively high number of agents with carboxyl content, are associated with the aroma of flue-cured tobacco. Other isoprenoids, and especially the composition of the acidic fraction, are related to the special aroma of air-cured tobaccos (Roberts and Rowland, 1962; Enzell, 1976; Spears and Jones, 1981; Tso, 1990). 3-Methylbutanoic acid (isovaleric acid) is considered to impart the most important flavor characteristic to oriental tobacco (Stedman *et al.*, 1963; Schumacher, 1970).

However, in regard to the toxicity and carcinogenicity of tobacco and tobacco smoke, the difference in the nitrate content of the tobaccos is of primary significance. Flue-cured tobacco can contain up to 0.9 percent of nitrate; yet, as it is used for regular cigarettes, it contains less than 0.5 percent of $NO_3$. In oriental tobaccos, one finds up to 0.6 percent of $NO_3$, in air-cured tobaccos between 0.9 percent and 5.0 percent, but generally below 3 percent in commercial cigarettes. The highest concentration of nitrate is present in the ribs, and the lowest concentration is in the laminae, especially in the laminae harvested from the top stalk positions of the tobacco plant (Neurath and Ehmke, 1964; Tso *et al.*, 1982). With the utilization of a greater proportion of air-cured tobacco in the U.S. cigarette tobacco blend, the nitrate content of the blended U.S. cigarette tobacco has risen from about 0.5 percent in the 1950s to 1.2–1.5 percent in the late 1980s (U.S. DHHS, 1989).

The concentrations of nitrogen oxides ($NO_x$) and methyl nitrite in smoke depend primarily on the nitrate concentrations in the tobacco, even though a portion of the nitrogen oxides is also formed during smoking from amino acids and certain proteins (Philippe and Hackney, 1959; Sims *et al.*, 1975; Norman *et al.*, 1983). Cigarettes made with flue-cured tobaccos deliver up to 200 µg of $NO_x$ and 20 µg methyl nitrite in the smoke. Smoking U.S. blended cigarettes produces up to 500 µg $NO_2$ and 200 µg methyl nitrite, and the smoke of air-cured tobacco cigarettes contains up to 700 µg $NO_x$ and 400 µg methyl nitrite. The major source of nitrate is air-cured tobacco and, thus, the major source of $NO_x$ in its smoke is the nitrogen fertilizers (Sims *et al.*, 1975). The stems of air-cured tobaccos are especially rich in nitrate ($\leq 6.8$ percent). Consequently, stems, as components of expanded and reconstituted tobaccos, contribute in a major way to $NO_x$ in the smoke (Brunnemann *et al.*, 1983).

Freshly generated smoke, as it leaves the mouthpiece of a cigarette, contains $NO_x$ virtually only in the form of nitric oxide (NO), and contains practically no nitrogen dioxide ($NO_2$). However, nitrogen dioxide is quickly formed upon aging of the smoke. It has been estimated that, within 500 seconds half of the NO in undiluted smoke is oxidized to $NO_2$ (Neurath,

1972). Of major importance is the high reactivity of $NO_x$ upon its formation in the burning cone and in the hot zones of a cigarette. The thermically activated nitrogen oxides serve as scavengers of C,H- radicals, whereby they inhibit the pyrosynthesis of carcinogenic polynuclear aromatic hydrocarbons. Table 5-8 presents data on the smoke yields of tar, nicotine, phenol, and BaP, and the tumorigenicities of the tars on mouse skin (Wynder and Hoffmann, 1963).

Freshly generated nitrogen oxides also react with secondary and tertiary amines to form volatile *N*-nitrosamines (VNA) and several *N*-nitrosamines from amino acids, as well as from additives. The $NO_x$ also form tobacco-specific *N*-nitrosamines (TSNA) by *N*-nitrosation of nicotine and of the minor tobacco alkaloids (Brunnemann *et al.*, 1977; Brunnemann and Hoffmann, 1981; Tsuda and Kurashima, 1991; Hoffmann *et al.*, 1994). BaP declined while NNK increased in the smoke of a leading U.S. non-filter cigarette between 1974 and 1997. Both trends correlate with the use of tobaccos with higher nitrate content. Recently, it was suggested that the formation of tobacco-specific nitrosamines in flue-cured tobacco in the United States is, in part, due to the use of propane gas heaters in the curing process. Oxides of nitrogen generated during the burning of the liquid propane react with nicotine in the tobacco leaf to form TSNA. This change in the curing method, introduced in the mid 1960s, is a likely contributor to the increase of TSNA levels in cigarette tobacco. Other important factors are the proportionally greater use of air-cured tobacco and the use of reconstituted tobaccos in the cigarette tobacco blend (Neurath and Ehmke, 1964; Brunnemann *et al.*, 1983; Peel *et al.*, 2001). Increased amounts of TSNA in tobacco compound the carcinogenic potency of the resulting cigarette smoke (Hoffmann *et al.*, 1994) and are considered to contribute to the rise of adenocarcinoma, which has become the dominant form of lung cancer in both male and female smokers during the last three decades (Vincent *et al.*, 1977; Cox and Yesner, 1979; el-Torkey *et al.*, 1990; Devesa *et al.*, 1991; Stellman *et al.*, 1997). Increasing concentrations of nitrate in tobacco have also led to an

Table 5-8

## Smoke Yields and Tumorigenicity of the Tars from the Four Major *N. tabacum* Varieties

| Factors | Flue-Cured Tobacco | Sun-Cured Tobacco | Air-Cured Tobacco Kentucky[a] | Maryland |
|---|---|---|---|---|
| **A: Yields/Cigarette** | | | | |
| Tar (mg) | 33.4 | 31.5 | 25.6 | 21.2 |
| Nicotine (mg) | 2.4 | 1.9 | 1.2 | 1.1 |
| Phenol (µg) | 95 | 120 | 60 | 43 |
| Benzo(*a*)pyrene (ng) | 53 (1.6)[b] | 44 (1.4)[b] | 24 (0.94)[b] | 18 (0.85)[b] |
| | | | | |
| **B: Tumorigenicity[c]** | | | | |
| Percentage of mice with skin tumors | 34 | 35 | 23 | 18 |

[a]*Low-nicotine, air-cured tobacco (Kentucky)*
[b]*Number in parentheses = µg BaP/g dry tar*
[c]*Bioassayed on a gram-to-gram basis of tar*
*Source: Wynder and Hoffmann, 1963.*

increase in cigarette smoke of the human bladder carcinogens 2-naphthy-lamine and 4-aminobiphenyl and of other aromatic amines (Patrianakos and Hoffmann, 1979; Grimmer *et al.*, 1995).

An important aspect relative to the toxicology of cigarette smoke is the correlation between the nitrate content of tobacco and the pH of cigarette smoke. Even though the different processes used to flue-cure and air-cure tobaccos have a significant impact on the smoke composition of the major types of tobacco, the role of nitrate is of major importance in determining the pH of the smoke. Whereas flue-cured tobacco and U.S. cigarette tobacco blends deliver weakly acidic smoke (pH 5.8–6.3), the smoke of cigarettes made from air-cured tobacco delivers neutral to weakly alkaline smoke (pH 6.5–7.5). A major reason for the range of pH values encountered in the smoke of the two major tobacco types is the concentration of ammonia in the smoke, which is directly tied to the concentration of nitrate in the tobacco. When pH levels of the smoke rise to greater than 6.0, the percentage of free, unprotonated nicotine increases to about 30 percent at pH 7.4 and to about 60 percent at pH 7.8 (Brunnemann and Hoffmann, 1974). Protonated nicotine is only slowly absorbed in the oral cavity; yet, unprotonated nicotine, which is partially present in the vapor phase of the smoke, is quickly absorbed through the mucosal membranes of the mouth (Armitage and Turner, 1970). The pH of cigar smoke rises with increasing puff numbers from pH 6.5 to 8.5; consequently, the rapid oral absorption of the free nicotine in the vapor phase gives a primary cigar smoker immediate nicotine stimulation so that he has no need for inhaling the smoke. Similarly, the smoker of black, air-cured cigarettes tends not to inhale the smoke at all, or only minimally (Armitage and Turner, 1970; NCI, 1998).

In 1963, the first comparative study on the tumorigenicity on mouse skin of tars from the four major types of *N. tabacum* revealed the highest activity for tars from flue-cured and sun-cured tobaccos, and the lowest for the two varieties of air-cured tobaccos (Table 5-8; Wynder and Hoffmann, 1963). The concentration of BaP, as an indicator of the concentrations of all carcinogenic PAH, is correlated with the tumor initiation potential of the tars. Upon topical application to mouse skin and human epithelia, carcinogenic PAH induces papilloma and carcinoma. In inhalation studies with Syrian golden hamsters, the smoke of a cigarette made with a particular tobacco blend was significantly more active in inducing carcinoma of the larynx than was the smoke of a cigarette with air-cured (black) tobacco (Dontenwill *et al.*, 1973).

To verify whether a reduction of carcinogenic PAH in the smoke due to the presence of high levels of nitrate in tobacco leads to reduced mouse skin tumorigenicity of the tar, sodium nitrate (8.3 percent) was added to the standard tobacco blend. On a gram-to-gram basis, the tar from the cigarette with added nitrate (0.6 µg BaP per gram tar) induced skin tumors in only 2 of 50 mice, whereas the tar from the control cigarette (without the addition of nitrate; 1.05 µg BaP per gram tar) induced skin tumors in 25 of 100 mice (Hoffmann and Wynder, 1967). In inhalation experiments with Syrian golden hamsters, smoke from the control cigarette plus 8.0 percent of sodium nitrate induced laryngeal carcinomas in only 25 of 160 animals (15.6 percent), compared to this type of neoplasm in 60 of 200 animals (30 percent) in assays with the control cigarette (Dontenwill *et al.*, 1973). Thus, all of these bioassays on the skin of mice and the inhalation studies with hamsters support the concept that increased nitrate content of the tobacco inhibits the pyrosynthesis of the carcinogenic PAH and that the tars of these cigarettes, and their smoke as a whole, have a reduced potential for inducing benign and malignant tumors in epithelial tissues when compared to the tar or whole smoke of cigarettes with tobacco that is low in nitrate.

**Reconstituted Tobacco and Expanded Tobacco**     In the early 1940s, the technology for making reconstituted tobacco (RT) was developed. Manufacturing RT enables the utilization of tobacco fines, ribs, and stems in cigarette tobacco blends (Halter and Ito, 1979). Prior to this technology, tobacco fines and stems had been discarded. With the utilization of RT as part of the tobacco blend, less top quality tobacco is needed and, thereby, the cost of making cigarettes has been reduced. Laboratory studies (Wynder and Hoffmann, 1967) have shown that cigarettes made entirely of RT deliver a smoke with significantly reduced levels of tar, nicotine, volatile phenols, and carcinogenic PAHs.

The two major technologies for making RT for cigarettes are the slurry process and the paper process. Either process leads to RT with low density. The advantage of RT lies in the creation of a high degree of aeration of the tobacco which enhances combustibility. Most of the tested tars from reconstituted tobaccos had significantly reduced carcinogenic activity on mouse skin (Wynder and Hoffmann, 1965; NCI, 1977a). In inhalation assays with Syrian golden hamsters, diluted smoke from cigarettes made of reconstituted tobacco induced significantly fewer carcinomas in the larynx (19/160) than the diluted smoke from control cigarettes (60/200). The cigarette with RT gave only 7 puffs per cigarette and yielded 20.8 mg tar and 16 ng of BaP compared to 10 puffs, 33.7 mg tar, and 35.4 ng BaP for the control cigarette (Dontenwill *et al.*, 1973). This result supports the concept that, at least in the experimental setting, the carcinogenic PAH, with BaP as a surrogate, are correlated with the induction of papilloma and carcinoma in epithelial tissues. The procarcinogenic TSNA, on the other hand, are not activated by enzymes to their reactive species in epithelial tissues; thus, they induce few, if any, tumors in such tissues. Tobacco ribs and stems, the major components of RT, are richer in nitrate (and this applies especially to the ribs and stems of air-cured tobaccos) than the laminae of tobacco (Neurath and Ehmke, 1964; Brunnemann *et al.*, 1983; Brunnemann and Hoffmann, 1991; Burton *et al.*, 1992). Therefore, in general, the nitrate content of today's blended U.S. cigarette, which may contain 20–30 percent RT, is at 1.2–1.5 percent—much higher than the nitrate level in cigarettes during the fifties and sixties when it was ≤0.5 percent (U.S. DHHS, 1989; Spears, 1974). Cigarettes with RT emit in their smoke significantly greater amounts of TSNA than cigarettes of the past. These TSNA include the adenocarcinoma-inducing NNK, which is metabolically activated to carcinogenic species in target tissues like the lungs (Hoffmann *et al.*, 1994). One major U.S. cigarette manufacturer was awarded a patent in December 1978 for developing a process that reduces more than 90 percent of the nitrate content of the RT made from ribs and stems (Kite *et al.*, 1978; Gellatly and Uhl, 1978). It is unclear to which extent this patented method has been applied to the RT manufacture for U.S. commercial cigarettes.

There are at least three methods for expanding tobacco by freeze-drying (NCI, 1977b). As a result of freeze-drying, expanded tobacco has greater filling power than natural tobacco, meaning that less tobacco is needed to fill a cigarette. An 85-mm filter cigarette, filled entirely with expanded tobacco, requires 630 mg tobacco; while a regular non-filter control cigarette of the same dimensions requires 920 mg tobacco. The tar yields in the smoke of both types of cigarettes amounted to 12.4 mg and 22.1 mg, respectively (NCI, 1977b, 1980). In 1982, incorporation of all possible modifications in the makeup of the cigarette required only 785 mg leaf tobacco; in contrast, in 1950, the blended U.S. cigarette required 1,230 mg leaf tobacco (Spears, 1974). Table 5-9 presents analytical data for the smoke of experimental cigarettes filled with puffed tobacco, expanded or freeze-dried tobacco, and a control cigarette. Levels of most components measured in the smoke of cigarettes with puffed tobacco, expanded tobacco, or freeze-dried tobacco were reduced, compared with data for the control cigarette (NCI, 1977b, 1980).

The changes that have occurred between 1950 and 1995 in the makeup of U.S. cigarettes, have significantly altered smoke composition. Table 5-10 compares data for individual components in the smoke of U.S. blended cigarettes of the 1950s with corresponding data for the cigarette smoke composition profiles that have been established between 1988 and 1995. All of these cigarettes were smoked using the FTC method (Pillsbury *et al.*, 1969).

**Additives**

**Humectants**

Humectants serve to retain moisture and plasticity in cigarette and pipe tobaccos. They prevent the drying of tobacco, which would lead to a harsh tasting smoke; importantly, they also preserve those compounds that impart flavor to the smoke. Today, the principal humectants in cigarette tobacco are glycerol (propane-1,2,3-triol) and propylene glycol (PG; propane-1-2-diol); of lesser importance are diethylene glycol (2.2'-di[hydroxyethyl]ether) and sorbitol (Voges, 1984). In the past, ethylene glycol (ethane-1,2,-diol) has been used as a humectant for cigarette tobacco. However, because this compound leads to the formation of ethylene oxide, which is carcinogenic to both animals and humans, its use has been prohibited (IARC, 1994a). In 1972, Binder and Lindner reported the presence of 20 μg ethylene oxide per cigarette in the smoke of the untreated tobacco of one cigarette brand (Binder and Lindner, 1972). In this context, it is noteworthy that Törnqvist and colleagues (1986) found significant levels of the *N*-hydroxyethylvaline moiety of hemoglobin in the blood of smokers ranging between 217 and 690 pmol/g Hb, averaging 389 ± 138 pmol/g, while levels in nonsmokers' blood ranged between 27 and 106 pmol/g Hb and averaged 58 ± 25 pmol/g Hb. The authors suggest that most of the ethylene oxide in the hemoglobin adduct is derived from endogenous oxidation of ethene in cigarette smoke (50–250 μg/cigarette) (Törnqvist *et al.*, 1986).

Humectants may comprise up to 5 percent of the weight of cigarette

Table 5-9

**Smoke Analyses of Cigarettes Made from Puffed, Expanded, and Freeze-Dried Tobacco and from a Control Cigarette**

| Smoke Component | Puffed Tobacco | Expanded Tobacco | Freeze-dried Tobacco | Expanded Stems | Control |
|---|---|---|---|---|---|
| CO (mg) | 9.33 | 11.8 | 12.3 | 23.1 | 18.0 |
| Nitrogen oxides ($\mu$g) | 247.0 | 293.0 | 235.0 | 349.0 | 269.0 |
| HCN ($\mu$g) | 199.0 | 287.0 | 234.0 | 248.0 | 413.0 |
| Formaldehyde ($\mu$g) | 20.7 | 21.7 | 33.4 | 58.0 | 31.7 |
| Acetaldehyde ($\mu$g) | 814.0 | 720.0 | 968.0 | 803.0 | 986.0 |
| Acrolein ($\mu$g) | 105.0 | 87.7 | 92.4 | 93.0 | 128.0 |
| Tar (mg) | 16 | 18 | 16 | 23 | 37 |
| Nicotine (mg) | 0.8 | 0.7 | 0.8 | 0.4 | 2.6 |
| BaA (ng) | 13.7 | 11.8 | 15.3 | 19.5 | 37.1 |
| BaP (ng) | 11.8 | 8.2 | 9.2 | 16.2 | 28.7 |

*Abbreviations: CO=carbon monoxide; HCN=hydrogen cyanide; BaA=banz(a)anthracene; BaP=benzo(a)pyrene.*
*Source: National Cancer Institute, 1980.*

Table 5-10

**Changes in the Yields of Selected Toxic Agents in the Smoke of U.S. Cigarettes (FTC Smoking Conditions)**

| Smoke Component | Earlier Cigarettes[a] | | Current Cigarettes[a] | |
|---|---|---|---|---|
| | Year | Concentration | Year | Concentration |
| Carbon monoxide (CO) | 1953 | 33-38 mg (NF) | 1994 | 11 mg (F) |
| Nitrogen oxides (HNO$_x$) | 1965 | 330 $\mu$g (NF) | 1994 | 500 $\mu$g (NF) |
| Benzene | 1962 | 30 $\mu$g (NF) | 1988 | 48 $\mu$g (NF) |
| | 1962 | 25-30 $\mu$g (F) | 1990 | 42 $\mu$g (F) |
| Acetaldehyde | 1960 | 1,000 $\mu$g (NF) | 1992 | 400 $\mu$g (F) |
| NDMA | 1976 | 43 ng (NF) | 1989 | 65 ng (NF) |
| Tar | 1953 | 38 mg (NF) | 1994 | 12 mg (F) |
| Nicotine | 1953 | 2.7 mg (NF) | 1994 | 0.85 mg (F) |
| | 1959 | 1.7 mg (F) | 1994 | 1.1 mg (F) |
| Phenol | 1960 | 100 $\mu$g (NF) | 1994 | 70 $\mu$g (NF) |
| | 1960 | 46 $\mu$g (F) | 1994 | 35 $\mu$g (F) |
| Catechol | 1965 | 390 $\mu$g (NF) | 1994 | |
| | 1976 | 790 $\mu$g (F) | 1994 | 140 $\mu$g (F) |
| 2-Naphthylamine | 1968 | 22 ng (NF) | 1985 | 35 ng (F) |
| BaP | 1959 | 50 ng (NF) | 1995 | 19 ng (NF) |
| | 1959 | 27 ng (F) | 1995 | 8 ng (F) |
| NNN | 1978 | 220 ng (NF) | 1995 | 300 ng (NF) |
| | 1978 | 240 ng (F) | 1995 | 280 ng (F) |
| NNK | 1978 | 110 ng (NF) | 1995 | 190 ng (NF) |
| | 1978 | 100 ng (F) | 1995 | 144 ng (F) |

[a]*Abbreviations: NF=non-filter; F=filter; NDMA=N-nitrosodimethylamine; BaP=benzo(a)pyrene; NNN=N'-nitrosonornicotine; NNK=4-(methylnitrosamino)-1-(3-pyridyl)-1-butanone*
*Source: Pillsbury et al., 1969.*

tobacco. In a 1964 study, 18 U.S. cigarette tobacco blends that were analyzed for humectants contained between 1.7 and 3.15 percent of glycerol,
which is to some extent decomposed to the ciliatoxic acrolein, and between
0.46 and 2.24 percent of PG (Cundiff *et al.*, 1964). The smoke of four
American cigarettes contained between 0.34 and 0.96 mg/cigarette of PG
(Lyerly, 1967). However, PG may be thermally degrading to yield propylene oxide. This would be of concern because propylene oxide is regarded as
possibly carcinogenic to humans (IARC, 1994b). Four U.S. cigarettes contained between 0.34 and 0.96 mg per cigarette (Lyerly, 1967). In 1999,
between 12 and 100 ng of propylene oxide were detected in the smoke of
cigarettes filled with PG treated tobacco. Several commercial samples of
PG, used as a humectant for cigarette tobacco, already contained traces of
propylene oxide (Kagan *et al.*, 1999).

**Flavor Additives**     Natural tobacco is composed of a wide spectrum of components
that, upon heating, release agents, which contribute to the flavor of the
smoke. These include tobacco-specific terpenoids, pyrroles, and pyrazines
among others (Roberts and Rowland, 1962; Gutcho, 1972; Senkus, 1976;
Leffingwell, 1987; Roberts, 1988). The effective reduction of smoke yields
by filter tips and by the incorporation of reconstituted tobacco also brought
about a reduction of flavor components in the smoke. To counteract this
loss of smoke flavor, the tobacco blends are treated with additives that are
essentially precursors to smoke flavors. They include natural agents contributing to minty, spicy, woody, fruity and flowery flavors. In some
instances, such additives also include synthetic agents as flavor enhancers.
While most of the flavor enhancers are chosen indiscriminately, it is realized that some of them may contribute to toxicity or carcinogenicity of cigarette smoke. A case in point was the cessation of the use of deer tongue
extract which contained several percent of the animal carcinogen coumarin
(Voges, 1984). It has been suggested that additives to cigarettes are used to
reduce the perception of environmental tobacco smoke (ETS; Connolly *et
al.*, 2001).

In 1993 and 1994, the tobacco industry convened an expert panel of
toxicologists to screen agents that were in use, or considered for use, as
tobacco additives. The panel established a list of 599 agents that were generally regarded as safe (GRAS), whereby the term 'safe' applied to each of
the additives as such without consideration of the fate and reactivity of
these agents during and after combustion (Doull *et al.*, 1994). An exception
was menthol, which was known to transfer into the smoke without yielding appreciable amounts of carcinogenic hydrocarbons (Jenkins *et al.*,
1970). A recent toxicologic evaluation of flavor ingredients dealt with 170
such agents that are commonly used in the manufacture of American
blended cigarettes, and examined their effects in four sub-chronic, nose-
only smoke inhalation studies in rats compared to effects of the smoke of
tobacco blends without additives. Control animals were exposed to filtered
air (Gaworski *et al.*, 1998). Smoke exposure was monitored with internal
dose markers, including carboxyhemoglobin, serum nicotine, and serum
cotinine. The mainstream smoke (MS) of flavored and nonflavored cigarette
types caused essentially the same responses in the respiratory tracts of the
rats; specifically hyperplasia and metaplasia in the nose and larynx. As this

study involved maximally 65 hours of exposure (while induction of tumors would not be expected until animals reach half their life span), one cannot deduce with certainty that the addition of these flavoring agents to tobacco blends has no impact on the development of tumors.

**New Types of** The tobacco companies have undertaken a substantial research
**Cigarettes** effort to develop new types of nicotine delivery devices. These devices were intended to generate an aerosol with nicotine in the range of the levels present in conventional cigarettes but with very low emissions of tar and other toxic agents. Toward the end of the 1980s, the first prototype of these new types of cigarettes was on the test market, a product named "Premier." It was a cigarette that "heats rather than burns tobacco" (R. J. Reynolds Tobacco Company, 1988; DeBethizy *et al.*, 1990; Borgerding *et al.*, 1990a & b, 1998). This 80-mm cigarette is comprised of three sections. The first 40-mm section of this cigarette is made with compressed charcoal, which is immediately linked to an inner aluminum tube containing tobacco, flavor additives, and glycerol. This tube is embedded in tobacco. Section 2 (~10 mm) is a cellulose acetate filter dusted with charcoal powder. The third section (~30 mm) is a cellulose acetate filter tip. Under FTC standard machine smoking conditions, the "Premier" delivers smoke containing 0.3 mg nicotine, 6.3 mg water, 4.6 mg glycerol, 0.4 mg propylene glycol, and 0.7 mg tar. Compared with the reference (conventional) cigarette, and disregarding nicotine, the majority of the known toxic and carcinogenic agents in the smoke are reduced by more than 90 percent. Known exceptions are carbon monoxide (CO) (+3.5 percent), ammonia (–5.6 percent), formaldehyde (–35.3 percent), resorcinol (–73.3 percent), quinoline (–56.6 percent), and acetamide (–18.2 percent). This new type of cigarette did not gain consumer acceptance, possibly because of difficulty in igniting the "Premier," the need for frequent puffing to ensure continuous burning, the lack of flavor, and the low nicotine delivery (0.3 mg/cigarette). Nicotine emission was below the level that would satisfy most smokers' acquired need for this agent even with compensatory smoking.

In 1996, a modified "Premier" came on the market. In the United States, it is known as "Eclipse"; in Germany it is called "HiQ," and in Sweden, it goes by the name "Inside." The "Eclipse" consists of four sections. Section 1, the heat source, is a specially prepared charcoal; section 2 consists of tobacco plus glycerol; section 3 contains finely shredded tobacco; and section 4 is a filter tip. Upon ignition, the special charcoal heats the air stream during puff drawing. The heated air stream enters the tobacco sections and vaporizes glycerol, as well as the volatile and semi-volatile tobacco components, including nicotine. Under FTC smoking conditions, the "Eclipse" delivers 8 mg CO (low-tar filter cigarette: 6–12 mg), 150 µg acetaldehyde (700 µg), 30 µg $NO_x$ (200–300 µg), 180 µg hydrogen cyanide (300–400 µg), 5.1 mg tar (11–12 mg), and 0.2–0.4 mg nicotine (0.7–1.0 mg). The remainder of the smoke particulates consists of 33 percent water, 47 percent glycerol, and 17 percent of various other compounds. The concentrations of the major carcinogens, such as BaP, 2-aminonaphthalene, 4-aminobiphenyl, and the TSNA are lowered by 85–95 percent (Rose and Levin, 1996; Smith *et al.*, 1996). Currently, the "Eclipse" is being test marketed and it appears that response is somewhat more favorable than it was to its predecessor, the "Premier." The products labeled, "Eclipse Full Flavor," "Eclipse Mild," and "Eclipse Menthol" produce FTC-standardized smoke yields of 0.2, 0.1, and 0.2 mg nicotine and 3, 2, and 3 mg tar per cigarette. Regular cigarette smokers were asked to switch for 2 weeks to "Eclipse." There were four study groups, each composed of 26–30 volunteers, for a total of 109 smokers. Smoking of "Eclipse" resulted in about a 30 percent larger puff volume, about 50 percent more puffs, which added up to a total puff volume per cigarette that was more than twice that of the total volume drawn from the control cigarettes (Stiles *et al.*, 1999). These data suggest that the volunteers smoked "Eclipse" more intensely than their non-filter cigarettes. This observation is also supported in the uptake of nicotine (Benowitz *et al.*, 1997). The mutagenic activities of the urine of smokers of four types of "Eclipse" were assayed on two bacterial strains and were reduced by 72% to 100%, compared with the mutagenic activities of the urine of the same volunteers after smoking their regular cigarettes (Smith *et al.*, 1996).

An Expert Committee from the Institute of Medicine of the National Academy of Sciences studied the scientific basis for a possible reduction of the "harm" induced by "Eclipse" relative to the "harm" induced by smoking conventional cigarettes. On the basis of the available data, the Committee came to the following conclusions: "Eclipse" offers the committed smoker an option that is currently not available. "Eclipse" does not add to the inherent biological activity of smoke from the range of cigarettes currently on the market. The elevated COHb levels should be regarded as a potential risk factor for cardiovascular diseases. The magnitude of this risk remains to be determined (Gardner, 2000).

The high concentration of glycerol in the "Eclipse" aerosol led to bioassays of glycerol in 2-week (1.0, 1.93, and 3.91 mg/L) and 13-week (0.033, 0.167, and 0.662 mg/L) "nose only" inhalation studies with Sprague-Dawley rats, testing for toxicity and especially for irritating effects. The investigators detected metaplasia of the lining of the epiglottis (Gardner, 2000). The 13-week inhalation studies with rats and hamsters had also resulted in some early histopathological changes in the upper respiratory tract in both laboratory animals. These observations signal the need for lifetime inhalation assays with the smoke of "Eclipse" in rats, preferably Fisher 344 rats, or better yet, in Syrian golden hamsters, possibly with an inbred strain of hamsters susceptible to carcinogens in the respiratory tract (Bernfeld *et al.*, 1974). Pauly *et al.*, from the Roswell Park Cancer Institute, Buffalo, New York, caution that harmful glass fibers have been found to migrate into the filter tip of the "Eclipse" and may be inhaled during puffing (Pauly *et al.*, 1998).

The Health Department of Massachusetts and the Society for Research on Nicotine and Tobacco disputed the claims made for "Eclipse." They requested that the FTC and the FDA institute regulatory procedures to ensure that insufficiently documented health claims are not made for tobacco products. Declaring "Eclipse" the "next best choice," or calling TSNA-reduced tobacco products "safer tobacco" (Anonymous, 2000; Society for Research on Nicotine and Tobacco, 2000) is deceiving.

In 1998, Philip Morris USA released a new type of cigarette (EHC) that is heated electrically to release an aerosol. On the basis of chemical analyses and short-term bioassays, it has significantly lower toxicity and mutagenicity than the smoke of the Kentucky reference filter cigarette, 1R4F. The prototype, containing a tobacco filler wrapped in a tobacco mat, is kept in constant contact with eight electrical heater blades in a microprocessor-controlled lighter. This cigarette contains about half the amount of the tobacco of a conventional cigarette. Under FTC-standardized smoking conditions, the cigarette delivers, with an average of 8 puffs, about 1 mg of nicotine, whereas all other smoke constituents analyzed were significantly lower than those in the smoke of the low-yield Kentucky reference cigarette, 1R4F (Terpstra *et al.*, 1998). However, formaldehyde yields were significantly higher in the smoke of the EHC and emissions of glycerol and 2-nitropropane were comparable to those recorded in the smoke of the 1R4F cigarette. Per gram of tar, the smoke of the EHC had significantly lower mutagenic activity than the smoke of the 1R4F reference cigarette in TA98 and TA100 tester strains with metabolic activation (Terpstra *et al.*, 1998).

**OBSERVATIONS ON CIGARETTE SMOKERS** In mice, rats, and hamsters, NNK induces adenomas and adenocarcinomas (AC) in the peripheral lung. This effect is independent of route and form of application (Hoffmann *et al.*, 1994). NNK is metabolically activated primarily to the unstable 4-(hydroxymethylnitrosamino)-1-(3-pyridyl) -1- butanone and to 4-($\alpha$-hydroxymethylene)-1-(3-pyridyl)-1-butanol, which decomposes into methane diazohydroxide and 4-keto-4-(3-pyridyl)butane diazohydroxide, respectively. The diazohydroxides react with DNA bases to form 7-methyl guanine, $O^6$-methyl guanine and $O^4$-methyl thymidine, respectively, and also form a pyridyloxobutyl adduct of presently unknown structure. Upon acid hydrolysis, this adduct releases 4-hydroxy-1-(3-pyridyl)-1-butanone. These adducts have been found in the lungs of mice and rats following treatment with NNK, and they have also been identified in human lungs. The origin of 7-methyl guanine in DNA from human lungs is unclear; conceivably, in addition to TSNA, nitroso compounds such as *N*-nitrosodimethylamine may also have been a source for this DNA-methylation. However, it is clear that higher levels of 7-methyl guanine have been found in the lung of smokers than in the lung of nonsmokers, thus strengthening the evidence that NNK is a major contributor to the methylation of the lung DNA of smokers (Hecht, 1998).

PAH induce squamous cell carcinoma of the lung in laboratory animals and in workers with exposures to aerosols that are high in PAH. NNK metabolites induce primarily AC of the lung in laboratory animals. Reactive PAH metabolites bind to DNA in epithelial tissues. In laboratory animals, metabolically activated forms of NNK react with the DNA of Clara cells in the peripheral lung (Belinsky *et al.*, 1990) to form methylguanine and methylthymidine, as well as pyridyloxobutylated adducts. 7-Methylguanine has been found in smokers' lungs at higher levels than in the lungs of nonsmokers.

Additional support for the observation that adenocarcinoma of the lung among cigarette smokers has increased relative to squamous cell carcinoma during the past 25 years, and for the concept that lung cancer risk of smokers of low-nicotine filter cigarettes is similar to that of smokers of non-filter cigarettes, comes from biochemical studies. In the mouse, the $O^6$-methylguanine pathway of metabolically activated NNK is clearly the major route for induction of lung tumors; this conclusion is consistent with the high percentage of GGT→GAT mutations in the K-*ras* oncogene induced by NNK (Hecht, 1998; Singer and Essigmann, 1991). A study from the Netherlands has shown that mutations on codon 12 of the K-*ras* oncogene are present in 24–50 percent of human primary adenocarcinoma. These mutations occur more frequently in AC of the lung in smokers than in nonsmokers. Twenty percent of the mutations in codon 12 involve GGT→GAT conversions, which supports the concept that NNK plays a role in the induction of AC of the lung in smokers. Histochemical examination of human lung cancer showed cyclooxygenase (COX)-2 expression in 70 percent of invasive carcinoma cases (Hida *et al.*, 1998). COX-2 expression was also identified in adenocarcinoma of the lung in rats treated with NNK (el-Bayoumy *et al.*, 1999). It is anticipated that future studies in molecular biology will fully elucidate the significance of TSNA, especially of NNK, and of the carcinogenic PAH in the induction of lung cancer in tobacco smokers.

**SUMMARY**    Major modifications in the makeup of the commercial cigarette were introduced between 1950 and 1975. Since then, there have been no substantive changes toward a further reduction of the toxic and carcinogenic potential of cigarette smoke beyond reducing MS yields of tar, nicotine, and carbon monoxide. Some of these modifications have also resulted in diminished yields of several toxic and carcinogenic smoke constituents.

Cigarettes with charcoal filter tips deliver MS with significantly lower concentrations of the major ciliatoxic agents, such as hydrogen cyanide and volatile aldehydes. However, except in Japan, South Korea, Venezuela, and Hungary, cigarettes with charcoal filter tips account for less than one percent (USA) and at most for a small percentage of all cigarettes sold worldwide (Fisher, 2000).

Cellulose acetate filters with or without perforation have the capacity for selective reduction of smoke yields of volatile *N*-nitrosamines and semi-volatile phenols. The latter are major tumor promoters in cigarette tar. In contrast to cigarettes manufactured in the 1950s, most of the cigarettes on the market today use a highly porous wrapper of paper treated with agents that enhance the burning, thus, contributing to the reduction of machine-measured yields of carbon monoxide, hydrogen cyanide, volatile aldehydes, volatile *N*-nitrosamines, PAH, and TSNA.

Reconstituted tobacco and expanded tobacco today amount to between 25 and 30 percent of the cigarette tobacco blend. Reconstituted tobacco reduces the yields of smoke components such as tar and CO. The tar from cigarettes made entirely of reconstituted tobacco is less carcinogenic on mouse skin and the smoke of these cigarettes reduces significantly the induction of carcinoma in the larynx of hamsters compared to the smoke of reference cigarettes made of natural tobacco. Reconstituted tobaccos and expanded tobaccos have a significantly greater filling power than natural tobacco. An 85-mm filter cigarette that is filled entirely with expanded tobacco requires 363 mg tobacco while a regular filter-tipped cigarette requires 667 mg tobacco. The smoke of cigarettes made of expanded tobacco has significantly lower MS yields of tar, nicotine, CO, hydrogen cyanide, PAH, and TSNA. On the basis of weight-to-weight comparisons, the tar from these cigarettes is significantly less tumorigenic on mouse skin than the tar of a reference cigarette made of the corresponding natural tobacco.

Since 1959, each year the levels of tar, nicotine, and benzo(*a*)pyrene in the mainstream smoke of a leading U.S. non-filter cigarette have been monitored. Beginning in 1977, the MS was also analyzed for NNK and in 1981, the determinations of CO in the mainstream smoke were added. For all of these analyses, the MS was generated with the standardized machine smoking parameters that are mandated by the Federal Trade Commission. Table 5-11 documents the decline of tar levels from 29.8 mg to 24.3 mg in the years between 1959 and 1984, while nicotine levels fell from 2.4 mg to 1.6 mg between 1959 and 1977. Since then, the smoke yields of tar and nicotine for this non-filter brand have not changed. Carbon monoxide remained stable at 16 to 18 mg per cigarette since it was first reported in 1981. By 1997, it was clear that significant changes in the smoke yields of the major lung carcinogens BaP and NNK have occurred since 1977 in that BaP levels declined from 49 ng to 19 ng, but NNK increased from 120 ng to 195 ng per non-filter cigarette.

It is important to note that we are lacking analytical data regarding the levels of these major carcinogens and toxins in the mainstream smoke of leading cellulose acetate filter-tipped cigarettes with and without filter perforation, as well as in the MS of charcoal filter cigarettes. These cellulose acetate filter cigarettes were actually the ones dominating the U.S. cigarette market as the use of non-filter cigarettes faded over the years and charcoal filter cigarettes had only a modest market share. Most importantly, we are also lacking data on biological activities of the tars of leading brands of filter cigarettes produced since the 1960s because tumorigenicity and carcinogenicity of tars have not been monitored on a regular basis. There is now also an urgent need for analytical profiles of the toxic and carcinogenic mainstream smoke constituents that are generated under conditions reflecting the puff drawing profiles actually exhibited by humans who smoke these cigarettes that give lower yields as per FTC measurements. Such analytical data would have to be established for major U.S. cigarette brands manufactured since 1960. They would serve as the scientific basis in support of epidemiological observations regarding the risk of cancer of the lung and upper aerodigestive tract for smokers who have exclusively smoked filter-tipped brands as compared to the risk for smokers who used non-filter cigarettes.

Changes in the agricultural, curing, and manufacturing processes of cigarettes have resulted in an increase in tobacco-specific nitrosamines in cigarette smoke that may have contributed to the increase in adenocarcinoma of the lung observed over the past several decades.

Table 5-11

**Tar, Nicotine, CO, BaP, and NNK in the Mainstream Smoke of a Leading U.S. NF Cigarette, 1959-1997[a]**

| Year | Tar (mg) | Nicotine (mg) | Carbon Monoxide[b] (mg) | Ba P (ng) | NNK[b] (ng) |
|------|------|----------|-----------------|------|------|
| 1959 | 29.8 | 2.4 | | 40 | |
| 1967 | 27.2 | 1.6 | | 49 | |
| 1971 | 29.0 | 1.8 | | 22 | |
| 1977 | 26.0 | 1.59 | | 19 | 120 |
| 1981 | 24.3 | 1.52 | 16.7 | 19 | 130 |
| 1988 | 24 | 1.5 | 16 | 19 | 140 |
| 1991 | 25 | 1.7 | 16 | 18 | 190 |
| 1997 | 26 | 1.7 | 18 | 19 | 195 |

*Abbreviations: NNK=4-(methylnitrosamino)-1-(3-pyridyl)-1-butanone; BaP= benzo(a)pyrene.*
*[a]The analytical data were generated by smoking the leading U.S. NF cigarette according to the FTC-mandated standard machine smoking method (Pillsbury et al., 1969).*
*[b]The open fields document the lack of analytical data for the years 1959, 1967, 1971, and 1977 for CO and 1959, 1967, and 1977 for NNK*
*Sources: Wynder and Hoffman, 1960; Federal Trade Commission, 1971, 1977, 1981, 1988, 1991, 1997; Hoffmann and Hoffmann, 1997.*

## CONCLUSIONS

1. Major modifications in the makeup of the commercial cigarette were introduced between 1950 and 1975, but since that time there have been few substantive changes toward a further reduction of the toxic and carcinogenic potential of cigarette smoke.

2. A variety of changes in cigarette design and filtration have resulted in chemical changes in cigarette smoke, some of which have also demonstrated decreased toxicity in animal assays. Toxicity or carcinogenicity in animal assays has not been monitored to allow evaluation of changes over time that have occurred for cigarette smoke produced by commercial brands of cigarettes.

3. Changes in the agricultural, curing, and manufacturing processes of cigarettes have resulted in an increase over the last several decades in the amounts of tobacco-specific nitrosamines in cigarette smoke. These changes are considered to have contributed to the increase in adenocarcinoma of the lung observed over the past several decades.

4. On the basis of the standard machine smoking method for cigarettes that has been mandated by the FTC, the sales-weighted average nicotine yields of U.S. cigarettes decreased gradually from 2.7 mg per cigarette in 1953 to 0.85 mg by the mid 1990s. Today, the smoker of filter cigarettes will greatly increase his/her smoking intensity to satisfy an acquired need for nicotine. Thus, the inhaled smoke of one cigarette contains 2 to 3 times the amount of tar, nicotine, and carbon monoxide and 1.6 to 1.8 times the level of biomarkers for the major lung carcinogens BaP, and NNK, compared to amounts in the smoke generated by the FTC method.

# Appendix

## Abbreviations

| | |
|---|---|
| AC | Adenocarcinoma |
| BaA | Benz(a)anthracene |
| BaP | Benzo(a)pyrene |
| FTC | Federal Trade Commission |
| Hb | Hemoglobin |
| IARC | International Agency for Research on Cancer |
| MS | Mainstream Smoke |
| NNK | 4-(Methylnitrosamino)-1-(3-pyridyl)-1-butanone |
| NNN | $N'$-Nitrosonornicotine |
| $NO_x$ | Nitrogen oxides (NO, $NO_2$, and $N_2O$) |
| PAH | Polynuclear Aromatic Hydrocarbons |
| RT | Reconstituted Tobacco |
| SCC | Squamous Cell Carcinoma |
| TSNA | Tobacco Specific $N$-Nitrosamines |
| VNA | Volatile $N$-Nitrosamines |

## REFERENCES

Anonymous. Massachusetts disputes claims about Eclipse cigarettes. *Tobacco Reporter* 127 (No. 11):11-13, 2000.

Armitage, A.K., Turner, D.H. Absorption of nicotine in cigarette and cigar smoke through the oral mucosa. *Nature (London)* 226:1231-1232, 1970.

Baker, R.R.. The effect of ventilation on cigarette combustion mechanisms. *Recent Advances in Tobacco Science* 10:88-150, 1984.

Battista, S.P. Ciliatoxic components in cigarette smoke. *Proceedings of the Third World Conference on Smoking and Health, New York, June 2-5, 1975. Vol. 1. Modifying the Risk for the Smoker.* Wynder, E.L., Hoffmann, D., Gori, G.B. (Editors). U.S. Department of Health, Education, and Welfare, Public Health Service, National Institutes of Health, National Cancer Institute, DHEW Publication No. (NIH) 76-1221, 1976.

Belinsky, S.A., Foley, J.F., White, C.M., Anderson, M.W., Maronpot, R. Dose-response relationship between O6-methylguanine formation in Clara cells and induction of pulmonary neoplasia in the rat with 4-(methylnitrosamino)-1-(3-pyridyl)-1-butanone. *Cancer Research* 50(12):3772-3780, 1990.

Benowitz, N.L. Biomarkers of cigarette smoking. *The FTC Cigarette Test Method for Determining Tar, Nicotine, and Carbon Monoxide Yields of U.S. Cigarettes. Report of the NCI Expert Committee.* Smoking and Tobacco Control Monograph No. 7. U.S. Department of Health and Human services, National Institutes of Health, National Cancer Institute, NIH Publication No. 96-4028, 1996.

Benowitz, N.L., Hall, S.M., Herning, S.I., Jacob, P. III, Jones, R.T., Osman, A.-L. Smokers of low yield cigarettes do not consume less nicotine during cigarette smoking. *New England Journal of Medicine* 309(3):139-142, 1983.

Benowitz, N.L., Henningfield, J.E. Establishing a nicotine threshold for addiction. The implications for tobacco regulation. *New England Journal of Medicine* 331(2):123-125, 1994.

Benowitz, N.L., Jacob, P.J., Slade, J., Yu, L. Nicotine content of the Eclipse nicotine delivery device. *American Journal of Public Health* 87(11):1865-1866. 1997.

Bernfeld, P., Homberger, F., Russfield, A.B. Strain differences in the response of inbred Syrian hamsters to cigarette smoke inhalation. *Journal of the National Cancer Institute* 53(4):1141-1157, 1974.

Binder, H., Lindner, W. Determination of ethylene oxide in the smoke of untreated cigarettes (in German). *Fachliche Mitteilungen Austria Tabakwerke* 13:215-220, 1972.

Bock, F.G., Moore, G.E., Dowd, J.E. Clark, P.C. Carcinogenic activity of cigarette smoke condensate. *Journal of the American Medical Association* 181:668-673, 1962.

Borgerding, M.F., Bodnar, J.A., Chung, H.L., Mangan, P.P., Morrison, C.C., Risner, C.H., Rodgers, J.C., Simmons, D.F., Uhrig, M.S., Wendelboe, F.N., Wingate, D.E., Winkler, L.S. Chemical and biological studies of a new cigarette that primarily heats tobacco. Part 1. *Chemical composition of mainstream smoke. Food and Chemical Toxicology* 36(7):169-182, 1998.

Borgerding, M.F., Hicks, R.D., Bodnar, J.E., Riggs, D.M., Nanni, E J., Fulp, G.W., Jr., Hamlin, W.C., Jr., Giles, J.A. Cigarette smoke composition. Part 1. Limitations of FTC method when applied to cigarettes that heat instead of burn tobacco. *Journal of the Association of Official Analytical Chemists* 73(4):605-609, 1990a.

Borgerding, M.F., Milhous, L.A., Hicks, R.D., Giles, J.A. Cigarette smoke composition. Part 2. Method for determining major components in smoke of cigarettes that heat instead of burn tobacco. *Journal of the Association of Official Analytical Chemists* 73(4):610-615, 1990b.

Bradford, J.A., Harlan, W.R., Hanmer, H.R. Nature of cigarette smoke; technique of cigarette smoking. *Industrial Engineering and Chemistry* 28:836-839, 1936.

Brunnemann, K.D., Hoffmann, D. Chemical studies on tobacco smoke. XXV. The pH of tobacco smoke. *Food and Cosmetics Toxicology* 12(1):115-124, 1974.

Brunnemann, K.D., Hoffmann, D. Analytical studies on N-nitrosamines in tobacco and tobacco smoke. *Recent Advances in Tobacco Science* 17:71-112, 1991.

Brunnemann, K.D., Hoffmann, D. Chemical studies on tobacco smoke. LXIX. Assessment of the carcinogenic N-nitrosodiethanolamine in tobacco products and tobacco smoke. *Carcinogenesis* 2(11):1123-1127, 1981.

Brunnemann, K.D., Hoffmann, D., Gairola, C.G., Lee, B.C. Low ignition propensity cigarettes: smoke analysis for carcinogens and testing for mutagenic activity of the smoke particulate matter. *Food and Chemical Toxicology* 32(10):917-922, 1994.

Brunnemann, K.D., Masaryk, J., Hoffmann, D. The role of tobacco stems in the formation of N-nitrosamines in tobacco and cigarette mainstream and sidestream smoke. *Journal of Agricultural and Food Chemistry* 31:1221-1224, 1983.

Brunnemann, K.D., Yu, L., Hoffmann, D. Chemical studies on tobacco smoke XVII. Assessment of carcinogenic volatile N-nitrosamines in mainstream and sidestream smoke from cigarettes. *Cancer Research* 37(9):3218-3222, 1977.

Burton, H.R., Dye, N.K., Bush, L.P. Distribution of tobacco constituents in tobacco leaf tissue. I. Tobacco-specific nitrosamines, nitrate, nitrite, and alkaloids. *Journal of Agricultural and Food Chemistry* 40:1050-1055, 1992.

Connolly, G.N., Wayne, G.D., Lymperis, D., Doherty, M.C. How cigarette additives are used to mask environmnental smoke. *Tobacco Control* 9: 283-291, 2000.

CORESTA Standard Smoking Methods 23: Determination of total and nicotine-free dry particulate matter using a routine analytical cigarette-smoking machine. Determination of total particulate matter and preparation for water and nicotine measurements. *CORESTA Information Bulletin* 1991-3:141-151, 1991.

Cox, J.D. and Yesner, R.A. Adenocarcinoma of the lung. Recent results from the Veterans Administration lung group. *American Review of Respiratory Disease* 120(5):1025-1029, 1979.

Cundiff, R.H., Greene, G.H., Laurene, A.H. Column elution of humectants from tobacco and determination by vapor chromatography. *Tobacco Science* 8:163-170, 1964.

Dalbey, W.E., Nettesheim, P., Griesemer, R., Caton, J.E., Guerin, M.R. Chronic inhalation of cigarette smoke by F344 rats. *Journal of the National Cancer Institute* 64(2):383-390, 1980.

Davis, B.R., Whitehead, J.K., Gill, M.E., Lee, P.N., Butterworth, A.D., Roe, F.J. Response of rat lung to tobacco smoke condensate or fractions derived from it ministered repeatedly by intratracheal installation. *British Journal of Cancer* 31(4):453-461, 1975.

DeBardeleben, M.Z., Claflin, W.E., Gannon, W.F. Role of cigarette physical characteristics on smoke composition. *Recent Advances in Tobacco Science* 4:85-111, 1978.

DeBethizy, J.D., Borgerding, M.F., Doolittle, D.J., Robinson, J.H., McManus, K.T., Rahn, C.A., Davis, R.A., Burger, G.T., Hayes, J.R., Reynolds, J.H., et al. Chemical and biological studies of a cigarette that heats rather than burns tobacco. *Journal of Clinical Pharmacology* 30(8):755-763, 1990.

Devesa, S.S., Shaw, G.L., Blot, W.J. Changing patterns of lung cancer incidence by histologic type. *Cancer Epidemiology Biomarkers and Prevention* 1(1):29-34, 1991

Djordjevic, M.V., Fan, J., Ferguson, S., Hoffmann, D. Self-regulation of smoking intensity, smoke yields of low-nicotine, low "tar" cigarettes. *Carcinogenesis* 16(9):2015-2021, 1995.

Djordjevic, M.V., Stellman, S.D., Zang, E. Doses of nicotine and lung carcinogens delivered to cigarette smokers. *Journal of the National Cancer Institute* 92(2):106-111, 2000.

Doll, R., Hill, A.B. Smoking and carcinoma of the lung. Preliminary report. *British Medical Journal* 2:739-748, 1950.

Dontenwill, W., Chevalier, H.J., Harke, H.-P., Lafrenz, U., Reckzeh, G., Schneider, B. Investigations on the effects of chronic cigarette smoke inhalation in Syrian golden hamsters. *Journal of the National Cancer Institute* 51(6):1781-1832, 1973.

Doull, J., Frawley, J. P., George, W. List of ingredients added to tobacco in the manufacture of cigarettes by six major American cigarette companies. Washington, D.C. Covington and Burling, 12 April, 1994 (reprinted: *Tobacco Journal International* 196:32-39, 1994).

Durocher, D.F. The choice of paper components for low-tar cigarettes. *Recent Advances in Tobacco Science* 10:52-71, 1984.

El-Bayoumy, K., Iatropoulos, M., Amin, S., Hoffmann, D., Wynder, E.L. Increased expression of cyclooxygenase-2 in rat lung tumors induced by the tobacco-specific nitrosamine 4-(methylnitrosamine)-4-(3-pyridyl)-4-(3-pyridyl)-butanone: Impact of a high-fat diet. *Cancer Research* 59(7):1400-1403, 1999.

el-Torkey, M., el-Zeky, F., Hall, J.C. Significant changes in the distribution of histologic types of lung cancer. A review of 4,928 cases. *Cancer* 65(10):2361-2367, 1990.

Enzell, C.R. Terpenoid components of leaf and their relationship to smoking quality and aroma. *Recent Advances in Tobacco Science* 2:32-60, 1976.

Essenberg, J.M. Cigarette smoke and the incidence of primary neoplasm of the lung in the albino mouse. *Science* 116:561-562, 1952.

Federal Trade Commission. *Report of "Tar" and Nicotine Content of the Smoke of 121 Varieties of Cigarettes*. Federal Trade Commission, Washington, D.C., 1971.

Federal Trade Commission. *Report of "Tar" and Nicotine Content of the Smoke of 166 Varieties of Cigarettes*. Federal Trade Commission, Washington, D.C., 1977.

Federal Trade Commission. *Report of "Tar", Nicotine and Carbon Monoxide of the Smoke of 187 Varieties of Cigarettes*. Federal Trade Commission, Washington, D.C., December 1981.

Federal Trade Commission. *Report of "Tar", Nicotine and Carbon Monoxide of the Smoke of 272 Varieties of Domestic Cigarettes*. Federal Trade Commission, Washington, D.C., 1988.

Federal Trade Commission. *Tar, Nicotine, and Carbon Monoxide of the Smoke of 475 Varieties of Domestic Cigarettes*. Federal Trade Commission, Washington, D.C., 1991.

Federal Trade Commission. *Tar, Nicotine, and Carbon Monoxide of the Smoke of 1,107 Varieties of Domestic Cigarettes*. Federal Trade Commission, Washington, D.C. 1995.

Federal Trade Commission. *Tar, Nicotine, and Carbon Monoxide of the Smoke of 1,206 Varieties of Domestic Cigarettes*. Federal Trade Commission, Washington, D.C., 1997.

Fisher, B. Filtering new technology. *Tobacco Reporter* 127(12):46-47, 2000.

Gaworski, C.L., Dozier, M.M., Heck, J.D., Gerhard, J.M. Rajendran, N., David, R.M., Brennecke, L.H., Morrissey, R. Toxicological evaluation of flavor ingredients added to cigarette tobacco: 13-week inhalation exposures in rats. *Inhalation Toxicology*10:357-381, 1998.

Gellatly, G., Uhl, R.G. Method for removal of potassium nitrate from tobacco extracts. U. S. Patent 4,131,118, December 26, 1978, 1978.

Gardner, D.E. (Editor). A safer cigarette? *Inhalation Toxicology* 12(Supplement 5):1-58, 2000.

Graham, E.A., Croninger, A.B., Wynder, E.L. Experimental production of carcinoma with cigarette tar. IV. Successful experiments with rabbits. *Cancer Research* 17:1058-66, 1957.

Green, C.R., Rodgman, A. The Tobacco Chemists' Research Conference. A half-century of advances in analytical methodology of tobacco and its products. *Recent Advances in Tobacco Science* 22:131-304, 1996.

Grimmer, G., Schneider, D., Naujack, K.-W., Dettbarn, G., Jacob, J. Intercept-reactant method for the determination of aromatic amines in mainstream tobacco smoke. *Beitrage zur Tabakforschung International* 16:141-156, 1995.

Gritz, E.R., Rose, J.E., Jarvik, M.E. Regulation of tobacco smoke intake with paced cigarette presentation. *Pharmacology, Biochemistry, and Behavior* 18:457-462, 1983.

Gutcho, S. *Tobacco Flavoring Substances and Methods*. Park Ridge, NJ: Noyes Data Corporation, 1972.

Haag, H.B., Larson, P.S., Finnegan, J.K. Effect of filtration on the chemical and irritating properties of cigarette smoke. *A.M.A. Archives of Otolaryngology* 69:261-265, 1959.

Halter, H.M., Ito, T.I. Effect of reconstitution and expansion processes on smoke composition. *Recent Advances in Tobacco Science* 4:113-132, 1979.

Hecht, S.S. Biochemistry, biology, and carcinogenicity of tobacco-specific N-nitrosamines. *Chemical Research in Toxicology* 11(6):559-603, 1998.

Herning, R.I., Jones, R.T., Bachman, G., Mines, A.H. Puff volume increases when low-nicotine cigarettes are smoked. *British Medical Journal (Clin Res Ed)* 283(6285):187-189, 1981.

Hida, T., Yatabe, Y., Achiwa, H., Muramatsu, H., Kozaki, K-I., Makamura, S., Ogawa, M., Mitsudomic, T., Sugiura, S., Takahashi, T. Increased expression of cyclooxygenase-2 occurs frequently in human lung cancers, especially in adenocarcinoma. *Cancer Research* 58(17):3761-3764, 1998.

Hoffmann, D., Brunnemann, K.D., Prokopczyk, B., Djordjevic, M.V. Tobacco-specific N-nitrosamines and Areca-derived N-nitrosamines. Chemistry, biochemistry, carcinogenicity, and relevance to humans. *Journal of Toxicology and Environmental Health* 41(1):1-52, 1994.

Hoffmann, D., Hecht, S.S. Advances in tobacco carcinogenesis. *Handbook of Experimental Pharmacology.* Cooper, C.S., Grover, P.L. (Editors.). New York: Springer Publications, 1989.

Hoffmann, D., Hoffmann, I. The changing cigarette, 1950–1995. *Journal of Toxicology and Environmental Health* 50(4):307-364, 1997.

Hoffmann, D., Hoffmann, I., Wynder, E.L. The changing cigarette: 1950-1997: facts and expectations. *"Report of Canada's Expert Committee on Cigarette Toxicity Reduction".* W.S. Rickert (Editor.). Health Canada, Toronto, Ontario, Canada, 1998, 94 p.

Hoffmann, D., Sanghvi, L.D., Wynder, E.L. Comparative chemical analysis of India bidi and American cigarette smoke. *International Journal of Cancer* 14(1):49-53, 1974.

Hoffmann, D., Wynder, E.L. Filtration of phenols from cigarette smoke. *Journal of the National Cancer Institute* 30:67-84, 1963.

Hoffmann, D., Wynder, E.L. The reduction in the tumorigenicity of cigarette smoke condensate by addition of sodium nitrate to tobacco. *Cancer Research* 27(1):172-174, 1967.

Hoffmann, D., Wynder, E.L. A study of tobacco carcinogenesis. XI. Tumor initiation, tumor acceleration, and tumor promoting activity of condensate fraction. *Cancer* 27(4):848-864, 1971.

Hoffmann, D., Wynder, E.L. Chemical analysis and carcinogenic bioassays of organic particulate pollutants. In: *Air Pollution,* A.L. Stern (Editor). Academic Press, New York, 1977, pp. 361-455.

International Agency for Research on Cancer. 1,3-Butadiene. *Occupational Exposures to Mists and Vapours from Strong Inorganic Acids; and Other Industrial Chemicals.* IARC Monographs on the Evaluation of Carcinogenic Risks to Humans. Lyon, France. 54:237-285, 1992.

International Agency for Research on Cancer. Acrylamide. *Some Industrial Chemicals.* IARC. Monographs on the Evaluation of Carcinogenic Risks to Humans. Lyon, France. 60:389-433, 1994e.

International Agency for Research on Cancer. Amino Acid Pyrolysis Products in Food. *Some Naturally Occurring and Synthetic Food Components, Furocoumarins, and Ultraviolet Radiation.* IARC Monographs on the Evaluation of Carcinogenic Risks to Humans. Lyon, France. 40:233-280, 1986b.

International Agency for Research on Cancer. Benzofuran. *Dry Cleaning, Some Chlorinated Solvents and Other Industrial Chemicals.* IARC Monographs on the Evaluation of the Carcinogenic Risks to Humans. Lyon, France. Vol. 63:431-441, 1995b.

International Agency for Research on Cancer. Coke Production. *Polynuclear Aromatic Compounds, Part 3: Industrial Exposure in Aluminum Production, Coal Gasification, Coke Production, and Iron and Steel Founding.* IARC Monographs on the Evaluation of the Carcinogenic Risk of Chemicals to Humans. Lyon, France. 34:101-131, 1984.

International Agency for Research on Cancer. DDT and associated compounds. *Occupational Exposures in Insecticide Application, and Some Pesticides.* IARC Monographs on the Evaluation of Carcinogenic Risks to Humans. Lyon, France. 53: 179-249, 1991.

International Agency for Research on Cancer. Di(2-ethylhexyl)phthalate. *Some Industrial Chemicals and Dyestuffs.* IARC Monographs on the Evaluation of Carcinogenic Risk of Chemicals to Humans. Lyon, France. 29: 257-280, 1982.

International Agency for Research on Cancer. Di(2-ethylhexyl)phthalate. *Some Industrial Chemicals.* IARC Monographs on the Evaluation of Carcinogenic Risk of Chemicals to Humans. Lyon, France. 77: 41-148, 2000.

International Agency for Research on Cancer. Ethylene oxide. *Some Industrial Chemicals.* IARC Monographs on the Evaluation of Carcinogenic Risks to Humans. Lyon, France. 60:73-159, 1994a.

International Agency for Research on Cancer. Furan. *Dry Cleaning, Some Chlorinated Solvents and Other Industrial Chemicals.* IARC Monographs on the Evaluation of the Carcinogenic Risks to Humans. Lyon, France. 63:393-407, 1995a.

International Agency for Research on Cancer. Isoprene. *Some Industrial Chemicals.* IARC Monographs on the Evaluation of Carcinogenic Risks to Humans. Lyon, France. 60:215-232, 1994c.

International Agency for Research on Cancer. Nitrobenzene. *Printing Processes and Printing Inks, Carbon Black and Some Nitro Compounds.* IARC Monographs on the Evaluation of the Carcinogenic Risks to Humans. Lyon, France. 65:381-408, 1996.

International Agency for Research on Cancer. *Overall Evaluation of Carcinogenicity: An Updating of IARC Monographs 1 to 42.* IARC Monographs on the Evaluation of Carcinogenic Risks to Humans. Lyon, France, Supplement No. 7, 1987.

International Agency for Research on Cancer. *Polynuclear Aromatic Compounds. Part 1. Chemical, Environmental and Experimental Data.* IARC Monographs on the Evaluation of the Carcinogenic Risk of Chemicals to Humans. Lyon, France, Vol. 33, 1983.

International Agency for Research on Cancer. Propylene oxide. *Some Industrial Chemicals.* IARC Monographs on the Evaluation of the Carcinogenic Risks of Chemicals to Humans. Lyon, France, 60:181-213, 1994b.

International Agency for Research on Cancer. Radon. *Man-Made Mineral Fibres and Radon*. IARC Monographs on the Evaluation of Carcinogenic Risks to Humans. Lyon, France. 43:173-254, 1988.

International Agency for Research on Cancer. Styrene. *Some Industrial Chemicals*. IARC Monographs on the Evaluation of Carcinogenic Risks to Humans. Lyon, France, 60:233-320, 1994d.

International Agency for Research on Cancer. *Tobacco Smoking*. IARC Monographs on the Evaluation of Carcinogenic Risks to Humans. Lyon, France. Vol 38, 1986a.

International Agency for Research on Cancer. 1,3-Butadiene. *Re-evaluation of Some Organic Chemicals, Hydrzine, and Hydrogen Peroxide*. IARC Monographs on the Evaluation of the Carcinogenic Risks to Humans. Lyon, France, 71:109-225, 1999a.

International Agency for Research on Cancer. Acetaldehyde. *Re-evaluation of Some Organic Chemicals, Hydrazine, and Hydrogen Peroxide*. IARC Monographs on the Evaluation of the Carcinogenic Risks to Humans. Lyon, France, 71:319-344, 1999b.

International Committee for Cigar Smoke Study: Machine smoking of cigars. *Bulletin du Information CORESTA* 1: 31-34, 1974.

International Standards Organization. *Routine Analytical Cigarette Smoking Machine: Part I. Specifications and Standard Conditions*. Geneva, Switzerland: ISO, 3308, 1991.

Ishiguro, S., Sugawara, S. *The Chemistry of Tobacco Smoke* (Japanese). (English translation 1981, 247 p.) Central Institute, Japanese Tobacco Monopoly Corporation, Yokahama, Japan, 1980, 202 p.

Jenkins, R.W.J., Neroman, P.H., Charms, M.D. Cigarette smoke formation. II. Smoke distribuion and mainstream pyrolytic composition of added 14C-menthol (U). *Beitrage zur Tabakforschung International* 5:299-301, 1970.

John, A.L. Japan. Always something new. *Tobacco International*, p. 30-35, August 1996.

Kagan, M.R., Cunningham, J.A., Hoffmann, D. Propylene glycol. A precursor of propylene oxide in cigarette smoke. 53rd Tobacco Science Research Conference, Abstract #41 and #42, 1999.

Kensler, C.J., Battista, S.P. Chemical and physical factors affecting mammalian ciliary activity. *American Review of Respiratory Disease* 93(3):93-102, 1966.

Kite, G.F., Gellatly, G., Uhl, R.G. Method for removal of potassium nitrate from tobacco extracts. U. S. Patent 4,131,117, December 26, 1978. 1978.

Leffingwell, J.C. (ed.). Chemical and sensory aspects of tobacco flavor. *Recent Advances in Tobacco Science* 14:1-218, 1987.

Leuchtenberger, C., Leuchtenberger, R. Effects of chronic inhalation of whole fresh cigarette smoke and of its gas phase on pulmonary tumorigenesis in Snell's mice. *Morphology of Experimental Respiratory Carcinogenesis. Proceedings of a Biology Division, Oak Ridge National Laboratory, Conference, Gatlinburg, Tennesee, May 13-16, 1970*. Nettesheim, P., Hanna, Jr., M.G., Deatherage, Jr., J.W. (Editors.). Washington, D.C.: U.S. Atomic Energy Commission, pp. 329-346, 1970.

Leuchtenberger, C., Leuchtenberger, R., Doolin, P.T. A correlated histological, cytological, and cytochemical study of tracheobronchial tree and lungs of mice exposed to cigarette smoke. *Cancer* 11:490-506, 1958.

Lewis, C.I. The effect of cigarette construction parameters on smoke generation and yield. *Recent Advances in Tobacco Science* 16:73-101, 1992.

Lyerly, L.A. Direct vapor chromatographic determination of menthol, propylene glycol, nicotine and triacetin in cigarette smoke. *Tobacco Science* 11:49-51, 1967.

Miller, J.E. Determination of the components of pipe tobacco smoke by means of a new pipe smoking machine. Proceedings of the 3rd World Tobacco Congress, Salisbury, Rhodesia, CORESTA, February 1963, p. 11.

Mohr, U., Reznik, G. Tobacco carcinogenesis. *Pathogenesis and Therapy of Lung Cancer*. C.C. Harris (Editor). Marcel Dekker, Inc., New York, pp. 263-361, 1978.

Moody, P.M. The relationships of qualified human smoking behavior and demographic variables. *Social Science & Medicine* 14A:49-54, 1980.

Mühlbock, O. Carcinogenicity of cigarette smoke in mice (Dutch). *Nederlands Tijdschrift voor Geneeskunde* 99: 2276-2278, 1958.

National Cancer Institute. *Tar and Less Hazardous Cigarettes. First Set of Experimental Cigarettes. Smoking and Health Program*. DHEW Publication No. (NIH) 76-905. 148 pages, 1977a.

National Cancer Institute. *Toward Less Hazardous Cigarettes. Second Set of Experimental Cigarettes. Smoking and Health Program*. DHEW Publication No. (NIH) 76-111. 153 pages, 1977b.

National Cancer Institute. *Smoking and Health Program. Toward Less Hazardous Cigarettes. Third Set of Experimental Cigarettes*. DHEW Publication No. (NIH) 77-1280, 152 pages, 1977c.

National Cancer Institute. *Toward Less Hazardous Cigarette. Fourth Set of Experimental Cigarettes. Smoking and Health Program*. DHEW Publication No. (NIH) 80. 213 pages, 1980.

National Cancer Institute. *Cigars: Health Effects and Trends*. Smoking and Tobacco Control Monograph No. 9. Burns, D.M., Hoffmann, D., Cummings, K.M. (Editors.). U.S. DHHS, Public Health Service, NIH-NCI. NIH Publ. No. 98-1302, Bethesda, MD. 232 pages, 1998.

Neurath, G.B. Nitrosamine formation from precursors in tobacco smoke. *N-Nitroso Compounds. Analysis and Formation.* Bogovski, P., Preussmann, R., Walker, E.A. (Editors.). International Agency for Research on Cancer. Lyon, France, IARC Sci. Publ. 3: 134-136, 1972.

Neurath, G., Ehmke, H. Studies on the nitrate content of tobacco. [German]. *Beiträge zur Tabakforschung International* 2:333-344, 1964.

Nil, R., Buzzi, R., Bättig, K. Effect of different cigarette smoke yields on puffing and inhalation. Is the measurement of inhalation volumes relevant for smoke absorption? *Pharmacology, Biochemistry, and Behavior* 24(3):587-595, 1986.

Norman, V., Ihrig, A.M., Larson, T.M., Moss, B.L. The effect of nitrogenous blend components on NO/NOX and HCN levels in mainstream and sidestream smoke. *Beiträge zur Tabakforschung International* 12:55-62, 1983.

Norman, V., Ihrig, A.M., Shoffner, R.A., Ireland, M.S. The effect of tip dilution on the filtration efficiency of upstream and downstream segments of cigarette filters. *Beiträge zur Tabakforschung International* 12:178-185, 1984.

Otto, H. Inhalation studies with mice exposed passively to cigarette smoke. (German) *Frankfurter Zeitschrift für Pathologie* 73:10-23, 1963.

Patrianakos, C., Hoffmann, D. Chemical studies on tobacco smoke. LXIV. On the analysis of aromatic amines in cigarette smoke. *Journal of Analytical Toxicology* 3:150-154, 1979.

Pauly, J.L., Lee, H.J., Hurley, E.L., Cummings, K.M., Lesser, J.D., Streck, R.J. Glass fiber contamination of cigarette filters: an additional health risk to the smoker? *Cancer Epidemiology, Biomarkers & Prevention* 7(11):967-979, 1998.

Peel, D.M., Riddick, M.G., Edwards, M.E., Gentry, J.S., Nestor, T.B. *Formation of Tobacco Specific Nitrosamines in Flue-cured Tobacco.* Presented at the 53rd Tobacco Science Research Conference. Montreal, Quebec, Canada. September 12–15, 1999.

Peele, D.M., Riddick, M.G., Edwards, M.E., Gentry, J.S., Nestor, N. Formation of tobacco-specific nitrosamines in flue-cured tobacco. *Recent Advances in Tobacco Science* 27: 3-12, 2001.

Peeler, C.L., Butters, G.R. Correspondence re: "It's time for a change: cigarette smokers deserve meaningful information about their cigarettes. *Journal of the National Cancer Institute* 92(10):842, 2000.

Philippe, R.J., Hackney, E. The presence of nitrous oxide and methyl nitrite in cigarette smoke and tobacco pyrolysis gases. *Tobacco Science* 3:139-143, 1959.

Pillsbury, H.C., Bright, C.C., O'Connor, K.J., Irish, F.W. Tar and nicotine in cigarette smoke. *Journal of the Association of Official Analytical Chemists* 52:458-462, 1969.

R. J. Reynolds Tobacco Company. *New Cigarette Prototypes That Heat Instead of Burn Tobacco. Chemical and Biological Studies.* Reynolds Tobacco Co., Winston-Salem, NC. 744 pages, 1988.

Roberts, D.L. Natural tobacco flavor. *Recent Advances in Tobacco Science* 14:49-81, 1988.

Roberts, D.L., Rowland, R.L. Macrocyclic diterpenes, a- and b- 4, 8, 13-duvatriene-1,3-diol from tobacco. *Journal of Organic Chemistry* 27:3989-3995, 1962.

Roe, J.F.C., Salaman, M.H. Cohen, J., Burgan, J.C. Incomplete carcinogens in cigarette smoke condensate. Tumor promotion by phenolic fraction. *British Journal of Cancer* 13:623-633, 1959.

Rose, J.E., Levin, E.D. (Eds.). *Eclipse and the Harm Reduction Strategy for Smoking.* Conference, Duke University, Bryan Center, Durham, N.C., August 23, 1996.

Russell, M.A.H. Low-tar, medium nicotine cigarettes: A new approach to safer smoking. *British Medical Journal* 6023:1430-1433, 1976.

Russell, M.A.H. The case for medium-nicotine, low-tar, low-carbon monoxide cigarettes. *Banbury Report 3.* Cold Spring Harbor, Cold Spring Harbor Laboratory, NY, pp. 297-310, 1980.

Schultz, W., Seehofer, F. Smoking behavior in Germany. The analysis of cigarette butts. In. *Smoking Behavior, Physiological and Psychological Influences.* Thornton, R.E. (Editor.). Edinburgh, Churchill Livingston, pp. 259-276, 1978.

Schumacher, J.N. The isolation of 6-O-acetyl-2, 3, 4-tri-O-[(+)-3 methylvaleryl]-b-D-glucopyranose from tobacco. *Carbohydrate Research* 13:1-8, 1970.

Senkus, M. (ed.). Leaf composition and physical properties in relation to smoking quality and aroma. *Recent Advances in Tobacco Science* 2:1-135, 1976.

Shepherd, R.J.K. New charcoal filters. *Tobacco Reporter* 121(2):10-14, 1994.

Sims, J.L., Atkinson, W.D., Benner, P. Nitrogen fertilization and genotype effects of selected constituents from all-burley cigarettes. *Tobacco Science* 23:11-13, 1975.

Singer, B, Essigmann, J.M. Site-specific mutagenesis: Retrospective and prospective. *Carcinogenesis* 12(6):945-955, 1991.

Smith, C.J., McCarns, S.C., Davis, R.A., Livingston, S.D., Bombick, B.R., Avolos, J.T., Morgan, W.T., Doolittle, D.J. Human urine mutagenicity study comparing cigarettes which burn or primarily heat tobacco. *Mutation Research* 361(1):1-9, 1996.

Society for Research on Nicotine and Tobacco. Policy committee urges regulation on Eclipse. *SRNT Newslett.* 6(2-3), 21-22, 2000.

Spears, A.W. Effect of manufacturing variables in cigarette smoke composition CORESTA Bull., Montreux, Switzerland, Symp. p. 6, 1974.

Spears, A.W. Selective filtration of volatile phenolic compounds from cigarette smoke. *Tobacco Science* 7:76-80, 1963.

Spears, A.W., Jones, S.T. Chemical and physical criteria for tobacco leaf of modern day cigarettes. *Recent Advances in Tobacco Science* 7:19-39, 1981.

Stedman, R.L., Burdick, D., Schmeltz, I. Composition studies on tobacco. XVII. Steam-smoke, volatile acid fraction of cigarette. *Tobacco Science* 7:166-169, 1963.

Stellman, S.D., Muscat, J.E., Thompson, S., Hoffmann, D., Wynder, E.L. Risk of squamous cell carcinoma and adenocarcinoma of the lung in relation to lifetime filter cigarette smoking. *Cancer* 80(3):362-368, 1997.

Stiles, M.F., Guy, T.D., Morgen, W.T., Edwards, D.W., Davis, R.W., Robinson, J.H. Human smoking behavior study. ECLIPSE cigarette compared to usual brand. *Toxicologist* 48:119-120, 1999.

Terpstra, P.M., Renninghaus, W., Solana, R.P. Evaluation of the electrically heated cigarette. S.O.T. 1998 Annual Meeting, The Toxicologist. *Abstract Issues Toxicological Sciences* 42(1S): 295; #1452, 1998.

Terrell, J.H., Schmeltz, I. Alteration of cigarette smoke composition. II. Influence of cigarette design. *Tobacco Science* 14:82-85, 1970.

Tiggelbeck, D. Vapor phase modification. An under-utilized technology. *Proc. 3rd World Conference on Smoking and Health. Vol. 1, Modifying the Risk for the Smoker.* DHEW Publication No. (NIH) 76-1221. pp. 507-514, 1976.

Törnqvist, M., Osterman-Golkar, S., Kautiainen, A., Jensen, S., Farmer, P.B., Ehrenberg, L. Tissue doses of ethylene oxide in cigarette smokers determined from adduct levels in hemoglobin. *Carcinogenesis* 7(9):1519-1521, 1986.

Tso, T.C. *Production, Physiology and Biochemistry of Tobacco Plant.* Beltsville, MD, Ideals, 753 pages, 1990.

Tso, T.C., Chaplin, J.P., Adams, J.D., Hoffmann, D. Simple correlation and multiple regression among leaf and smoke characteristics of burley tobaccos. *Beiträge zur Tabakforschung International* 11:141-150, 1982.

Tsuda, M., Kurashima, Y. Tobacco smoking, chewing and snuff dipping. Factors contributing to the endogenous formation of N-nitroso compounds. *Critical Reviews in Toxicology* 21(4):243-253, 1991.

U.S. Consumer Product Safety Commission. *Practicability of Developing a Performance Standard to Reduce Cigarette Ignition Propensity.* Vol. 1, U.S.C.P.S.C., Washington, D.C., 30 pages, 1993.

U.S. Department of Health and Human Services. *Reducing the Health Consequences of Smoking. 25 Years of Progress. A Report of the Surgeon General.* Anonymous. Massachusetts disputes claims about Eclipse cigarettes. Tobacco Reporter 127 (No. 11):11-13, 2000.

Vincent, R.G., Pickren, J.W., Lane, W.W., Bross, I., Takita, H., Haten, L., Gutierrez, A.C., Rzepka, T. The changing histopathology of lung cancer. *Cancer* 39(4):1647-1655, 1977.

Voges, E. Tobacco Encyclopedia. *Tobacco Journal International,* Mainz, Germany. 468 pages, 1984.

Waltz, P., Häusermann, M. Modern cigarettes and their effects on the smoking habits and on the composition of cigarette smoke (in German). *Zeitschrift fur Präventivmedizin* 8:3-98, 1963.

Wilkenfeld, J., Henningfield, J., Slade, J., Burns, D., Pinney, J. It's time for a change: cigarette smokers deserve meaningful information about their cigarettes. *Journal of the National Cancer Institute* 92(2):90-92, 2000a.

Wilkenfeld, J., Henningfield, J., Slade, J., Burns, D., Pinney, J. Response to correspondence re: "It's time for a change: cigarette smokers deserve meaningful information about their cigarettes". *Journal of the National Cancer Institute* 92(2):842-843, 2000b.

Wittekindt, W. Changes in recommended plant protection agents for tobacco. *Tobacco Journal International* 5:390-394, 1985.

Wynder, E.L., Graham, E.A. Tobacco smoking as a possible etiologic factor in bronchiogenic carcinoma. A study of six hundred and eighty-four proved cases. *Journal of the American Medical Association 143:329-336, 1950* (reprinted *Journal of the American Medical Association* 253(20)2986-94).

Wynder, E.L., Graham, E.A., Croninger, A.G. Experimental production of carcinoma with cigarette tar. *Cancer Research* 13:855-864, 1953.

Wynder, E.L., Hoffmann, D. Some practical aspects of the smoking—Cancer problem. *New England Journal of Medicine* 262:540-545, 1960.

Wynder, E.L., Hoffmann, D. A study of tobacco carcinogenesis. VIII. The role of acidic fractions as promoters. *Cancer* 14:1306-1315, 1961.

Wynder, E.L., Hoffmann, D. A study of air pollution carcinogenesis. III. Carcinogenic activity of gasoline engine exhaust. *Cancer* 152:103-108, 1962.

Wynder, E.L., Hoffmann, D. A contribution to experimental tobacco carcinogenesis. (In German). *Deut. Med. Wochenschr.* 88:623-628, 1963.

Wynder, E.L., Hoffmann, D. Reduction of tumorigenicity of tobacco smoke. An experimental approach. *Journal of the American Medical Association* 192:85-94, 1965.

Wynder, E.L., Hoffmann, D. Tobacco and Tobacco Smoke. *Studies in Experimental Carcinogenesis.* New York: Academic Press, 730 pages, 1967.

Wynder, E.L., Hoffmann, D. Smoking and lung cancer: scientific challenges and opportunities. *Cancer Research* 54(20):5284-5295, 1994.

Wynder, E.L., Kopf, P., Ziegler, H. A study of tobacco carcinogenesis. II. Dose-response studies. *Cancer* 10:1193-1200, 1957.

Wynder, E.L., Mann, J. A study of tobacco carcinogenesis III. Filtered cigarettes. *Cancer* 10:1201-1205, 1957.

# Public Understanding of Risk and Reasons for Smoking Low-Yield Products

Neil D. Weinstein

**INTRODUCTION** Few members of the public understand the probabilities and odds that form the vocabulary scientists use to discuss risk (Weinstein, 1999). Thus, lay people rely upon other cues, such as the cigarette labels 'Light' and 'Ultra Light', to help them make decisions about smoking and other hazards (see Chapter 7). This chapter examines public perceptions of Light cigarettes, reasons for smoking Lights, and the relationship between smoking Lights and quitting.

**PERCEPTIONS OF LIGHT CIGARETTES** The labels 'Light' and 'Ultra Light', when applied to cigarettes, imply a variety of benefits. These include lower levels of tar and nicotine, less risk to health, and milder taste. Cigarette advertising, including the way in which these labels are used in the advertising, further modifies and shapes public perceptions of these products. What 'Light' and 'Ultra Light' come to mean to members of the public is an empirical question that can be revealed by careful survey research.

A substantial portion of smokers believe that low-tar cigarettes are less risky than Regular cigarettes. For example, a nationwide 1987 survey (Giovino *et al.*, 1996, p. 49) found that 45.7 percent of Ultra-Light smokers, 32.2 percent of Light smokers, and 29.4 percent of Regular smokers said that low-tar cigarettes reduce the risk of cancer. Nevertheless, smokers' knowledge about low-tar cigarettes is quite limited.

In 1995, a random sample of 12,371 Canadians adults were asked by telephone interviewers what the word "light" means in relation to cigarettes (Health Canada, 1995). The most frequently mentioned topics were: "less tar" (20.1 percent), "less nicotine" (36.2 percent), "safer" or "less addictive" (3.2 percent), "milder taste" (6.7 percent), "different filter" (2.3 percent), and "nothing" or "ad gimmick" (14.1 percent). A further 21.2 percent had no idea what the term meant. The meanings ascribed to "light" were generally similar among various subgroups of smokers, although former and never smokers were more likely than current smokers to say that they had no idea what the term meant (17.8 percent and 28.7 percent versus 12.2 percent, respectively), and former smokers were more likely than current and never smokers to state that "light" was a meaningless advertising term (22.2 percent versus 16.0 percent and 10.6 percent, respectively).

A 1994 national random telephone survey found that 95% of regular smokers could identify that they were "somewhat certain" or "very certain" that they smoked a Regular, Light, or Ultra-Light cigarette (Kozlowski *et al.*, 1998a & b). However, when asked how much tar their cigarettes contained, few smokers knew the answer to this question. For example, Cohen (1996a, p. 128) reported that 79% of smokers answered that they did not know the answer to the question. Comparing the estimates given by smokers to the actual figures for their brands, Kozlowski and colleagues (1998b) found that only 3% of smokers could correctly state (within 2 mg) the amount of tar in their cigarettes. In fact, few knew where to look to learn the tar content (Kozlowski *et al.*, 1998b). Although 67% of smokers said that they would look on their cigarette package to find the tar content, only 6.3% of cigarettes sold have this information on the package. When asked how many Light cigarettes someone would have to smoke to get the same amount of tar as from one Regular cigarette, the most common response from about half of those surveyed was, "don't know"; about 40 percent said two cigarettes or more and less than 10 percent said one cigarette (Kozlowski *et al.*, 1998a).

There are significant differences in knowledge and reported use of tar numbers among different types of smokers. For example, when Ultra-Light, Light, and Regular cigarettes were compared, the members of the first group were found to be somewhat more accurate about their cigarette's tar number (Kozlowski *et al.*, 1998b). Accuracy was shown by 17% of Ultra-Light smokers, 2% of Light smokers, and 1% of Regular smokers. Ultra-Light smokers were also much more likely to say they used this number in making judgments about cigarette safety (Cohen, 1996a, p. 132). Thus, although only 14% of Cohen's overall sample said that they used tar numbers to make such judgments, 56% of the smokers of 1- to 5-mg tar cigarettes said that they determined safety from advertised tar values. Ultra-Light smokers also saw a much bigger difference between the risk of Regular and Light cigarettes than did other smokers (Cohen, 1996a, p. 130). A large majority (83%) of Ultra-Light smokers said that switching from a 20-mg to a 5-mg tar cigarette would significantly reduce health risks, whereas only about 50% of other smokers shared this belief.

Clearly, knowledge about the reported tar values of their chosen brands, about where these values can be found, and about vent holes in cigarettes is largely absent among smokers. Of particular importance is the finding that a large proportion of smokers believe that switching to a lower tar cigarette reduces one's health risks, and since most smokers are only aware of a cigarette's advertised type—'Regular', 'Light', or 'Ultra Light'— and not its tar number, this classification is used as a surrogate to indicate risk. Attention to tar numbers is particularly true among Ultra-Light smokers, a majority of whom say they use these numbers to judge a cigarette's safety.

**REASONS FOR SMOKING OR SWITCHING TO LIGHT CIGARETTES**  A variety of studies have asked smokers about their reasons for choosing to smoke Light or Ultra Light cigarettes or their reasons for switching to such cigarettes. The results show that the desire to reduce disease risk is one of the main factors guiding these choices. Although it would be desirable to distinguish in this section between initial cigarette choices, switching as a prelude to quitting, switching as a substitute for quitting, and switching following an unsuccessful quit attempt, the available data do not permit such a fine-grained analysis. In the 1987 National Health Interview Survey

(Giovino *et al.*, 1996, p. 45), 44 percent of current smokers said that they had at some time switched to a low-tar/low-nicotine cigarette in order to reduce their health risk. Similarly, a national survey found that about 60 percent of Ultra-Light smokers and approximately 40 percent of Light smokers said that they smoked reduced-tar cigarettes "to reduce the risks of smoking without having to give up smoking" (Kozlowski *et al.*, 1998a)

In this same national telephone survey, the reasons given by current daily smokers for why they chose to smoke Ultra-Light/Light cigarettes were: step toward quitting (49/30 percent), reduce risk (58/39 percent), reduce tar (73/57 percent), reduce nicotine (72/50 percent), and prefer the taste (69/80 percent) (Kozlowski *et al.*, 1998a). Very similar figures were obtained in telephone interviews of 266 randomly selected Massachusetts smokers (Kozlowski *et al.*, 1998a). In a recent experiment involving a randomly selected sample of 568 smokers of Light cigarettes, the reasons given for smoking Light cigarettes by people in the control or delayed intervention groups were: step toward quitting (25 percent), reduce risk (43 percent), reduce tar or nicotine (70 percent), and prefer taste (81 percent) (Kozlowski *et al.*, 1999). In these same groups, 39 percent said that Light cigarettes decreased their risk of having health problems.

A national survey of adolescents and young adults in 1993 found somewhat less of an emphasis on health issues, with smokers of Light or Ultra-Light cigarettes saying that they chose their brand because of taste (33 percent), because they were less irritating (29 percent), because they were healthier than other brands (21 percent), and because they "just liked them" (19 percent) (Giovino *et al.*, 1996, p. 49).

Not surprisingly, national survey of adults in 1986 showed that those who have ever switched in order to reduce tar or nicotine are more likely than those who never switched to believe that some brands are more hazardous than others (54 percent versus 40 percent, respectively) and to believe that their current brand is less hazardous than other brands (33 percent versus 16 percent, respectively) (Giovino *et al.*, 1996, p. 50). Although most smokers recognize that smoking is risky to one's health, those who chose Light and Ultra-Light cigarettes are more likely to acknowledge the risk than smokers of Regular cigarettes. For example, 85 percent of those who had switched to lower tar/nicotine brands said they were concerned about the health effects of smoking, compared to 70 percent of those who had never made this switch (Giovino *et al.*, 1996, p. 50). People who had switched were also more likely to say that their health had been affected by smoking and that a doctor had advised them to quit (Giovino *et al.*, 1996, p. 48).

Similarly, when the previously mentioned Canadian smokers were asked about the likelihood of developing health problems such as emphysema, asthma, lung cancer, or stroke from smoking for many years, those who had switched from Regular to Light cigarettes cited more problems as very likely than those who started and continued smoking Regular cigarettes (2.13 v. 1.94 problems, respectively) (data from Health Canada, 1995).

Overall, the data are consistent in showing that smokers of Light and Ultra-Light cigarettes are especially concerned about protecting their health. The majority of these smokers choose Light or Ultra-Light cigarettes in the belief that this will reduce their health risks and/or make it easier to quit.

**THE RELATIONSHIP OF SWITCHING TO QUITTING** Smokers of low-yield cigarettes not only express greater concern about the risks of smoking, but they also show more interest in quitting. In fact, 38 percent of the smoker respondents to the 1987 National Health Interview Survey who switched to Light cigarettes saw this change as a step toward quitting (Giovino *et al.*, 1996, p. 49), and people who smoked Light or Ultra-Light cigarettes tended to have tried more quitting strategies than those who smoked Regular cigarettes (Giovino *et al.*, 1996, p. 51). Among those smokers who had never attempted to quit, smokers of low-tar cigarettes were more likely to say that they had considered quitting.

Similar interest in both quitting and healthy behavior comes from a study of U.S. Air Force trainees (Haddock *et al.*, 1999). These researchers reported that individuals who said that they had "switched to a lower tar/nicotine cigarette just to reduce their health risk" were more likely to have experienced a successful 24-hour quit attempt in the past, had more healthy diets, and were less likely to take other kinds of risks. These switchers were also less likely to say that they were addicted to cigarettes.

However, there are no data that show switching to reduced-tar cigarettes increases the likelihood of quitting. In fact, given the perceived reduction in risk from smoking Light cigarettes, a switch to such brands may well weaken the motivation to quit. In the Health Canada survey, 32.0 percent of those who started with, and continued to, smoke Light cigarettes made a quit attempt in the previous 3 months, compared to 15.1 percent of those who started with, and continued to, smoke Regular cigarettes. But of those who started with Regular cigarettes and were currently Light cigarette smokers, only 16.7 percent had tried to quit recently (data from Health Canada, 1995).

A large 1986 national study of adults in the United States who had ever smoked found that those who smoked low-yield cigarettes, regardless of whether they had ever switched to lower yield cigarettes, were less likely to have quit than those who smoked high-yield brands (Giovino *et al.*, 1996, p. 49). Persons who had ever switched brands to reduce their level of tar and nicotine also were less likely to have quit than those who had never switched brands to reduce their level of tar and nicotine.

When Air Force trainee smokers—who had been required to abstain from smoking throughout their basic military training—were contacted 12 months later, only 12.5 percent of switchers and 11.1 percent of nonswitchers were still abstinent (Haddock *et al.*, 1999). Controlling for demographic factors and smoking history, this difference was not statistically significant (odds ratio = 1.04, $p > .5$). Among Air Force trainees, switchers did report smoking fewer cigarettes than nonswitchers. However, in the 1995 Health Canada survey, people who had started smoking Regular cigarettes and currently smoked Light cigarettes did not smoke fewer cigarettes per day than those who stayed with Regular cigarettes.

Thus, even among individuals who had switched specifically because they were concerned about health risks, who had been assisted in long-term quitting by a mandatory abstinence period, or who said they were less addicted to cigarettes than did the nonswitchers, the switch to Light cigarettes prior to the abstinence period did not help them stay abstinent. Switching to Light cigarettes does not seem to be any more of a route toward quitting than simply staying with Regular cigarettes.

Thus, no data exist that indicate switching to Light or Ultra-Light cigarettes actually assists smokers in quitting.

**SUMMARY**     Overall, the accumulated data are quite consistent. They show that many consumers use the terms 'Light' and 'Ultra Light' as a guide to the riskiness of particular brands of cigarettes. To a considerable extent, smokers choose Light and Ultra-Light brands because they think that these cigarettes are not as harmful and cause fewer health problems. Particularly, individuals who are most concerned about smoking risks and most interested in quitting adopt low-yield brands.

To determine whether switching helps people to smoke less or to quit, one would ideally examine two groups with the same interest in quitting and the same smoking history. One would compare the group that switched with the group that did not, looking at both cessation and smoking rates over time. In reality, however, those who switch are different from nonswitchers in numerous ways, all of which should facilitate their quitting and reduce the amount that they smoke. Despite these facilitating factors, the data show that switchers to a Light or Ultra-Light cigarette are not more likely to become nonsmokers than are nonswitchers.

Surveys indicate that switching to low-yield cigarettes is viewed by many smokers as a healthier choice. Given the interest in quitting among those who make this choice, their failure to quit at rates any higher than those who do not switch suggests that switching reduces the motivation to stop smoking. Thus, the advertising of brands designated as 'Light' or 'Ultra Light' misleads smokers as to the benefits these brands offer.

The data collected since publication of the 1996 NCI monograph only reinforce the conclusion reached by Giovino and colleagues (1996) in that volume that the existence of so called 'Light' and 'Ultra Light' cigarettes has kept many smokers interested in protecting their health from quitting. "The net effect of the introduction and mass marketing of these brands, then, may have been and may continue to be an increased number of smoking-attributable deaths."(Giovino *et al.*, 1996.)

## CONCLUSIONS

1. Many consumers use the terms 'Light' and 'Ultra-Light' as a guide to the riskiness of particular brands of cigarettes.

2. Many smokers choose Light and Ultra-Light brands because they believe that such cigarettes are less likely to cause health problems.

3. Individuals who are most concerned about smoking risks and most interested in quitting adopt low-yield brands.

## REFERENCES

Cohen, J.B. Consumer/smoker perceptions of Federal Trade Commission Tar Ratings. *The FTC Cigarette Test Method for Determining Tar, Nicotine, and Carbon Monoxide Yields of U.S. Cigarettes. Report of the NCI Expert Committee.* Smoking and Tobacco Control Monograph No. 7. U.S. Department of Health and Human Services, National Institutes of Health, National Cancer Institute, NIH Publication No. 96-4028, 1996a.

Cohen J. B. Smokers' knowledge and understanding of advertised tar numbers: Heath policy implications. *American Journal of Public Health* 86:18-24, 1996b.

Giovino, G.A., Tomar, S.L., Reddy, M.N., Peddicord, J.P., Zhu, B., Escobedo, L.G., Eriksen, M.P. Attitudes, knowledge, and beliefs about low-yield cigarettes among adolescents and adults. *The FTC Cigarette Test Method for Determining Tar, Nicotine, and Carbon Monoxide Yields of U.S. Cigarettes. Report of the NCI Expert Committee.* Smoking and Tobacco Control Monograph No. 7. U.S. Department of Health and Human Services, National Institutes of Health, National Cancer Institute, NIH Publication No. 96-4028, 1996.

Haddock, C.K., Talcott, G.W., Klesges, R.C., Lando, H. An examination of cigarette brand switching to reduce health risks. *Annals of Behavioral Medicine* 21(2):128–134, 1999.

Health Canada. *Survey on Smoking in Canada. Cycle 4.* Ottawa: Health Canada, June, 1995.

Kozlowski, L.T., Goldberg, M.E., Yost, B. A., White, E.L., Sweeney, C. T., Pillitteri, J.L. Smokers' misperceptions of light and ultra-light cigarettes may keep them smoking. *American Journal of Preventive Medicine* 15:9–16, 1998a.

Kozlowski, L.T., Goldberg, M.E., Yost, B.A., Ahern, F.M., Aronson, K.R. Smokers are unaware of the filter vents now on most cigarettes: Results of a national survey. *Tobacco Control* 5:265–270, 1996.

Kozlowski, L.T., Goldberg, M.E., Sweeney, C.T., Palmer, R.F., Pillitteri, J.L. Yost, B.A., White, E.L., Stine, M.M. Smoker reactions to a "radio message" that Light cigarettes are as dangerous as regular cigarettes. *Nicotine and Tobacco Control* 1:67-76, 1999.

Kozlowski, L.T., Pillitteri, J.L., Ahern, F.M., Yost, B.A., Goldberg, M.E. Advertising fails to inform smokers of official yields of cigarettes. *Journal of Applied Biobehavioral Research* 3:55-64, 1998b.

Kozlowski, L.T., White, E.L., Sweeney, C.T., Yost, B.A., Ahern, F.M. Goldberg, M.E. Few smokers know their cigarettes have filter vents. *American Journal of Public Health* 88:681–682, 1998c.

Weinstein, N.D. What does it mean to understand a risk? Dimensions of risk comprehension. *Journal of the National Cancer Institute—Monograph* 25:15–20, 1999.

# Marketing Cigarettes With Low Machine-Measured Yields

Richard W. Pollay, Timothy Dewhirst

**INTRODUCTION**　　During the early 1950s, scientific and popular articles that presented lung cancer research findings initiated what the tobacco industry termed the "health scare," as consumers became increasingly concerned about the potential health risks incurred from smoking. Companies initially responded to this health scare by introducing filtered products that were accompanied by advertisements with explicit health-related statements. For example, Viceroy® maintained that it provided "Double-Barreled Health Protection" and also claimed that it was "Better for Your Health" in ad copy.

In time, the industry became aware that explicit health claims had the undesirable effects of making health concerns salient or predominant in the minds of consumers, and encouraged consumers to use "healthfulness" as the criterion by which they judged cigarettes. Motivation researchers and other trade analysts advised the industry to shift from explicit verbal assertions of health toward implied healthfulness, an approach that incorporated the use of visual imagery (Pollay, 1989a).

January of 1964 marked the release of the first Surgeon General's Report on smoking, and this event reawakened public concerns about the potential health consequences of smoking. Tobacco manufacturers needed to reduce consumer concerns and the ensuing anxious feelings. Quitting was not an easy option for smokers because nicotine is highly addictive. Switching to a lower (tar and nicotine) yield cigarette became an attractive alternative for many smokers once they were convinced by advertising that this would be a meaningful step toward health and away from risk. Thus, there was a ready market for "new and improved" cigarettes, or at least for those that seemed to be that way.

This chapter will review recently released documents from the tobacco industry and its consultants, produced during litigation, as well as excerpts from the relevant trade press, for insights into the firms' intentions and actions in marketing their products. Particular attention will be paid to the period of the mid-1970s, the launch period for most of the new generation of low-yield products. It will be shown that advertising for reduced-yield products led consumers to perceive filtered and low-tar delivery products as safer alternatives to regular cigarettes.

**THE 1950s**

**Filters Debut as
Health Protection**

Advertising during the 1950s promoted filters as the technological fix to the health scare. Filters were heralded with various dramatic announcements featuring 'news' about: scientific discoveries; modern pure materials; research and development breakthroughs; certification by the United States Testing Company; implied endorsement by the American Medical Association (see Figure 7-1); "miracle tip" filters; and descriptions of "20,000 filter traps" or filters made of activated charcoal, "selectrate," "millecel," "cellulose acetate" or "micronite" that were variously described as effective, complete, superior, and producing mildness, gentleness, smoothness, etc.

In 1958, for example, a press conference was held at New York's Plaza Hotel to launch Parliament® and its new filter, called "Hi-Fi" ("high filtration," as in high-fidelity state-of-the-art sound reproduction of the 1950s).

"In the foyers, test tubes bubbled and glassed-in machines smoked cigarettes by means of tubes. Men and women in long white laboratory coats bustled about and stood ready to answer any questions. Inside, a Philip Morris executive told the audience of reporters that the new Hi-Fi filter was an event of 'irrevocable significance'. The new filter was described as 'hospital white'." (See Whelan, 1984, p.90)

The purported product benefit of this new filtration was obviously the perceived reduction, if not elimination, of cancer and other health risks. Health benefits were implied through various slogans, such as "Just What the Dr. Ordered" (L&M®), "Inhale to your Heart's Content" (Embassy®), "The Secret to Life is in the Filter" (Life®), "Extra Margin" (of safety protection; analogy to helmets, seat belts, and other safety gear— Parliament®), and "Thinking Man's Filter" (Viceroy®). Other slogans were more implicit, but still provided health inferences to consumers (See Pollay, 1989b).

If nothing else, the high technology attributes of filtration, and its ability to produce healthful conditions in other media such as water, were communicated (see Figure 7-2).

"The speed with which charcoal filters penetrated the health cigarette market shows the effectiveness of a new concept. The public had been conditioned to accept the filtering effects of charcoal in other fields, and when charcoal was added to cigarette filters it proved to be an effective advertising gimmick." (See Johnston, 1966, p.16)

"Claims or assurances related to health are prominent in the (cigarette) advertising. These claims and assurances vary in their explicitness, but they are sufficiently patent to compel the conclusion that much filter and menthol-filter advertising seeks to persuade smokers and potential smokers that smoking cigarettes is safe or not unhealthful." (See the Federal Trade Commission, 1964, p. 72)

The result in the marketplace was a dramatic conversion from 'regular' (short length; unfiltered) products to new product forms (filtered; king sized; 100 mm). Spending on advertising nearly tripled from 1952 to 1959, largely through promoting the virtues of the new filtered products, thereby enticing smokers to switch from their regular unfiltered products to filtered and, presumably, safer brands or product-line variants.

"He had abandoned the regular cigarette, however, on the ground of reduced risk to health. . . . A further consequence of the 'tar derby' was the rapid increase in advertising expenditures during this period. Advertising expenditures in selected media jumped from over $55 million in 1952 to approximately $150 million in 1959." (See Pepples, 1976, p. 1)

Figure 7-1

**Kent—Implied AMA Endorsement (Circa 1953)**

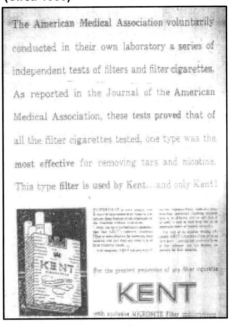

**Females and Older Smokers as Early Filter Smokers**  Gender and age were predictors of who adopted the new filtered products. Females converted more readily than males, and older concerned smokers adapted more readily than young starters (O'Keefe and Pollay, 1996). Thus, Philip Morris anticipated that females would be the largest potential market for a "health cigarette" following the release of the 1964 Surgeon General's Report:

"Women, and particularly young women, would constitute the greatest potential market for a health cigarette." (See Johnston, 1966, p. 1)

Psychology-based consumer research conducted for Brown & Williamson implied that the females who smoked filters were normal, whereas the males seemed unusually anxious. In 1967, this research described women who smoked filter cigarettes as "neither rebels (like women who smoke plain cigarettes), nor insecure (like females who smoke menthols)." The males who smoked filter cigarettes were described as ". . . apprehensive and depressive. They think about death, worry over possible troubles, are uneasy if inactive, don't trust others." (See Oxtoby-Smith, Inc., 1967, pp. 24-25.)

**Filter Cigarette Marketing to Males**  Once the public accepted filters as an adequate response to at least assuage their worst fears, there was a market opportunity in providing males with filtered products that delivered 'full flavor':

"... [O]nce the consumer had been sufficiently educated on the virtues of filters, a vacuum was created for a filter with taste; this vacuum was filled by Winston and Marlboro." (See Latimer, 1976, p. 5.)

Some internal industry documents from the 1970s portray the filters of the 1950s and the associated risk reduction as essentially 'cosmetic':

"... [T]he public began to accept filters as a way to reduce the *cosmetic risks* of smoking and the attendant 'ego-status' risk of appearing to have an immoral, unclean habit." [Emphasis added.] (See Latimer, 1976, p. 3.)

**The Early Tar Wars**    The period from the mid-1950s until the mid-1960s was tumultuous for the industry. Various new filter products were launched, many competitive advertising claims used different standards of measurement, and the Federal Trade Commission (FTC) guidelines concerning what was permissible in cigarette advertising changed as well. Episodes of intense competitive rivalry of claims and counter-claims about cigarette yields were dubbed the "tar derby" or "tar wars" within the trade, and the ensuing publicity in the popular press affected the marketplace. Some manufacturers took advantage of these dynamics to present their cigarettes as "healthy" to the public during a period of intense advertising claims, then capitalized on such reputations while selling products that were actually quite high in tar and nicotine yields.

Figure 7-2

**Tareyton—Charcoal Filter (1972)**

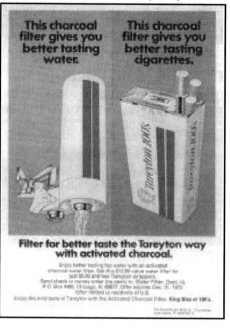

"In 1955, the FTC, reacting to conflicting claims as to tar and filtration, has imposed 'Cigarette Advertising Guides' banning all mention of tar, nicotine and filtration 'when not established by competent scientific proof'. This put a stop to such claims in advertising. In July and August of 1957, the *Reader's Digest* published two articles with figures on tar and nicotine mentioning Kent by name. The August article, written with Kent's assistance was practically an ad for Kent. In 90 days, Kent's sales leaped from 300 million to 3 billion per month. This article broke the dike and set off the famous Tar Derby. Over the next 4 years, tar levels were drastically cut. Marlboro dropped from 34 mg. tar in 1957 to 25 mg. in 1958 and 19 mg. in 1961." (See Cunningham and Walsh, 1980, p. 11)

Kent®, whose advertising of its asbestos-based "Micronite" filter had been very effective, engaged in a series of product revisions in the 1950s. With each iteration, the Kent® product yielded more and more tar and nicotine, and this pattern continued into the 1960s. Similar filter "loosening" was the subject of U.S. Congressional inquiry (Blatnik, 1958).

> "In mid 1960, the FTC called off the Tar Derby, rigidly prohibiting tar and nicotine claims. Some of the new low tar brands disappeared. Soon thereafter, the brands stopped reducing tar levels and, indeed, began to raise them. Kent, for example, went from 14 mg. in 1961 to 16 mg. in 1963 and 19 mg. in 1966. The FTC prohibition ended March 25, 1966 initiating a new phase in Hi-Fi development. Lorrillard [sic] decided not to reduce Kent's tar level again. Instead it put out True." (See Cunningham and Walsh, 1980, p.12.)

**Medicinal Menthol**  During this tar derby period, new menthol-filtered products were introduced, such as Salem®, Newport®, and Oasis®. Manufacturers of these new products capitalized on the reputation that menthol already had, due to its use in cold remedies and related medicinal applications, and the history of "pseudo-health" claims made in earlier menthol cigarette advertising. The Kool® brand had long been promoted as a medicinal product with would-be remedial properties that could make the cigarette suitable when smokers were suffering from coughs, colds, sore throats, etc.:

> "Kool not only remained, but was actively positioned as a remedial/medicinal type product throughout the 1950's." (See Cunningham and Walsh, 1980, p. 9.)

Salem® was introduced in 1956 as the "first truly new smoking advance" (see Figure 7-3).

> "Salem created a whole new meaning for menthol. From the heritage of solves-the-negative-problems-of-smoking, menthol almost instantly became a positive smoking sensation. Menthol in

Figure 7-3
**Salem—First Truly New Smoking Advance (1956)**

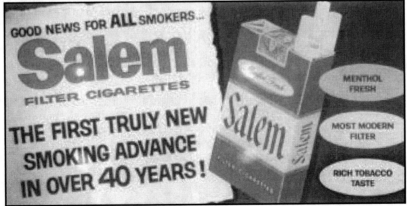

the filter form in the Salem advertising was a 'refreshing' taste experience. It can be viewed as very 'reassuring' in a personal concern climate. Undoubtedly, the medicinal menthol connotation carried forward in a therapeutic fashion, but as a positive taste benefit." (See Cunningham and Walsh, 1980, p. 9.)

"During the 'tar derby', menthol styles were perceived as healthier, low 'tar' smokes due to the quasi-medical health claims in menthol advertising. . . the first true menthol hi-fi was True Green, introduced in 1967. . . By 1974, menthol hi-fi styles had a 27% share of the hi-fi category—close to the proportion of menthols to all styles." (See Chambers, 1979.)

**THE 1960s**

**Implications of the 1964 Surgeon General's Report**

The first Surgeon General's Report on smoking and health in 1964 established cigarette smoking as a cause of lung cancer, at least in males. Philip Morris expressed some regret that the 1964 report did not strongly endorse the filtered products that had been sold to the public as a technological fix:

"The health value of filters is undersold in the report and is the industry's best extant answer to its problem. The Tobacco Institute obviously should foster the communication of the filter message by all effective means." (See Wakeham, 1964, p. 8.)

**Consumer Guilt and Anxiety**    Brown & Williamson's advertising agency and market research contractors recognized consumers' mass sense of being addicted, as well as the ensuing conflict, guilt, anxieties, and need for reassurance:

"Most smokers see themselves as addicts . . . the typical smoker feels guilty and anxious about smoking but impotent to control it." (See Oxtoby-Smith, Inc., 1967, p. 6.)

"Psychologically, most smokers feel trapped. They are concerned about health and addiction. Smokers care about what commercials say about them. Advertising may help to reduce anxiety and guilt. . . Brand user image may be critical in influencing shifts in brand loyalty." [Emphasis in original.] (See Oxtoby-Smith, Inc., 1967, p. 14.)

[People who smoke filter cigarettes] ". . . may be receptive to advertising which helps them escape from their inner conflicts about smoking." (See Oxtoby-Smith, Inc., 1967, p. 23.)

"While unquestionably smokers are concerned about the tar and nicotine contents and the filtration effectiveness of their brands, nevertheless, both on the surface and even to some extent unconsciously, they appear to be resisting open involvement with this 'frightening' element of smoking."(See Alex Gochfeld Associates, Inc., 1969, p. 9.)

Some brands were less successful than others when trying to directly address consumer conflicts. Kent®, for example, used a visual portrayal of a smoker's conscience, and risked their ad being experienced as a nagging message (see Figure 7-4).

"... [T]he psychological blinders that smokers have donned, consciously or unconsciously ... advertising which stresses tar and nicotine content was received less enthusiastically ... even in the Silva Thins commercial where this theme was the major aspect of the spoken message, a large number of people effectually [sic] blocked it out of their consciousness retaining only the total image of the story shown on the screen." (See Alex Gochfeld Associates, Inc., 1969, pp. 72-73.)

**Segments of Concerned Consumers**  In order to provide a "foundation upon which marketing and advertising executions can be built," Lorillard did a market segmentation analysis.

"One of the most important revelations of the present study was the identification of four market segments in the smoker market who are distinct in terms of their desires in cigarettes and their psychological profile.

The fundamental basis upon which the market segments were divided was their desires in the 'ideal cigarette'. After the market segments were divided in terms of their smoking needs, they were then further analyzed in terms of their demography, smoking behavior, and their personality profile." [Emphasis in original.] (See Kieling, 1964, p. 2.)

The consumer segment most appropriate for Kent® was described in substantial psychological detail. Despite the label of "social conformist," of central concern to these smokers were health consequences:

"Segment B, the social conformists, represents the prime potential market for development of Kent's share.

Compared with the rest of the market, Segment B is less concerned about smoking enjoyment and more concerned about the health aspect of cigarettes. He cares particularly about a cigarette's filter, its king size, and its association with health.

Type B is a self-controlled person who is willing to compromise and give up immediate physical gratification for longer range objectives; he is a thinking person who acts deliberately, and is most likely to sacrifice some of the enjoyment of smoking in the interest of health, about which he is highly concerned. . . These requirements appear to be compatible with Kent's current image.

The other psychological requirement of Type B is the need for social benefits through association with 'educated moderns'. . . 'educated moderns' include the active, modern people, college graduates, and professionals such as lawyers, doctors, etc." [Emphasis in original.] (See Kieling, 1964, pp. 3-5.)

205

Given that Kent® had a long-established association with 'health' from more than a decade's worth of health-themed advertising, the advertising deliberately offered reassurances to targeted consumers of being seen as "educated moderns," with the health promises subtly made:

> "In the present climate of opinion after the Surgeon General's Report, it may be desirable to offer reassurance on 'association with health' in Kent's advertising." [Emphasis in original.] (See Kieling, 1964, p. 14.)

**The "Illusion of Filtration"**    In their 1966 analysis of the market potential for a 'health' cigarette, Philip Morris recognized that while a large proportion of smokers had health concerns, they could be assuaged by products with largely illusory filtration systems. This was helpful since Philip Morris also knew that they had to keep delivering nicotine to those already addicted, as well as to those that they hoped would become addicted. The report's conclusions include the following:

**Figure 7-4**
**Kent—Voice of Wisdom (1955)**

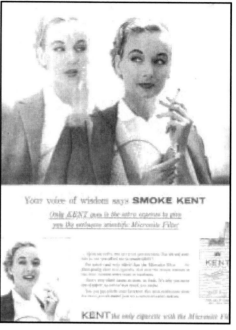

> "1. A large proportion of smokers are concerned about the relationship of cigarette smoking to health. . .
>
>   9. Mere reduction in nicotine and TPM [total particulate matter] deliveries by conventional methods of filtration would not be a sufficient basis for launching a new cigarette.
>
> 10. The illusion of filtration is as important as the fact of filtration.
>
> 11. Therefore any entry should be by a radically different method of filtration but need not be any more effective." (See Johnston, 1966, pp. 1-2.)

Within this report, Philip Morris' analyst captured the dilemma between health concerns and nicotine delivery felt by both smokers and manufacturers:

> ". . . [A]ny health cigarette must compromise between health implications on the one hand and flavor and nicotine on the other . . . flavor and nicotine are both necessary to sell a cigarette. A cigarette that does not deliver nicotine cannot satisfy the habituated smoker and cannot lead to habituation, and would therefore almost certainly fail." (See Johnston, 1966, p. 5.)

Many early brands had been sold with filters that were essentially cosmetic, without meaningful filtration. U.S. Congressional investigations in 1958 found reversals in which some firms' filtered products delivered even more tar and nicotine than their unfiltered traditional products. Reversals occurred even within brand families, with Brand X filtered versions yielding higher tar and nicotine than the unfiltered Brand X products that they ostensibly improved upon (Blatnik, 1958, pp. 45-49).

**Fear that Low-Yield Cigarettes Would Allow the Consumer to Wean from Nicotine**
In 1969, R. J. Reynolds articulated concerns about reducing nicotine delivery and also maintaining a continuing profitable enterprise. The company saw nicotine as the *sine qua non* of smoking satisfaction and worried that reducing the delivery of nicotine to consumers might have the "self-defeating consequences" of weaning them away from smoking and letting them off the nicotine hook:

> "In its search for 'safer' cigarettes, the tobacco industry has, in essentially every case, simply reduced the amount of nicotine . . . perhaps weaning the smoker away from nicotine habituation and depriving him of parts of the gratification desired or expected. . . Thus, unless some miraculous solution to the smoking-health problem is found, the present 'safer' cigarette strategy, while prudent and fruitful for the short term, may be equivalent to long term liquidation of the cigarette industry." (See Teague, 1969, pp. 9-10.)

This concern with possible 'weaning' was still being expressed later by the British American Tobacco Co. when looking ahead to the 1980s:

> "Taking a long-term view, there is a danger in the current trend of lower and lower cigarette deliveries—*i.e.*, the smoker will be weaned away from the habit. . . Nicotine is an important aspect of 'satisfaction', and if the nicotine delivery is reduced below a threshold 'satisfaction' level, then surely smokers will question more readily why they are indulging in an expensive habit." (See British American Tobacco Company, 1976, p. 2)

**THE 1970s**

**Early High-Filtration (Hi-Fi) Brands**
"Carlton and True appeared in the mid 1960's, and Doral and Vantage followed shortly after. . . Lights and milds [sic] versions of full-taste brands proliferated in the early '70's, accounting for 31.6% of hi-fi business by 1975." (See Chambers, 1979.)

By 1973, it was clear to industry participants that a significant number of brands shared certain characteristics that led them to be described as a "new low-delivery segment." Precise relevance to tar and nicotine levels was elusive, in part because some brands like Kent® and Parliament® were perceived by consumers as being low in delivery due to their product and advertising histories, even though they were no longer in fact low in delivery. Listed below are some of the guidelines used by Philip Morris to define low-delivery brands for that company's internal purposes:

"2. All brands in the segment have advertising, if any, focussed on low delivery. No other brand has advertising focused on low delivery.

3. Some brands in the segment have tar and nicotine numbers on their packs. No brand not in the segment has tar and nicotine numbers on its pack.

4. Some brands in the segment have unusual construction filters or dilution holes. No brand not in the segment has either of these characteristics. . .

6. Brands in the segment which are extensions of 'flavor' brands have names which imply low delivery: Marlboro <u>Light</u>, Kool <u>Mild</u>, Pall Mall <u>Extra Mild</u>, Lucky <u>Ten</u>, etc.

Note that Kent and Parliament do not qualify for this new low delivery segment on any of the criteria above. One can still argue, however, that in the minds of consumers Kent and Parliament are low delivery cigarettes . . . consumer opinion should be the ultimate criterion for market segmentation." [Emphasis in original.] (See Tindall, 1973, p. 16.)

**Nicotine as a Product Design Feature**  During the early 1970s, Philip Morris was internally expressing confidence in its ability to selectively reduce tar yield while continuing to deliver the all-important nicotine:

". . . [T]he tar deliveries of the currently best selling cigarettes might be reduced somewhat, leaving nicotine as it is, without any significant overall decrease in the cigarettes' acceptability." (See Schori, 1971, p. 1.)

R. J. Reynolds was following a similar line of thought in focussing its product development on nicotine delivery:

"If nicotine is the <u>sine</u> <u>qua</u> <u>non</u> of tobacco products and tobacco products are recognized as being attractive dosage forms of nicotine, then it is logical to design our products—and where possible, our advertising—around nicotine delivery rather than 'tar' delivery or flavor." [Emphasis in original.] (See Teague, 1972b, p. 3.)

"In today's market it is reasonable to believe that, given the choice, the typical smoker will chose [sic] and use the cigarette which delivers the desired, required amount of nicotine, with satisfactory flavor, mildness and other attributes, accompanied by the <u>least</u> amount of 'tar'." [Emphasis in original.] (See Teague, 1972a, p. 4.)

By 1976, the R. J. Reynolds Market Research Department (MRD) had joined the research and development (R&D) effort with a clear statement of their intent to maximize the nicotine satisfaction while maintaining high profitability by using conventional filters and packaging:

"MRD and R&D have been working on a sophisticated consumer product testing program to help us ensure that we select the best blend alternative for our brands to optimize physiological satisfaction." (See Fitzgerald *et al.*, 1976, p. 1.)

"Our top priority is to develop and market low 'tar' brands (12 mg. 'tar' and under) that: Maximize the physiological satisfaction per puff—the single most important need of smokers. . . [and] yield higher profitability which means conventional filters and soft packaging for high speed production efficiencies." (See Fitzgerald *et al.*, 1976, p. 38.)

A few years later in 1981, British American Tobacco, the parent company of Brown & Williamson, maintained that, ". . . effort should *not* be spent on designing a cigarette which, through its construction, denied the smoker the opportunity to compensate or oversmoke [sic] to any significant degree." [Emphasis added.] (See Oldman, 1981, p. 2.)

**Consumer Reactions and Behavior**

Consumer Ignorance and Confusion

During the 1970s, additional evidence of consumer confusion, misinformation, rationalizations, and the corresponding role played by advertising was gathered by multiple firms. Market researchers for industry members and their advertising agencies were not even confident that consumers knew what they were talking about when referring to the 'taste' of a cigarette:

". . . [I]t is almost impossible to know if the taste smokers talk about is something which they, themselves attribute to a cigarette or just a 'play-back' of some advertising messages." (See Marketing and Research Counselors, Inc., 1975, p. 2.)

Apparently, even the so-called 'taste' of a product is greatly influenced by the brand and its reputation. Merit®, as a free-standing brand, had difficulties in being perceived as flavorful, whereas in contrast, product line extensions like Marlboro Light® had the advantage of being perceived as more flavorful due to the taste reputation of the 'parent' brand:

". . . [W]e talked to consumers about Merit's image and advertising. They told us that Merit, like other free standing low tar brands such as Kent, Vantage, Carlton, etc., were perceived to be weaker and have less taste than the line extension low tars: like Marlboro Lights, Winston Lights, Camel Lights. Apparently, these line extension low tars share the taste heritage of their parent full flavor brands." (See Philip Morris, 1990, pp. 13–14.)

In 1974, Kenyon & Eckhardt Advertising studied "recently starting smokers" for Brown & Williamson:

"The purpose of this research was to gain insight into the perceptions, attitudes and behavior of younger, recently starting smokers regarding initial product usage, current smoking and health concerns. In addition, an effort was made to determine reactions to alternative product positionings [sic]." (See Kenyon & Eckhardt, 1974, p. 1).

"Health concerns exist among younger smokers. . . One type of smoker rationalized smoking as a pleasure that outweighed the risks. Another felt that they didn't smoke enough to be dangerous.

209

A third type rationalized his use of cigarettes by feeling he would quit before it was 'too late'. A final smoker group said that science would come to his rescue." (See Kenyon & Eckhardt, 1974, p. 2).

"In talking to these young smokers about the different brands of cigarettes they have smoked, we found that they have little knowledge and, in fact, a great deal of misinformation on brand yields. In all of the sessions, not a single respondent know [sic] the tar and nicotine level of the cigarette he or she smoked." (See Kenyon & Eckhardt, 1974, p. 7).

Lorillard and their ad agency had the same experience when studying consumers for Kent®. Lorillard, along with Foote, Cone & Belding, encouraged scores of targeted smokers to talk about their lives, their cigarettes, their perceptions, and their feelings about tar content for Kent Golden Light®. They, like Brown & Williamson, found that "practically no one knew" the tar content of their own regularly smoked brands. This implied to these firms the need for ads showing comparative packages and data (O'Toole, 1981, pp. 94-95).

Philip Morris also knew about smokers' ignorance of yield levels in the 1970s. Most consumers were not only ignorant of the facts, but even their general impressions were "not too accurate," despite their faith in the technology of filters as displayed by shifts to filters and hi-fi products:

"As yet, there is low awareness among smokers of the tar content of their brand. When asked if they knew the specific milligram tar content of their brand, the vast majority (89%) said they didn't know. . . smokers' <u>impressions</u> of whether their brand has high, moderate or low tar content is more on the mark—although still not too accurate." [Emphasis in original.] (See The Roper Organization, Inc., 1976, p. 14.)

**Filters Are Still Perceived As Feminine**

As in the 1950s and 1960s, females and older, health-concerned smokers most readily adopted the new, seemingly low-yield products of the 1970s:

"The modern low 'tar' market began in the 1960's with such brands as True, Carlton, and Doral . . . initial gains were from females and older smokers." (See Brown & Williamson, circa 1977, p. 4.)

"The hi-fi smoker demographics tend to be female, older, and have switched from a full flavor style to its counterpart in the hi-fi segment." (See Brown & Williamson, circa 1977, p. 13.)

This was so much the case that the males who smoked these products were suspected of being 'weak' and somehow wimpish or unmasculine in the eyes of consumers who were studied for Brown & Williamson:

"Only women and weak men smoke True or any of those low tar and nicotine cigarettes." (See Marketing and Research Counselors, Inc., 1975, p. 9.)

210

In 1974, advertising agency advisors to Lorillard tried to counter this problem with a style of advertising for the True® brand that they felt was more masculine in its tonality (see Figure 7-5).

"In order to obtain a greater share of males. . . logical, rational approaches. . . a 'reasoning' empathetic approach. . . masculine, 'macho' tonality and appeal. Vantage's tonality can be described as 'laying it on the line' in an aggressive, possibly masculine, open fashion." (See DeGarmo, Inc., 1974.)

This problem of low-yield products being perceived as highly feminine seems to have led R. J. Reynolds to design a marketing strategy that attracted males to a low-yield cigarette that they were developing in 1976:

"What we want is to portray the feeling and image projected by Marlboro and Kool advertising on a Vantage/Merit type of cigarette. In other words, put 'balls' (two of them) on a low 'tar' and nicotine cigarette and position." [Parenthetical clarification of the male genitalia meaning of "balls" as in original.] (See Hind *et al.*, 1976, p. 63.)

While young male consumers understood that filters seemingly offered improved health prospects, this was in conflict with their desires to appear bold and daring:

"In discussing how a smoker can limit the risks of serious disease without actually giving up smoking, the respondents clearly recognized the role of high filtration cigarettes. . . the underlying mechanism working against acceptance of high filtration brands in this age group is that the image of these cigarettes is contrary to one of the initial motivations for smoking—to look manly and strong." (See Kenyon & Eckhardt Advertising, 1974, p. 10.)

Continuing Consumer Conflicts

Consumers' conflicted feelings about smoking cigarettes were such that they became poor respondents to Brown & Williamson's research efforts:

". . . [S]mokers themselves falter badly when asked to comment on the rewards accruing to them from smoking. . . Smokers are so overwhelmed by the addictive properties of cigarettes and the potential health hazard that they wax virtually inarticulate when asked to present a case for the other side. They become guilty and shame-faced." (See Kalhok and Short, 1976, p. 8.)

Smokers were not even aware and/or willing to admit how much they smoked:

"Smokers' own estimates of their daily consumption levels are extremely unreliable. Many smokers underestimate their actual consumption and certain segments of many populations, notably young people and women, are often reluctant to admit they smoke." (See British American Tobacco Co., 1979, p. 1.)

Brown & Williamson blamed consumer confusion on advertising, in part. When contemplating a possible "index of safety" for cigarettes, Brown & Williamson commented that:

"Such an index would have merit for the health-conscious smoker, who otherwise may well become confused and increasingly dismayed if one alleged hazard follows another, coupled with the manufacturers' 'prescription for health' through advertising." (See Kalhok and Short, 1976, p. 11.)

Additional market research conducted for Brown & Williamson and its advertising agency, Ted Bates, indicated that ads needed to be carefully designed, lest they challenge consumer denials and rationalizations and trigger consumer defensiveness:

**Figure 7-5**

**Vantage "Don't Cop Out"—Macho Tonality (1971)**

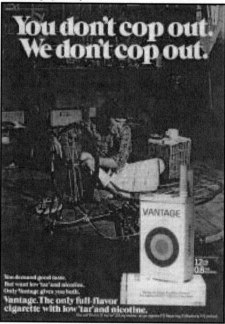

". . . [S]mokers have to face the fact that they are illogical, irrational and stupid . . . <u>while an ad that depicts an exciting, invigorating situation could be interesting to the smoke-viewer, the very thin line separating positive excitement from negative-creating situation should never be crossed.</u>" [Emphasis in original.] (See Marketing and Research Counselors, Inc., 1975, pp. 1-2.)

". . . [C]ommunication with the smoker that either directly or indirectly violates and belittles this rationalized need will meet smoker's objection—it destroys the rationalization and the smoker would feel naked and rather stupid." (See Marketing and Research Counselors, Inc., 1975, p. 5.)

One of the problems that advertising could address was the declining social esteem of smokers, helping them to avoid shame and guilt:

"Over the period of 20 years, the public and the private image of the smoker (though exceptions may be found among teenagers starting to smoke) has changed from being one of an individual exulting in his positive strength, masculinity and acceptance in the community, to that of a weak and dependent slave, with prospects of illness, however distant these may be, unnerved by his children's forebodings [sic], and without strength to quit." (See Kalhok and Short, 1976, p. 14.)

In discussing the "elements of good cigarette advertising or how to reduce objections to a cigarette," this point was reiterated while stating that "there are not any real, absolute, positive qualities and attributes in a cigarette," as noted in the following:

> "Most advertising for other products presents real, or at least accepted, benefits, values, attributes, end-results, etc., of the product it 'pushes,' sells. Cigarette advertising can not do the same. There are not any real, absolute, positive qualities and attributes in a cigarette and no one, even the most devout smokers, could believe any glorification or lies about it. . . The more a cigarette ad is disbelieved, the more it 'fights' the defense mechanism of the smoker— the more the smoker feels challenged. . . The picture, situation presented and the copy should be ambiguous enough to allow the reader to fill-in his/her illogical-logic which are the results of each individual defense-mechanism." (See Marketing and Research Counselors, Inc., 1975, pp. 12-13.)

**Image of Health**     It was important to the industry that certain cigarette brands continued to appear to be 'healthy', even if this was an image or illusion, and even if the manufacturing technology did not yet allow for the control of smoke toxicity:

> "Looking further down the road, the possibility exists that . . . filters might offer a selective means of controlling smoke toxicity. Well before that date, however, **opportunities exist for filter and cigarette designs which offer <u>the image</u> of 'health re-assurance'.**" [Emphases added.] (See British American Tobacco Co., 1976, p. 6.)

**New Product Activity**     Philip Morris had seen the competitive value of a so-called "health cigarette" following the first Surgeon General's Report on cigarettes in 1964. Over the course of the next 12 years, Philip Morris worked on such a product, culminating in the 1976 product launch of the Merit® brand. Just as with Philip Morris' earlier efforts in the 1950s to develop and consumer-test the Marlboro® product, packaging, and promotion, the product development process for Merit® was as much focused on consumer and market testing as on product technologies, per se. The final market launch strategies used in 1976 gave particular emphasis to the choice of the name Merit®, obviously communicating apparent virtue, and used an advertising style that made this product development seem eminently scientific and newsworthy and less like an ad (see Figure 7-6). The product launch strategy included a very high level of advertising investment ($45 million in 1976) to support a "multi-media blitz."

> "The objective of the advertising campaign was to establish enough credibility to overcome smoker skepticism towards low-tar good taste claims. The name 'MERIT' was chosen because it was short, to the point, and it reflected the consumer appeal of good taste at low tar." (See John and Wakeham, 1977, p. 13.)

"Merit was the primary focus of the sales force for a full year. . . We spent $45 million on advertising—remember $45 million in 1976! This was a record amount for a new brand introduction. . . Creatively, we used provocative headlines and important looking copy which looked like it had real news value. <u>Tar/taste theory exploded!—Smoke cracked!—Taste barrier broken!</u>" [Emphasis in original.] (See Philip Morris, 1990, p. 4.)

This Merit® launch effort, and its stunning success, led to a rash of similar competitive efforts:

**Figure 7-6**

**Merit Science Works—"Enriched Flavor" (1979)**

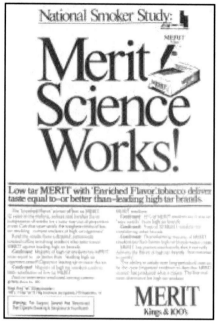

"Merit's introduction gave birth to a series of me-too's. . . 'Fact' was introduced in 1976. . . RJR tried to counter Merit's technological enriched flavor story with their all natural 'Real' launched in mid 1976. . . 'Decade', which was launched on the platform of 'the cigarette that took 10 years to create'. . . Later, Barclay was introduced." (See Philip Morris, 1990, p. 5.)

**Marketing of Reduced Gas Phase Cigarettes**

Brown & Williamson's introduction of the Fact® brand was described by a company spokesman as "a typical new product introduction as compared to Philip Morris' sudden national blitz for Merit. . . Fact is directed to the educated, concerned smoker. Our copy is straightforward and direct, and there is no gender differentiation or symbolism." (See Brand Report 12, 1976, p. 146.) Fact® was using the "Purite" filter to filter gases, but needed to first inform consumers that gases were an issue. Their initial effort (see Figure 7-7) was test-marketed in New England and the North Central States, but did not perform well in the marketplace, despite advertising support of about $30 million over 1976-1977. The senior brand manager of Brown & Williamson explained:

"The low gas benefit of the product wasn't of interest to the public, and wasn't understood. The advertising and packaging failed to reinforce the flavor aspect of the brand. . . The package was perceived by customers as medicinal, like a prescription bottle of Geritol. The tar level wasn't low enough by mid-1976 to allow it to be a talking point in advertising." (See Brand Report 23, 1977, p. 152.)

Brown & Williamson's reconsideration of its Purite gas filter showed a recognition that in having to educate consumers about gas in smoke, they might raise more anxiety than they could resolve with this type of product:

> "While low gas does offer the opportunity to make positive health statements to active and passive smokers alike, it does run the category risk of raising another health issue and perceptively offering lower taste/satisfaction. . . past experiences with Lark and FACT (*i.e.*, good taste and greater health reassurance via a new method) demonstrate the inability to immediately proceed with either of these options." (Brown & Williamson, circa 1977, p. 1.)

**Figure 7-7**

**Introducing Fact—Low Gas (Before—1976)**

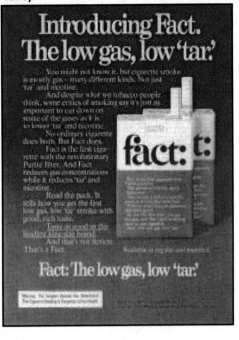

**Marketing Cigarettes Without Additives**

R. J. Reynolds' 1976 assessment for their 3-year action plan acknowledged that they were not yet technologically capable of producing products that had reduced tar without the undesirable effect of also having reduced nicotine:

> "In general, methods used to reduce 'tar' delivery in cigarettes lead to a proportionate reduction in nicotine. . . It would be more desirable from our standpoint, *i.e.*, providing satisfaction to the smoker and maintaining his allegiance to smoking if we could reduce 'tar' to whatever target we choose without a proportionate drop in nicotine. . . It will take some time to get there by the approaches we visualize." (See Fitzgerald *et al.*, 1976, p. 91.)

Nonetheless, R. J. Reynolds wanted to participate in the rapidly expanding category of concerned consumers, referred to as "worriers" by the company:

> "[The]. . . 'worrier' segment of the market (17% of smokers are so classified). . . 'Numbers' products have a growing appeal to these smokers. Products in the 1-6 mg. 'tar' range will continue to build successful long-term franchises (*e.g.*, Carlton's growth rate, NOW's immediate acceptance—fostered by the intense industry commitment in 1976 to hi-fi brands)." (See Fitzgerald *et al.*, 1976.)

**Figure 7-8**
**Real Natural (1977)**

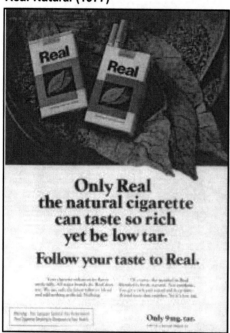

Only Real
the natural cigarette
can taste so rich
yet be low tar.

Follow your taste to Real.

Only 9 mg. tar.

R. J. Reynolds' product offering was the Real® brand, with a "natural—no additives" claim (see Figure 7-8). This 'natural' position was thought to convey positive features to both full-flavor smokers and those seeking effective filtration and health protection. The Real® concept was described as having, "Broad appeal based primarily on 'natural'/no additives claim. Connotes taste to full flavor smokers, low numbers to hi-fi smokers. No significant negatives." (See Fitzgerald *et al.*, 1976.)

When the Real® brand was launched by R. J. Reynolds in 1977, it had a budget of $40 million for "boxcar loads of display materials, more than 25 million sample packages, the biggest billboard overlooking Times Square, the summer long services of 2,000 salesmen. . . and advertising, according to the agency running the campaign, on everything but painted rocks." (See Crittenden, 1977, p. 1ff.)

That same year, Brown & Williamson was scheduled to spend $50 million through the Ted Bates advertising agency on just the product-line extension of Kool Super Light®. The Kool Super Light® campaign was to appear "in every conceivable non-broadcast medium, and even an inconceivable one"—1,500 Beetleboards, *i.e.*, painted up Volkswagen Beetle® cars (Dougherty, 1977).

**Promotional Patterns**

Disproportionate
Advertising Budgets

The enormous advertising budgets used to launch the new low-yield products commanded a very disproportionate share of the firms' total advertising budgets (share of voice, or SOV), and were seen as creating marketplace demand for low-yield products. The advertising spending for new products in 1976-1978 was awesome. New brands and product-line extensions (variations on familiar brands) were introduced with major budgets as follows (Source: Lorillard, Inc., 1980):

| Product | Budget | Year |
|---|---|---|
| Merit® | $44 million | (1976) |
| Now® | $23 million | (1976) |
| Fact® | $20 million | (1976) |
| Real® | $29 million | (1977) |
| Decade® | $24 million | (1977) |
| Camel Light® | $25.3 million | (1978) |
| Carlton® | $15.3 million | (1976) |
| Vantage® | $20.6 million | (1976/1977) |
| Kent Golden Light® | $21.0 million | (1976-1978) |
| Marlboro Light® | $20.1 million | (1976-1978) |

"The phenomenal growth of hi-fi brands is, in part, a self-fulfilling prophecy. Hi-fi expenditures have grown from 7% SOV in 1972 to 45% in 1977, much faster than actual segment growth. Spending per share point now equals $8.3MM." (See Brown & Williamson, circa 1977, p. 14.)

"[The]. . . low tar revolution [of 1976ff] is not ignited by a particular event, such as a *Reader's Digest* article, a Surgeon General's Report, etc.; it happens quietly based on technologically improved products and consumers' desire for a reasonable compromise and the industry's massive advertising support leading category development." (See Cunningham and Walsh, 1980, p. 55.)

"Lo Fi advertising now (Feb 1980) accounts for only 21% of total—less than a third of 1974's share of voice. Reduced tar brands have increased to 79% share of voice—with ULT's (Ultra Low Tar's) now accounting for 19% of the total. ULT advertising is growing at a faster rate than any other category." (See Lorillard, Inc., 1980.)

**Executional Aspects**    The advertising executions that communicated the "lightness" theme were 'light' in many dimensions:

" 'Light-lighter-lightest' were achieved by insistance [sic] on lighter presentations—product story imagery—white packs—pale colours—mildness dominated copy." (See British American Tobacco Company, circa 1985, p. 13.)

This tactic of using color and imagery to connote product 'lightness' had been used earlier with the introduction of Marlboro Light® in 1971 (see Figure 7-9).

"... [W]hen Marlboro Lights was first introduced in 1971. . . the advertising was dramatically different. . . first using water color executions, then, big pack shots, a lot of white space and a small cowboy visual." (See Philip Morris, 1990, p. 6.)

This means of communicating 'lightness' with white or pale-colored props, settings, and pristine environments wasn't new with Marlboro Light®, and has proven to be a durable execution tactic. For example, Kent® in the early 1960s showed models all dressed in white, with both white props and in a pure white, interior studio environment (see Figure 7-10).

**Figure 7-9**
**Marlboro Lights (1972)**

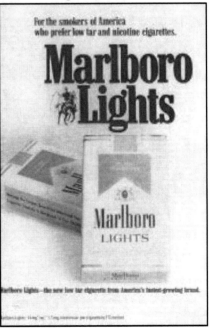

217

Figure 7-10
**Kent—Black Smokers in Pure White Environment (1964)**

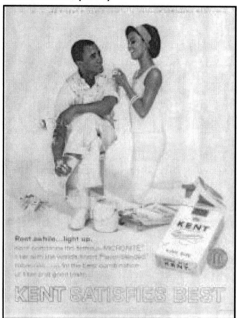

Through most of the 1990s, the Parliament® campaign consistently used models dressed all in white placed in white environments as well as in outside pristine environments (see Figure 7-11).

Artwork for Marlboro Ultra Light® has featured a pristine environment dominated by fresh air and water, with only minimally sized cowboys or horses (see Figure 7-12).

Even the packaging design is important in affecting perceptions of relative safety, as well as taste:

"Red packs connote strong flavor, green packs connote coolness or menthol and white packs suggest that a cigaret [sic] is low-tar. White means sanitary and safe. And if you put a low-tar cigaret [sic] in a red package, people say it tastes stronger than the same cigaret [sic] packaged in white." (See Koten, 1980, p. 22)

Because of its importance, Brown & Williamson tested 33 packages before choosing the blue, gold, and red design used for its Viceroy Rich Light® brand. Philip Morris heightened the social status appeal of its Benson & Hedges® brand by printing the company's Park Avenue address on the front and back of each pack. R. J. Reynolds gave Now® a "modern, chrome-and-glass look designed to appeal to upscale city and suburban dwellers." Philip Morris' successful Merit® connotes a "flamboyant, young-in-spirit image" (to offset low tar's dull image) with big yellow, brown, and orange racing stripes (Koten, 1980). Most "Light" and "Ultra Light" cigarettes are presented in pure white packaging with minimal adornments.

To supplement and reinforce their advertising efforts, Brown & Williamson conceived of public relations and political activities that encouraged consumers to perceive apparently independent endorsements of low-yield products. This would reinforce advertising impressions about the virtues of low-tar products with seemingly independent "news" from credible sources.

"B&W will undertake activities designed to generate statements by public health opinion leaders which will indicate tolerance for smoking and improve the consumer's perception of ultra low 'tar' cigarettes (5 mg. or less). . . Through political and scientific friends, B&W will attempt to elicit. . . statements sympathetic to the concept that generally less health risk is associated with ultra low delivery cigarette consumption. . . B&W would seek to generate spontaneous mainstream media articles dealing with component deliveries, much as the old <u>Readers Digest</u> [sic] articles." (What are the obstacles/enemies of a swing to low "tar" and what action should we take? Minnesota Trial Exhibit 26,185, 1982.)

**Capturing Consumer Concerns**    The continuation of intensive promotion into 1977 involved "a numbers game that boggles the mind while promising to relieve the lungs" (Brand Report 23, 1977, p. 150). Competition was intense, due in part to the high stakes and the relatively few number of switchers. Said Lorillard's Tom Mau several years later:

Figure 7-11

**Parliament Lights White on White in Pristine Environment (1998)**

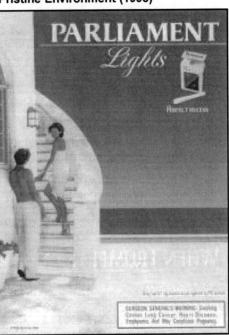

> "The vast majority of the cigarette consumers are brand loyal. . . Only somewhere around 10% of people switch brands annually. That's not a lot of people. . . To come out with something new and successful is difficult." (See Gardener, 1984, p. 176.)

It was clear to industry observers that the pace of new product launches in the mid-1970s was seeking to capitalize on the health concerns of smokers:

> "The current duel between True and Vantage and between Carlton and Now are other examples of competitive efforts to capitalize on the smoking/health controversy." (See Pepples, 1976, p. 9.)

When the motivations for smoking ultra-low-tar cigarettes were studied by Philip Morris' contractors in 1978, representatives of the Brand Management Group, Marketing Research Department, and the advertising agency all observed the discussion groups from behind a two-way viewing mirror and tape recordings were made available. The discussions were guided by a detailed outline with extensive probing. The findings were that all of the reasons for selecting this product form were health-related:

> ". . . [W]ith respect to ultra low tar brands there appear to be particular additional motivations for smoking this type of cigarette. These include:

A - Voluntary desire for a safer cigarette.

B - Increasing awareness and concern about possible hazards of smoking.

C - Health problem forcing a change to a safer cigarette (as an alternative to not being able to quit).

D - Peer and family pressure to smoke a safer cigarette (as an alternative to not being able to stop smoking).

E - Mental commitment to do something about smoking habits." (See Goldstein/Krall Marketing Resources, Inc., 1979.)

Many consumers considered, tried, and even switched to the nominally lower yield products, and did so primarily in pursuit of better health:

"More people have switched brands in the past year, and the largest group of switchers have gone to low tars. Even among those who have not switched to a low tar brand, there is fairly high disposition among smokers to consider switching to one. This is probably attributable to the continuing concern over smoking and health." (See The Roper Organization, Inc., 1976, p. 3.)

"Results show that almost two-thirds of smokers are 'impressed' by the talk of how cigarettes can seriously affect their health. . . Women are more concerned about smoking and health than men, young people more than older people, whites more than blacks, and the college educated more than those less well educated." [The growth among low tar brands was] ". . . particularly strong among two groups who have traditionally been trend setters in the cigarette market—women and the college educated." (See The Roper Organization, Inc., 1976, pp. 8, 12.)

When asked if and why some brands were thought to be better for health, smokers had believed the idea that the nominally low yields were meaningful:

"The low tar brands have cornered opinion that to the extent any brands are better for your health, they are. All smokers were asked whether they thought any

**Figure 7-12**

**Marlboro Ultra Light Pristine Environment (1998)**

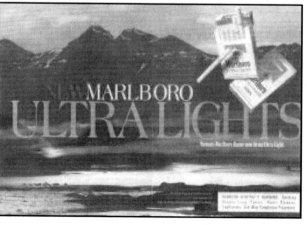

particular brands were better for your health than others, and if so, which brands. Three in ten of all smokers said some brands were better for health than others, and almost half of the low tar brand smokers said this. The brands named were almost exclusively low tar brands, with the older low tar brands (Vantage, True and Carlton) getting most mentions. Considering the short length of time they have been on the market, both Merit and Now had comparatively good mention." (See The Roper Organization, Inc., 1976, p. 19.)

". . . [I]t is the lower tar content of these brands that make people say they are better for health. When asked why the brands they named were better for your health, answers overwhelmingly were concerned with lower tar content." (See The Roper Organization, Inc., 1976, p. 20.)

The reassurance of apparent low yields led many smokers to switch rather than quit:

"Smokers <u>needed</u> light brands for tangible, practical, understandable reasons. . . It is useful to consider lights more as a third alternative to quitting and cutting down—a branded hybrid of smokers' unsuccessful attempts to modify their habit on their own." [Emphasis in original.] (See British American Tobacco Co., circa 1985, pp. 9, 13.)

[Many said] ". . . they had tried to quit smoking at some point in time, they do not appear to have cut down the number of cigarettes they are smoking. The only concession that has been made is the switch to an ultra low tar brand. These smokers seemed to be either resigned to the fact or satisfied that they will probably never quit smoking. In point of fact, smoking an ultra low tar cigarette seems to relieve some of the guilt of smoking and provide an excuse not to quit." (See Goldstein/Krall Marketing Resources, Inc., 1979, p. 12.)

The True® campaign in the 1970s spoke directly to the desire to quit, portraying quitting and smoking True® as equivalent alternatives (see Figure 7-13).

An important strategic reason for adding low-yield products to a product line, also known as a brand family, was to retain the patronage of consumers as they aged and became more concerned about their health:

[Developing] ". . . new products in the higher end of the reduced tar category. . . is especially important for Lorillard's long term growth. Younger smokers (less than 35) are smoking products in the higher end of the reduced tar segment and lo-fi. These consumers will move down the tar spectrum, as they get older, with the probability of staying with the line extensions of products consumed in their youth." (See Mau, 1981, p. 7.)

**Lessons Learned About Advertising** Tobacco manufacturers saw advertising, and marketing efforts more generally, as vital to how consumers perceived the products and themselves; these efforts ultimately determined how well various firms succeeded. Lorillard listed marketing's psychological import right alongside of the product's capacity to deliver the physiological stimulation of nicotine.

Figure 7-13

**Quit or Smoke True as Equivalent Options (1976)**

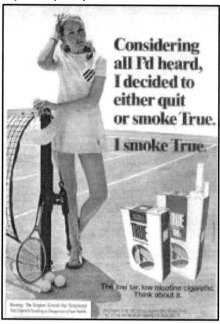

". . . [L]et me try to define the elements of product acceptance (given sales distribution and trial) as they relate to tobacco products. . . The value or price of the product is a factor. . . The second element in acceptance is psychological. One principle component of this element arises from our marketing effort. . . The third element in acceptance is physiological, being comprised largely of the nicotine-induced stimulation." (See Spears, 1973, pp. 2-3.)

With experience, members of the industry realized that the best advertising gave filter smokers ego reinforcement, and didn't focus solely on nominal filter effectiveness. This might be appropriate when introducing new product concepts (*e.g.*, filters), but once the concept was understood, it was better to avoid any direct addressing of health aspects.

"1964-1972—The beginning of the high filtration derby. . . In this type of environment, good new product copy directly addressed the health arguments by focusing on lowered tar and nicotine while also claiming to retain real tobacco taste." [Emphasis in original.] (See Latimer, 1976, p. 4.)

"Less effective copy during this period continued to focus on the filtration process (*e.g.*, selectrate filter, charcoal filters, accu-ray, etc.) or vacillated between emphasis on taste and emphasis on filter." (See Latimer, 1976, p. 3.)

Brown & Williamson articulated the dual objectives of good advertising—providing reassurance about healthfulness (without, of course, doing so in a heavy-handed way to induce defensiveness) and also providing a socially attractive brand image that the smoker could acquire when buying and displaying the package:

". . . [T]he average smoker often seeks self-justification for smoking. Good cigarette advertising in the past has given the average smoker a means of justification on the two dimensions typically used in anti-smoking arguments: 1. <u>High performance risk dimension</u>. . . . 2. <u>Ego/status risk dimension</u>.

<u>Cigarette advertising</u>. . . <u>provides only justification/rationalization for those who already smoke</u>. . . The smoker's cigarette brand choice process is largely an exercise in risk reduction. For some smokers reduction in physical performance risk is paramount, for others reduction in 'ego/status' risk comes first. . . All good cigarette advertising has either directly addressed the anti-smoking arguments prevalent at the time or has created a strong, attractive image into which the besieged smoker could withdraw." [Emphasis in original.] (See Latimer, 1976, pp. 1-2.)

The international headquarters of Brown & Williamson's parent firm, the British American Tobacco Co., counseled that new marketing approaches should:

". . . [C]reate brands and products which reassure consumers, by answering to their needs. Overall marketing policy will be such that we maintain faith and confidence in the smoking habit." (See Short, 1977, p. 1.)

The advertising campaigns and related communications were central to how this was to be done:

"All work in this area [communications] should be directed towards providing <u>consumer reassurance</u> about cigarettes and the smoking habit. . . by claimed low deliveries, by the perception of low deliveries and by the perception of 'mildness'. Furthermore, advertising for low delivery or traditional brands should be constructed in ways so as not to provoke anxiety about health, but to alleviate it, and enable the smoker to feel assured about the habit and confident in maintaining it over time." [Emphasis in original.] (See Short, 1977, p. 3.)

This attempt to reassure, but not so bluntly as to raise defensiveness, and to simultaneously offer positive, ego-satisfying, brand imagery, seems to have been a key to the success of some of the pioneering filter products. Even the firms being dominated by the more successful marketing efforts of other firms recognized this. In 1969, American Tobacco noted that:

". . . [T]hose ads which make a special point of stressing low tar and nicotine appear to enjoy less attention and seem to have less positive impact than those whose advertising has an enjoyment, fun, or 'story' orientation." (See Alex Gochfeld Associates, Inc., 1969, p. 18.)

**THE 1980s**

**Policing Deceptive Advertising**

Carlton®

Some very deceptive practices went totally unchecked. Carlton® had the technology for delivering very low machine-measured tar yields, and used these low-yield test results in its advertising. A very desirable brand image was created while promoting Carlton® in a hard box, emphasizing its very low numbers (see Figure 7-14). Unfortunately, the boxed product seems to have been a "phantom brand" and consumers who bought Carlton® in the store got soft packs. Although consumers might well have expected that they were getting the same product in a different box, it was in fact a very different product—one that at times was delivering many, many more times the tar and nicotine than indicated in the ads.

"FTC's present system further contributes to consumer deception because it allows some cigarette companies to promote heavily a 'box' brand, <u>without adequately distinguishing it from the soft pack of the same brand name</u>, which delivers considerably more 'tar'. In fact, however, the companies produce such a small volume of the box brand as to make it a phantom brand that is rarely found in the marketplace. On the other hand, the soft-pack version bearing the identical brand name and package design but testing at a considerably higher 'tar' level, is the version readily available to the consumer." [Emphasis in original.] (See Pepples, 1982, p. 4.)

Now®, like Carlton®, also featured its very low-yield hard box product in the advertising, while its other product forms delivered many, many more times higher yield rates (see Figure 7-15).

The only effective policing of deceptive advertising of low-tar products came from competitors, rather than the FTC or any other agency. In one case, Lorillard used their data from a taste comparison test to imply a consumer preference for its Triumph® brand over Merit® (see Figure 7-16) and other brands. Both Philip Morris and R. J. Reynolds objected, and had data of their own to support their claims. In the court proceedings, it was learned that the Lorillard survey showed 36 percent favored Triumph® over Merit®, 24 percent rated them even, and 40 percent favored Merit®; these preferences were obtained after subjects

Figure 7-14
Carlton Box "Phantom Brand" (1985)

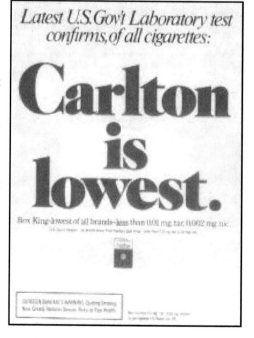

had been informed of the products' tar levels. Although nearly a quarter of the subjects had no preference, the enjoined statement took advantage of this and stated, "An amazing 60% said 3 mg Triumph tastes as good or better than 8 mg Merit." (See Philip Morris, Inc., v. Loew's Theatres, Inc., 1980, p. 1.)

Figure 7-15

**Now Box with Substantially Lower Yield Than Soft Pack (1980)**

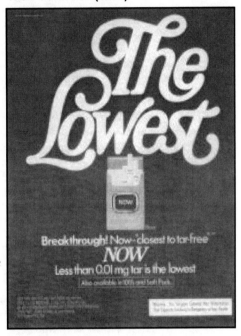

Barclay®    With the FTC yield data providing an apparent accreditation, consumers were likely to perceive these yield numbers as valid and meaningful. When Brown & Williamson brought the Barclay® product to market in 1981, it did so with an ad campaign that called the product 99 percent tar free (see Figure 7-17). The product's structure, which was described as "extremely easy to design and produce," allowed for so much dilution of the smoke column when tested on machines that it generated phenomenally low-yield data in the FTC test. This caused alarm among Brown & Williamson's competitors, who petitioned the FTC for help. Because of the competitive threat posed by Barclay®, its competitors disclosed to authorities their awareness that the FTC testing procedure was flawed and that the yield data were invalid for human smokers.

"The next generation of 'Barclay competitors' will be spawned (indeed has already been spawned) in the minds of R&D and marketing people throughout the industry and its suppliers. This generation of products, or the next, could easily be products which will deliver NO 'tar' or nicotine when smoked by the FTC method, and yet when smoked by humans essentially be unfiltered cigarettes. Such products could (and would) be advertized [sic] as 'tar-free', 'zero milligrams FTC tar', or the 'ultimate low-tar cigarette', while actually delivering 20-, 30-, 40-mg or more 'tar' when used by a human smoker! They will be extremely easy to design and produce. . . . Such cigarettes, while deceptive in the extreme, would be very difficult for the consumer to resist, since they would provide everything that we presently believe makes for desirable products: taste, 'punch', ease of draw and 'low FTC tar'." [Emphasis in original.] (See Reynolds *et al.*, 1982, p. 1.)

[As to the threat Barclay represented:] "Here was a 1 mg. tar product that delivered the taste of a much stronger cigarette. Of course we know how they did it, but to consumers the 99% tar free claim was intriguing. . . Merit responded by supporting Merit Ultra Lights with an $80 million media budget." (See Philip Morris, 1990, p. 8.)

**Figure 7-16**
**Triumph Beats Merit with Deceptive Data (1980)**

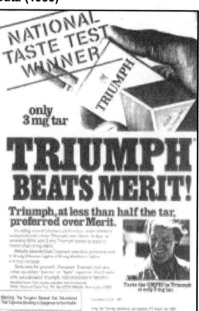

**Important Imagery**    Once the product concept of low-yield filtration had been communicated, and the previously discussed brands had established some corresponding reputation, their advertising strategies tended toward more visual, image-oriented forms, as these could convey enviable lifestyles, healthy behavior, rewarded risk-taking, and the social class and 'intelligence' of brand users.

When Merit Ultra Light® was introduced in 1983, the advertising program had an $80 million media budget, which did not account for retail promotional efforts. This advertising series featured imagery of large sailing ships in what was termed the "sea" campaign (see Figure 7-18). The executions not only showed young people in an enviable, carefree, affluent lifestyle amidst a pristine environment, they also were careful to avoid any suggestions of danger.

**Vantage®—An Intelligent Choice**    Images and ad copy had to be carefully selected, lest the ads reinforce fears rather than offer reassurance. In 1980, one Vantage® ad made direct reference to "what you may not want" from a cigarette, only to discover that it alarmed some readers about cancer:

> "The fact that a Vantage ad dares to raise the issue of 'what you may not want' generates defensiveness toward smoking in general, and a feeling of discomfort. The reference to the taste of Vantage is lost; overpowered by the implications of tar, nicotine and cancer." (See R. J. Reynolds-MacDonald, 1980.)

The target Vantage® smoker was "female, white collar, extremely concerned about their health, and would like to quit smoking." A Vantage® ad headlined "To Smoke or Not to Smoke" (see Figure 7-19) ran in both the United States and Canada. It stated that, "Vantage is the cigarette for people who may have second thoughts about smoking and are looking for a way to do something about it." According to an R. J. Reynolds operational plan

(1983) and strategic plan (1983-1987), the basic strategy was to present Vantage® as an intelligent choice, "positioning Vantage as the only contemporary choice for intelligent smokers." (See Pollay, 2000.) The tactic was to influence consumer perceptions. A 1983 R. J. Reynolds media plan sought "to establish a consumer perception that Vantage is a contemporary cigarette for intelligent smokers." (See Pollay, 2000.) Apparently, this aim was accomplished because, in 1987, an R. J. Reynolds media plan briefing document stated that the goal for a target audience with a "high amount of quitters" was "to maintain consumer perception that Vantage is a contemporary cigarette for intelligent smokers." (See Pollay, 2000.)

Figure 7-17
**Barclay—99% Tar Free (1981)**

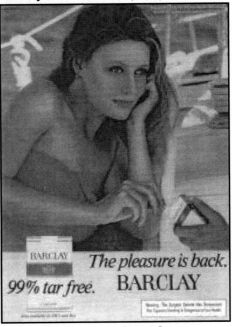

**Psychoanalyzing Merit®
and Vantage® Smokers**

No doubt envious of the success of Merit® among "concerned smokers," as well as that of Marlboro® among starters, R. J. Reynolds commissioned in-depth psychological research from Social Research, Inc., in 1982. The purpose of the survey was to compare the smokers of Vantage® and Merit® based on their smoking histories, their beliefs about the filter and other responses to advertising, and their personalities. In-depth interviews elicited insights into some of the psychological subtleties of respondents from Atlanta, Indianapolis, Denver, Phoenix, and San Francisco. R. J. Reynolds gleaned some useful information from the research:

> "Both Vantage and Merit smokers have similar early smoking histories. . . moving from non-filters to filters, switching to lighter cigarettes to relieve physical symptoms and as an acknowledgement of increased concerns about alleged health hazards." [Emphasis in original.] (See Levy and Robles, 1982, p. 5.)

> "Vantage smokers believe that the filter itself is strong enough to catch these impurities and that the hole structure is such that they will not see so much of the resulting discoloration. These ideas make them think the end product is a milder and more 'healthful' smoke." (See Levy and Robles, 1982, p. 16.)

> "Merit smokers. . . have been influenced by Merit advertising which so single-mindedly proclaims the brand's lowered tar and nicotine. . . Vantage smokers. . . the advertising influenced them by

promising real smoking satisfaction from a cigarette, by
not focusing so much on
the low tar aspect." (See
Levy and Robles, 1982, p.
89.)

**Figure 7-18**
**Merit Ultra Light "Sea" Campaign (1986)**

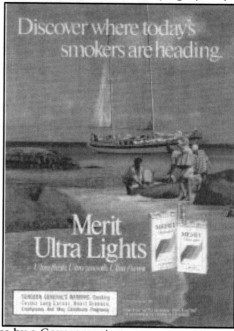

## DISCUSSION

### The Value of Official Government Ratings

Some members of the industry have long found the appearance of Federal Government vetting to be a desirable factor usable in advertising. For example, the 1958 advertising for Parliament® boasted that it was "the first filter cigarette in the world that meets the standards of the United States Testing Co." (see Figure 7-20). The ad showed the organization's official seal, which included a microscope, and although the ad was generated by a private firm, the seal was readily perceived as acceptance by a Government agency.

Note, too, the Carlton® use of a headline stating that the "Latest U.S. Gov't [sic] Laboratory test confirms. . . Carlton is lowest" in 1985, as seen earlier in Figure 7-14.

The Federal Government's adoption of a "uniform and reliable testing procedure" consistent with the methodology of Philip Morris also seemed beneficial to that corporation. Philip Morris foresaw in 1964 that such test results could be used in advertising copy, as they could communicate that an official Government agency had vetted the products, as well as the possibility that data with a competitive advantage angle could be provided:

> "Apart from possible legal requirements, such a policy would enhance advertising opportunities." (See Wakeham, 1964, p. 6.)

Later, Brown & Williamson saw the benefit to them, even if not to the public, in using Government evaluations and rating procedures. While the industry preferred to go unregulated, regulation offered some benefits, namely prospects for greater stability and the appearance of Government approval of their products by official testing procedures.

> "The tobacco industry, of course, would prefer no regulation at all. If there must be regulation, the industry is probably better off to have it at the federal level. . . Even expanded regulatory efforts may be shared by the industry to [illegible word] stability in the market

or by individual manufacturers
to bolster market positions—
for example, by capitalizing
on official tar and nicotine
ratings in cigarette advertising." (See Pepples, 1976, p. 8.)

The promotional value of the
FTC data meant that the industry
recognized protecting the credibility of the FTC procedure was
in its own interests:

> "Inherent limitations of
> the FTC cigarette testing pro-
> gram, and borderline low-'tar'
> advertising practices resulting
> from the way the test results
> are reported have contributed
> to substantial consumer con-
> fusion and misunderstanding.
> This situation threatens to
> erode public confidence in
> both the FTC's test reports
> and the industry's advertising
> claims." (See Pepples, 1982, p.
> 1.)

Figure 7-19

**Vantage "To Smoke or Not To Smoke" (1974)**

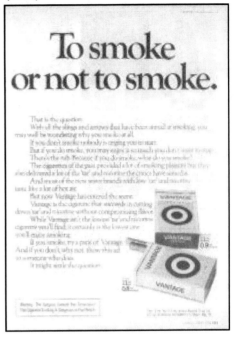

**Poor Information, But Rich Imagery**

Cigarette advertising is notoriously uninformative, with characteristic forms using veiled health implications and pictures of 'health' along with vague promises of taste and satisfaction (Pollay, 1994, pp. 179-184). Occasionally, ads for new technological developments in filter design called attention to the filter, with allusions to filter effectiveness, but almost always without being specific about what constituents of tobacco or its smoke were being filtered, what degree of filtration effectiveness was being realized, or what health or safety consequences were warranted. Only the tar and nicotine information—as mandated by regulation and generated by conventional test methods—is given, without interpretation. For example, Carlton® now encourages smokers to start "thinking about number 1" and smoke its "Ultra Ultra Light" cigarette (see Figure 7-21).

Many cigarette ads contain no information whatsoever, save for the implicit reminder that a brand exists, *e.g.*, many Marlboro® ads. Some contemporary ads, like a recent campaign for Merit Ultra Light®, take a humorous visual approach to convey that it might be lighter than expected (see Figure 7-22).

**Consumer Information**

The cigarette industry has not voluntarily employed its advertising to inform consumers in a consistent and meaningful way about any of the following: 1) the technologies employed in fabricating the products, 2) the constituents added in the manufacturing processes, 3) the residues

229

and contaminants that may be present in the combustible column, 4) the constituents of smoke that may be hazardous, 5) the addictiveness of nicotine, or 6) the health risks to which its regular consumers and their families are inevitably exposed. Instead, their advertising for low-yield products has relied on pictures of health and images of intelligence, and has misled consumers into believing filtered products in general, and low-tar products in specific, to be safe or safer than other forms without explaining exactly why.

Figure 7-20

**Parliament—Endorsement of United States Testing Co. (1958)**

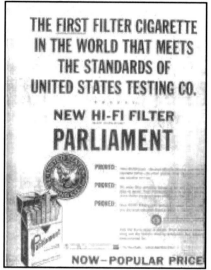

**Marketing/Advertising Gives Cigarettes Vitality** While the technological means to produce low-yield products might seem important, to industry insiders it was the marketing sophistication that was even more crucial in determining the relative success of various firms:

> [In contrast to the import of marketing] ". . . technology in the tobacco industry has had virtually no effect on the relative success of the six companies. . . the industry has *become so sophisticated in marketing* that nontechnical developments, while they might have a large influence on the industry in terms of the types of cigarettes available, would probably do little to shift shares from one company to another." [Emphasis added.] (See Ennis *et al.*, 1984.)

Michael Miles, Chairman and Chief Executive Officer of Philip Morris, defended advertising eloquently in a trade ad:

> "Those of us in the business of building brands don't have to be sold on the importance of advertising or on the necessity for advertising. For me, there is still nothing more exciting in business than to watch effective advertising work its magic in the marketplace. For when a brand is acknowledged and accepted by the consumer, it becomes something much more than what it really is. . . we invest $2 billion annually in advertising. It's worth every penny. For we believe that a strong brand gives the consumer another whole set of reasons—emotional and personal—to act." (See Miles, 1992, p. 16.)

**SUMMARY** This chapter has reviewed many tobacco industry documents and marketing trade sources. The review revealed the importance of marketing and advertising to the vitality of this industry, and the many means used to create an appearance of healthfulness for various cigarette products, especially those with nominally low yields. Several tactics were employed by the tobacco industry that misled consumers to perceive filtered and low-tar delivery products as safe or safer and as a viable alternative to quitting.

Nicotine delivery is a design feature of cigarette products, and an essential part of the design. Tobacco company documents reflect a fear of consumers becoming weaned from smoking if they are not maintained with sufficient nicotine. Consumer acceptance of products that fail to deliver adequate nicotine satisfaction is also difficult to maintain.

Health concerns of a serious nature have been present among some smokers since at least the 1950s. Females, older, and more highly educated smokers have long been more likely to mani-

Figure 7-21

**Carlton—"Isn't It Time You Started Thinking About Number One?" (1999)**

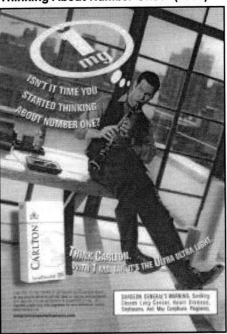

fest health concerns. The ramifications of these health concerns are anxieties, conflicts, shame, and guilt, leading to a need for reassurance from advertising. In the 1950s, the promotion of filters provided this reassurance with very explicit verbal representations about the health protection that they offered. Once the nominal purpose of filtration was well understood by the consuming public, the healthfulness of filters was represented by more implicit means. For example, thinly veiled language ("hospital white" filters; "Alive with Pleasure") and visual "pictures of health" images were used, displaying bold and robust behavior in pristine environments.

The image or illusion of filtration is essential to the selling of cigarettes, whereas the fact of filtration is not. Consumer (smoker) opinion and perceptions are what governs their behavior, not the medical or technological facts known to manufacturers and experts.

Many deceptive practices have been employed over the years (some continue to this date) that foster and perpetuate the illusion that various cigarette brands and product forms are relatively healthy. These tactics include:

- Using Medicinal Menthol. Menthol was introduced into some products capitalizing on its "pseudo-health" benefit, a consumer perception derived from experiencing menthol elsewhere in the medicinal context of cough and cold remedies.

231

- Loosening Filters. Once established in the public's mind as having effective filtration, Kent® offered several successive generations of product in the 1950s and 1960s that were heralded as "new and improved," but in fact contained ever more tar and nicotine.

- Using High-Tech Imagery. New filters were offered that seemed to be the fruits of scientific research and to have meaningful technological innovations, such as charcoal filters, dual filters, chambered filters, recessed "safety zoned" filters, gas trap filters, etc. Almost none of these specified the hazardous elements being filtered.

- Using Virtuous Brand Names and Descriptors. Brands were given names to imply state-of-the-art technology and/or a virtuous product, *e.g.*, Life®, Merit®, Now®, True®, or Vantage®. Product variations are described in technically meaningless, but seemingly quantitative, descriptors like "Mild," "Ultra," "Light," or "Super-Light."

- Adding a Very Low-Yield Product to a Product Line. Some product lines had wide-ranging tar and nicotine deliveries in the same brand family. The best of these levels was used for adver-

**Figure 7-22**
**Merit Ultra Lights—Sumo Ballet Lighter Than Expected (1999)**

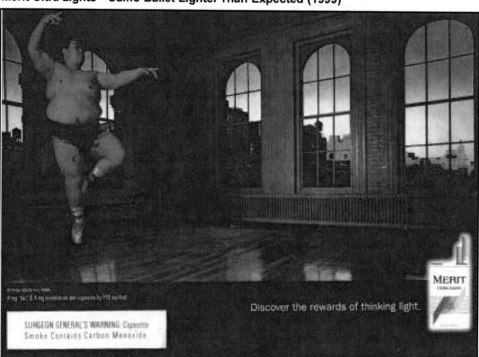

tising purposes to reassure consumers while selling other product varieties. In some cases, the best product variant was rarely sold and was known as a phantom brand.

- Fooling the Machines and Using the Data to Fool Smokers. Filters and cigarette papers were developed starting in the 1950s that "air-conditioned" the smoke by diluting the smoke column with side-stream air. When smoked by machines as in the FTC tests, low-tar and low-nicotine numbers resulted, a desirable outcome for promotional purposes—but higher yields were ingested by real smokers, a desirable outcome for maintaining nicotine addiction.

Low-yield cigarettes were heavily promoted. Promotional programs for cigarettes have been lavishly funded in general, with advertising in multiple media. A disproportionate amount of this funding promoted low-yield products when they were introduced in the 1970s.

Little or no meaningful information is contained in promotions for a given cigarette, such as its ingredients and additives, the technology of filtration, the hazardous constituents of smoke, or the health consequences of smoking. Consumer ignorance and confusion has been persistent over many decades. While smokers who switch to low-yield brands manifest faith in their relative healthfulness, few consumers know the true delivery characteristics of the brands that they smoke, and even their general impressions are not very accurate.

Finally, testing of products by official Government agencies, such as the FTC, imbues the industry with a certain level of credibility, while providing Government-rated data that can be used for promotional purposes.

## CONCLUSIONS

1. Advertisements of filtered and low-tar cigarettes were intended to reassure smokers (who were worried about the health risks of smoking) and were meant to prevent smokers from quitting based on those same concerns.

2. Advertising and promotional efforts were successful in getting smokers to use filtered and low-yield cigarette brands.

3. Internal tobacco company documents demonstrate that the cigarette manufacturers recognized the inherent deception of advertising that offered cigarettes as "Light" or "Ultra-Light," or as having the lowest tar and nicotine yields.

## REFERENCES

*Dr. R. W. Pollay explains the bracketed numbers following some of the World Wide Web/trail-related References: The two numbers (A, B, [e.g., 026, K0358]) following the descriptive information (author, title, date, etc.) are: (A) a sequence number for the authors' unique set of documents, and (B) the number that the National Cancer Institute or others used for identifying documents. This latter sequence is the more helpful for the reader, as it should link to a database at the National Cancer Institute. The Institute provided the authors with a lengthy inventory of documents from which items were selected by these numbers.*

*Note as to source of sources: Items 001-064 were supplied by KBM Group as the contractor for National Cancer Institute project on "Cigarettes with Low Machine-Measured Yields of Tar and Nicotine," and bear both the "TIPS" and "K" numbers in parentheses (e.g., 001, K0474). Items 065-081 were from sundry alternative sources, including the (Canadian) Physicians for a Smoke Free Canada Web site. Items 101-114 were from various corporate and trial Web sites, and were provided on request by Ms. Nadine Leavell, archivist of the Roswell Park Cancer Institute, Buffalo, New York.*

Alex Gochfeld Associates, Inc. The present competitive position of Pall Mall Gold 100's and Silva Thins: A motivational research study. Prepared for The American Tobacco Company, March, 1969. Bates No. ATXO5 0278907-ATX05 0278953. [101]

Blatnik, J. Making cigarette ads tell the truth. *Harper's Magazine* 217:45-49, 1958.

Brand Report 12: Cigarettes. *Media Decisions* 11(10):141-158, 1976.

Brand Report 23: Cigarettes. *Media Decisions* 12(10):149-164, 1977.

British American Tobacco Co., Ltd. The product in the early 1980s. March 29, 1976. [080, PSC 42b]

British American Tobacco Co., Ltd. Year 2000. April 4, 1979. [039, K0137]

British American Tobacco Co., Ltd. Research & development/marketing conference. Circa 1985. [081, PSC 60]

Brown & Williamson. Purite filter. Circa 1977.

Chambers, R.L. U.S. cigarette history. Brown & Williamson, September 21, 1979. [038, K0481]

Crittenden, A. $40 million for a real smoke. *The New York Times*, May 15, 1977, Section 3, p. 1 ff.

Cunningham and Walsh. [Advertising] Kool: 1933-1980. A retrospective view of Kool. Brown & Williamson, November 10, 1980. [041, K0478]

DeGarmo, Inc. Conclusions and implications of True portfolio research. DeGarmo, Inc., Research Department; prepared for Lorillard, August, 1974. [102]

Dougherty, P.H. Advertising, new low-tar, high budget smoke. *The New York Times*, p. 44, June 20, 1977.

Ennis, D.M., Tindall, J.E., Eby, L.C. Product testing short course. Product Evaluation Division, Research & Development Department, Philip Morris U.S.A., January 23-24, 1984. [058, K0081]

Federal Trade Commission. *Trade Regulation Rule for the Prevention of Unfair and Deceptive Advertising and Labelling of Cigarettes in Relation to the Health Hazards of Smoking and Accompanying Statement of Basis and Purpose of Rule.* Federal Trade Commission, Washington D.C., June 22, 1964.

Fitzgerald, C.W., Senkus, M., Laurene, A., Kecseti, F.M. (presenters). New product/merchandising directions: A three year action plan. R. J. Reynolds, August 19, 1976. [023, K0203]

Gardner, F. Under siege, cigarette marketers fight back. *Marketing and Media Decisions* 19(9):34-37, 175-177, 1984.

Goldstein/Krall Marketing Resources, Inc. A qualitative exploration of smoker potential for a new entry in the ultra low tar market category (two focused group interviews). Prepared for Philip Morris, January, 1979. [037, K0041]

Hind, J.F., Fitzgerald, C.W., Ritchy, A.P. New brand orientation for Ogilvy & Mather, Inc. R. J. Reynolds Tobacco Company, August 10, 1976. [103]

John, J., Wakeham, H. Breakthrough of the high taste, low tar cigarette—A case history of innovation. Philip Morris Research Center. 1977. [075]

Johnston, M.E. Market potential of a health cigarette. Special Report No. 248, Philip Morris, June, 1966. [004, K0126]

Kalhok, A.I., Short, P.L. The effect of restrictions on current marketing on marketing in the future. Brown & Williamson, May, 1976. [024, K0365]

Kaplan, M. Inside advertising: Perfect match. *American Photographer* October:100-102, 1986.

Kenyon & Eckhardt Advertising. Young adult smoker life styles and attitudes. Prepared for Brown & Williamson, 1974. [018, K0028]

Kieling, R.F. Implications for Kent. Director of Market Research. August 31, 1964. [002, K0016]

Koten, J. Tobacco marketers' success formula: Make cigarets [sic] in smoker's own image. *The Wall Street Journal*, p. 22, February 29, 1980.

Latimer, F.E. Cigarette advertising history. Brown & Williamson, November 29, 1976. [026, K0358]

Levy, S.J., Robles, A.G. Vantage and Merit smokers. Social Research, Inc., prepared for R. J. Reynolds, April, 1982. [112]

Lorillard, Inc. Triumph planning seminar: Competitive advertising. February 25, 1980. [111]

Marketing and Research Counselors, Inc. What have we learned from people? A conceptual summarization of 18 focus group interviews on the subject of smoking. Prepared for Brown & Williamson, May 26, 1975. [020, ASH]

Mau, T.H. August 11, 1981. Lorillard memo. Replies to 5-year plan questionnaire. [044, K0383]

Miles, M. 4 A's advertisement. *The New York Times*, p. 16, November 24, 1992.

O'Keefe, A.M., Pollay, R.W. Deadly targeting of women in promoting cigarettes. *Journal of the American Medical Womens Association* 51(1-2):67-69, 1996.

Oldman, M. Products/consumer interaction. British American Tobacco Co., Ltd., May 19, 1981. [043, K0373]

O'Toole, J.E. *The Trouble with Advertising.* New York: Chelsea, 1981.

Oxtoby-Smith, Inc. A psychological map of the cigarette world. Prepared for the Ted Bates advertising agency and Brown & Williamson, August, 1967. [005, K0107]

Pepples, E. February 4, 1976. Brown & Williamson memo. Industry response to cigarette health controversy. [027, K0125]

Pepples, E. Low-"tar" cigarette advertising and the FTC cigarette testing program: A time for reexamination. Brown & Williamson memo, June 9, 1982.

Philip Morris, Inc. v. Loew's Theatres, Inc., 511 F. Suppl. 855 (SDNY 1980).

Philip Morris, Inc. Merit history (script for slide presentation). August 17, 1990. [065]

Pollay, R.W. Promotion and Policy for a Pandemic Product: Notes of the History of Cigarette Advertising (US). Tobacco Litigator's Bookshelf 4.7 TPLR, 1989a.

Pollay, R.W. Filters, flavors . . . flim-flam, too! Cigarette advertising content and its regulation. *Journal of Public Policy and Marketing* 8:30-39, 1989b.

Pollay, R..W. Historical content analyses of cigarette advertising. *Preventing Tobacco Use Among Young People: A Report of the Surgeon General.* U.S. Department of Health and Human Services, Centers for Disease Control and Prevention, Office on Smoking and Health, 1994.

Pollay, R.W. Targeting youth and concerned smokers: Evidence from Canadian tobacco industry documents. *Tobacco Control* 9(2):136-147, 2000.

R. J. Reynolds-MacDonald (Canada). Vantage Lights Media Brief, 1980.

Reynolds, J.H., Norman, A.B., Robinson, J.H. March 4, 1982. R. J. Reynolds interoffice memo. Possible consequences of failure of the FTC to act against the Barclay cigarette filter and its mimics. [050]

The Roper Organization, Inc. A study of smokers' habits and attitudes with special emphasis on low tar cigarettes. Prepared for Philip Morris U.S.A., May, 1976. [025, K0286]

Schori, T.R. Tar, nicotine and smoking behavior. Philip Morris U.S.A. Research Center, November, 1971. [010, K0327]

Short, P.L. Smoking & health item 7: The effect on marketing. British American Tobacco Co., Ltd., April 14, 1977. [030, Minnesota Litigation]

Spears, A. Untitled (Re: Costs of making tobacco products). Lorillard, November 13, 1973. [015, K0134]

Teague, C.E. Proposal of a new, consumer-oriented business strategy for RJR tobacco company. September 19, 1969. [007, K0083]

Teague, C.E. A gap in present cigarette product lines and an opportunity to market a new type of product. March 28, 1972a. [012, K0416]

Teague, C.E. Research planning memorandum on the nature of the tobacco business and the crucial role of nicotine therein. R. J. Reynolds, April 14, 1972b. [011, K0121]

Tindall, J.E. A new low delivery segment. Philip Morris U.S.A. Research Center, May 22, 1973. [014, K0324]

Wakeham, H. Smoking and health—Significance of the report of the Surgeon General's committee to Philip Morris, Incorporated. Philip Morris Research Center, February 18. [001, K0474]

What are the obstacles/enemies of a swing to low "tar" and what action should we take? Anonymous—July 2, 1982, Trial Exhibit 26,185, Minnesota Litigation. [053]

Whelan, E.M. *A Smoking Gun: How the Tobacco Industry Gets Away With Murder.* Philadelphia: Geo. Stickley, 1984.

Zoler, J.N. Research requirements for ad claims substantiation. *Journal of Advertising Research* 23: 9-15, 1983.

CPSIA information can be obtained
at www.ICGtesting.com
Printed in the USA
FSOW02n1048290415
6807FS